SUPERIMMUNITY

Paul Pearsall, Ph.D.

SUPER

IMMUNITY

Master Your Emotions
& Improve Your Health

McGRAW-HILL BOOK COMPANY

New York   St. Louis   San Francisco   Hamburg
Mexico   Toronto

If you are sick or have symptoms of illness, or even before you get sick, go to a physician. Form a mutually trusting relationship with her or him. This book is not intended to replace medical advice, but to remind us that we should not allow doctors or hospitals to do things to us or for us, but with us. All healing is a team effort. No bridge can be built from the new field of psychoneuroimmunology to more traditional medicine if we forget those people who are building on the other bank.

5 6 7 8 9 D O C D O C 8 7

ISBN 0-07-049028-7

Library of Congress Cataloging-in-Publication Data

Pearsall, Paul.
   Superimmunity : master your emotions and improve
your health.

   1. Medicine and psychology. 2. Mind and body.
3. Immune response. I. Title.
R726.5.P4   1987   613   86-15262
ISBN 0-07-049028-7

Editing Supervisor: Margery Luhrs
Book design by Kathryn Parise

In memory of my father, Frank,
and for my mother, Carol.

CONTENTS

ACKNOWLEDGMENTS

This book is the result of decades of research by people who will never write a popular general book about the new field of psychoneuroimmunology. They will continue to devote lifetimes to the study of small pieces of the infinitely complex puzzle of human sickness, immunity, and healing. We will never see them on talk shows, but they will sacrifice anonymously for our survival. Some of their names are listed in the reference section of this book, and there are numerous others working on tomorrow's miracles. I can only hope that my attempt to offer a progress report on their diverse detective work will not offend them through its generalizations or misrepresent them through its optimism. I thank them for all of us.

My own work in this new field began 14 years ago. Dr. Norman Rosenzweig, Chairman of the Department of Psychiatry at Sinai Hospital of Detroit, gave me the opportunity and trust to design one of the first programs for the prevention of major mental illness. This program, the Problems of Daily Living Clinic, attracted patients suffering from the challenges to the immune system described in this book. They are the characters of the true-life minidramas you will read in the following chapters. I have disguised their names, but I am awed by their courage and inspired by the lessons they have taught me.

In the summer of 1984, I heard a presentation by Dr. Steven Locke of Harvard University. I thank him for his pioneering work as an integrator and educator in this new field of mind and immunity. I thank the Institute for the Advancement of Health for promoting the scientific study of the relationship between feelings and health and for providing me with important leads to researchers on the cutting edge in this new field.

I thank Norman Cousins and Dr. Robert Eliot, whose personal strength and professional skill in sharing their experiences made public the news that research was catching up with what we instinctively know, that how we think, relate, and feel profoundly influences our health and healing.

Finally, this book is the product of 7 years of support, tolerance, encouragement, patience, and endurance on the part of those people forced to relate with me as I struggled to present an accurate yet interesting, documented yet encouraging, popular yet valid early report on the most important research in history. My secretary, or should I say my boss, Ellen Schlafer, deserves a medal for her support and patience. I could never have finished this book without my agent, Susan Cohen, whose balance of personal and professional concern is remarkable. My editor, Tom Miller, took the risk of turning radical new ideas into a book. My friends and colleagues, Michael Salesin, M.D., at Sinai Hospital, Michael Aronoff, M.D., at Indiana University, John Helfrick, D.D.S., at the Houston Medical Center, and Nancy Burrell, M.S.N., at the Oklahoma Medical Center, read and reviewed the original manuscript.

As you read this book, you will understand that the most important elements in its production were my own supersystem and my wife, Celest, and my sons, Roger and Scott, who provided the love that energized my superimmunity. To all of you, I say, "Thank you, you did it!"

FOREWORD

When I first met Paul Pearsall twelve years ago, we talked about contemporary health care—we wondered why people become ill when they do, and how the doctor-patient relationship affects wellness. A few years later, we discussed the biochemistry of sexual response. In *Superimmunity*, Dr. Pearsall has found a way to tie together these and other questions with the theories of many of our greatest researchers in physics, biochemistry, and the neurosciences.

I have never before seen such a complete networking of research that crosses so many disciplines. Anatomists, biochemists, physiologists, and clinicians rarely write or make presentations for each other; however, Dr. Pearsall has done our library work, leaving us free to use our imagination.

Superimmunity postulates a great system within the body, capable of recognizing and repairing injury. This same system is capable of inflicting injury when certain conditions permit. There is no question that the brain is directly connected with, and in charge of, this system. Physicians and patients alike should consider the unity of brain and body to draw upon the strengths of the mind in our battle with disease.

Eighty to ninety percent of my patients recover from their illnesses in spite of, not because of, me. The hardest part of my job is to identify the ten to twenty percent who will require the intervention of modern medical technology. I have found that when patients tell me what they believe is wrong with them, most of the time they are correct. Dr. Pearsall reminds us that patients can also be very good at telling us what is *right* with them. Fortunately, a very large percentage of my patients want to learn about their illnesses and take the responsibility for their improvement.

The connection of mind and body is certainly not a new idea to Western medicine; Dr. Pearsall's theory of a superimmunity, based upon that concept, should not threaten our traditional wisdom. Almost eight hundred and fifty years ago, Maimonides, the physician-philosopher, said, "Most doctors err in their treatment; in endeavoring to assist nature, they weaken the body with their prescriptions." Perhaps this is because we have concentrated on *how* people become ill.

Dr. Pearsall illustrates the importance of asking the other question: "*Why* do we become ill?" In my own practice, I'm regularly asked why herpes is recurrent, why some people infected with the AIDS virus develop AIDS while others do not, and why doctors don't contract the contagious diseases of their patients. Readers of this book will find some reasonable answers to these questions.

After reading *Superimmunity*, I have found that I no longer see my patients, colleagues, family, or friends as I had before. We are all in this together.

Michael S. Aronoff, MD
Indiana University

INTRODUCTION

Superimmunity is the capacity to think and feel in ways that can protect us from disease, heal us when we are sick, and help us attain new levels of wellness—a level far beyond the mere absence of symptoms. No longer need we be helpless victims of random viruses, artery-clogging foods, cell-destroying chemicals, and environmental toxins. Neither do we really have to exercise vigorously, eat a spartan, partially cooked diet, or struggle to achieve the latest fashionable weight. We can develop superimmunity, a revolutionary new way of accepting the responsibility for our health.

Physicians don't have the ultimate say about our state of health. In a very real way, we can become our own physicians, our own doctors. The word "doctor" derives from the Latin word for teach. We can teach our bodies—every cell and fluid within us—to function at the maximum, drawing from the miracles of modern medicine only when we need to augment our natural healing system. This book will tell you how to use imagination, to innoculate yourself with the natural chemicals of the body, drawing on a wonderful and natural apothecary within.

Each thought and feeling is accompanied by a shower of brain chemicals that affects and is affected by billions of cells. This is our immune system, the constant surveillant of intrusion, of even the most minute malfunction of a cell within our bodies. The immune system identifies the invader, compares it to a constantly updated memory bank that knows friend from foe, and prepares an appropriate defense. It attacks the intruder, defeats it, cleans up after itself, and rids the body of wastes. While all this is going on, the immune system learns, preparing itself for future challenges.

Until recently, we have behaved as if the immune system were somehow separate from us, doing its job secretly, automatically, beyond our control. To be immune was to be safe, separate, secure in the feeling that a covert system was ever on the alert. Research now tells us that the immune system functions within a *supersystem* of the mind and body. When the supersystem is left alone, it functions like a well-prepared army that has lost its general. It may become overactive, underactive, attack itself—even suffer from bad morale.

While new and exciting research is teaching us more about our supersystem, the remarkable findings have ancient roots. Around 50 B.C., the most comprehensive document in China, the *Huangdi Neijing, The Yellow Emperor's Inner Book,* described health as an ever-changing system of interactions between the cells and the universe. According to this book, illness occurs when a person loses balance between *yang* and *yin*. Overdominance of yin results in what was described as the "cold diseases" of deficiency; overdominance of yang results in diseases of "overfullness," the hot diseases. The aim of the ancient physician was to help the patient reestablish a natural flow between yin and yang, to eliminate overfullness and to make up for the deficiencies.

So it is with the supersystem. I will tell you about two styles of the supersystem—"hot styles" and "cold styles." I will help you determine which style characterizes your day-to-day life and will help you assume control of your supersystem to develop superimmunity, a natural flow of life, wellness, and healing.

I may be accused of premature speculation, of going beyond the limits of research data currently available. I believe that the evidence I have integrated for this book offers sufficient support to document my theories. Certainly, new data are constantly emerging, and the link between the mind and immunity is far from clear. But there is *no question* that the link exists. Whatever the research may unearth, we must begin to recognize the impact of self on sickness and do something for ourselves now.

An important caution is in order. People are sometimes accused of causing their own illnesses, of character flaws or personality traits that have resulted in health problems. At the most vulnerable times in our lives, we are sometimes made to feel guilty. When illness becomes a flaw, a failing, a sign of weakness, we misunderstand the unity of the mind and the immune system.

The extent of this misunderstanding is illustrated by the labeling of people with letters of the alphabet. "Type A" becomes an accusatory label for anyone who is more competitive, more active, or more successful than we are. "Type B" is viewed as a gurulike, peaceful person of extreme emotional control and serenity, enjoying immunity from the ultimate cardiovascular punishment awaiting Type A colleagues. Now we even have "Type C," the cancer personality (as if cancer were actually one disease rather than the several forms of misgrowth and overgrowth of cells it actually is). The Type C personality is seen as somehow punished by cell disease, the ultimate end for a person unable to be close to others or to express his or her feelings openly.

All this is pure myth. No research has proved that any type of person, behavior, thought, or feeling directly causes any one disease.

A beautiful, vibrant, energetic woman came to my office. Cancer was spreading through her body, to her liver, brain, and lungs, but she had rallied in the face of this crisis and was fighting her disease on all fronts. She felt she had selected competent doctors, whose advice and guidance was in keeping with her personal philosophy and spiritual orientation. I asked why she had come to see me, a psychologist specializing in the problems of daily living. She seemed to be doing so well within her own support system.

"Well, I thought so, too," she said. "That is, until I met a therapist who said I had to figure out why I got this cancer and learn to see sharks eating my cancer cells. I just hate sharks. I hate meditating about them even more. I thought my disease was just some kind of combination of bad luck, genetics, and a whole bunch of other factors."

I reassured her. I said she did not need sharks, meditation, or a therapist at this time. I invited her to continue within her family support system, to attend her church as she did regularly—to love, pray, hope, and fight in her own way, to continue with her own strategy of learning and growing from her experience.

"Do you think I really caused this thing? Am I a Type C? The therapist seems to think I really am. If I don't do something, I might pay for this in the end," she said.

"Yes," I responded. "You are a Type C. You are a C for caught—caught in the trap of overinterpretation of too little data by a person eager to help but ill informed. You have mobilized your own powerful system from within. Keep on using it."

"What a relief," she responded. "You know, I was starting to feel sick just thinking about that Type C thing, all that meditation, and all those sharks. But you know, underneath it all, it just didn't seem right to me." The woman looked down, hesitated, and then continued, "There is one other problem, though. The therapist said that I was denying things, and maybe I am denying some of the factors in my life that have caused this disease."

"The only thing you are denying is bad information," I said. "You have your own style. Keep working at it. Work with your doctors and call me if you need any help. Maybe if we work together in the future, I can suggest some ideas that can augment your own system, but for now things seem to be going just beautifully."

This patient continues to struggle with her disease in her own way. Her orientation to life is helping her mobilize her supersystem. Her oncologist tells me she is one of the strongest patients he has ever dealt with and she is totally in charge of her own treatment regimen. She has even arranged special flights on corporation jets so that she can fly to treatment centers, and she has coordinated flights for other patients who use otherwise empty seats on privately owned jets.

My interest is to help others find strength within themselves, understand their own styles, and maximize their styles for their own benefit. Health is not something you do, it is how you are. It is not something proved or achieved; it is received.

I provide my patients with a magic formula. I call it the *B-A-FITER* formula. It seems to work for almost everybody. I present it as a guideline for the book you are about to read.

B stands for *b*elief. If you believe in your own health, your capacity for survival, you are helping boost your immune system's morale. If you believe, so will your supersystem.

A stands for *a*ttitude. If your attitude is one of hope, positive orientation, and high self-esteem, you give confidence to your immune system and make it proud of itself, eager to defend and enhance the body system.

F stands for *f*eelings. If you allow yourself to experience a rainbow of evolving feelings rather than attempt to force feelings upon yourself, you also strengthen your immune system. The constructive feelings for immunity are not just the positive feelings. By remembering that, you free your supersystem to do its work.

I stands for *i*magination. If you are able to maintain a freedom of association, to transcend the confines of the mechanical world, to see miracles where others see the everyday, you give your supersystem permission to transcend the limits of our present knowledge, to heal where healing may have seemed impossible. As Albert Einstein once pointed out, imagination is more important than knowledge. All perception is hypothesis, and a positive, creative hypothesis about life enhances the immune system.

T stands for *t*hinking. If you are able to think more rationally—to realize that our uniquely human gift is a noncatastrophic, rational, responsible orientation to daily living—you unburden your supersystem of the clutter of destructive chemicals involved with irrational, self-accusatory, self-demeaning thought.

E stands for *e*xperience. If you assume more control for your life, if you free yourself from habits that unnecessarily and destructively inhibit the supersystem, you give a major gift to the immune system. Do not overeat. Avoid toxic substances such as alcohol, sugar, artificial additives, and tobacco. Invigorate the supersystem by providing it with a healthy ecology, with exercise and fresh air that nurture all living things. When you do these things, you provide your supersystem with a major head start against any invasion.

R stands for *r*emembrances. If you focus your memories on the beauty of your life—if you look back for the joy, not just the blame; for the love, not just the loss—you provide your supersystem with the positives it needs to promote wellness, not just to survive. If you remember that denial destructively distorts reality, but that avoidance can help free us for action beyond ruminating on unchangeable or uncontrollable events, you will realize that even though memories may be sad, they are a key part of your continuing growth. If you remember that modern medicine complements your own natural healing power—translates rather than validates truths about the capacity for health beyond the mere absence of symptoms—you avoid dichotomizing the human experience.

To "B-A-FITER" does not mean to struggle courageously *against* disease, but to fight *for* life, for your natural, healing supersystem. It also means hopefully to transcend the narrow limits of our lives and move on to a perspective of responsibility and caring for others. We are fighting for a world that is a healing place for all its people. I will share ideas from some of the world's great thinkers about the world view that must be applied to healing.

This book is divided into five parts. In Part One I will describe the supersystem, consisting of two major components, the brain and the immune cells, which interact to form the most complex and effective of all health maintenance systems.

In Part Two I will identify the two styles of supersystem, the hot and cold daily living strategies that relate to the ancient yang and yin orientation. I will relate these styles to the major diseases of civilization—heart and cell disease. I will provide several tests to help you understand your own supersystem style at a given time in your life.

Part Three will show you how you can assume more control for your supersystem, how you can develop a mind-over-immunity approach that offers new ways of enhancing your health and the health of those around you.

Part Four explores some radical new ways of thinking about your life experiences. I will discuss myths regarding stress and disease and will explore how physics relates to the supersystem.

Part Five will show how ancient truths can be applied to your modern life, how you can transcend health and move toward a high-level wellness.

Throughout, I emphasize a healing environment, both within and without. I focus not on disease prevention, but rather on learning from disease; not fearing it, but understanding; not finding blame, but rather hope.

Each part of this book represents an integration of findings and ideas from professionals who do not typically read each other's journals, work in the same laboratories, or attend the same meetings. I hope to serve as an integrator, organizer, progress reporter, and interpreter of new research on the relationship between the brain and the immune system. I take full responsibility for the interpretations and integration, none of the credit for the ideas and the creativity behind the research.

I suggest that you read through the reference section for each chapter. I have attempted to suggest further reading and study sources for those areas in which you may have a specific interest. I also include diverse opinions on interpretation of the findings in this complex field, and I elaborate on points stated in simplified form in the body of the chapters.

I hope my book will be an inspiration and a guide for a continuing dialogue for wellness, for superimmunity, for a new healing place. I suggest you use *Superimmunity* as a primer for your supersystem. This book is just the beginning. The true miracles of our supersystem still await discovery in the laboratory, in the doctor's office, and in our own spirit.

Part One

THE SUPERSYSTEM

The distinctive human problem from time immortal has been the need to spiritualize human life, to lift it on to a special immortal plane, beyond the cycles of life and death that characterize all of the organisms.

ERNEST BECKER

The supersystem is that magnificent total of interactions between brain, immune cells, behavior, environment, feelings, thought, and other people. This part describes the most complex health maintenance system in the universe, the human immune system. To understand it, we must remember that to be immune is not to resist, but to be able to strike a balance for growth of mind, body, and spirit.

Chapter One

THE MIND AND BODY CONNECTION

Neurophysiologists will not likely find what they are looking
for, for that which they are looking for is that which is looking.

KEITH FLOYD

TEST TERROR AND THROAT TICKLES

The pencil was moist from the sweat from his fingertips. His heart
pounded in his ears. His stomach seemed to be talking to him in low,
mumbling gurgles. He tried unsuccessfully to disguise the sound by
shifting in his chair and clearing his throat. In spite of the sweat on his
hands, he felt cold, almost to the point of shivering. The old lecture
hall looked larger than the day before, and he felt somehow insignificant
sitting among the dozens of other students who seemed more confident
and comfortable than he. He felt that his score on this examination was
a measure of his competence now and in the future, a measure of his
reputation as an effective, bright, competent person.

His few close friends had nagged that he was becoming more
withdrawn, distracted, and impatient. He complained about the unfair-
ness of some of his instructors, the ineptness of other students, even
the inefficiency of enrollment procedures, seemingly designed specifically to frustrate his career plans. And now it was all on the line. In

spite of taking a deep breath and stretching his fingers, he suffered a private terror as the examination form slid onto his desk.

Another student in the same lecture hall heard the rumblings of a nervous stomach. Somehow such sounds inevitably signaled his own stomach to join in a gastric duet. He was anxious to start taking the test, but his palms were sweaty and his heart seemed to be skipping beats. He was rolling his pencil back and forth, giving himself points every time the words "Velvet No. 2" rolled face up. His friends had scheduled what they called a "survivors' party" at the campus hamburger house. He always enjoyed the nonsense and complete waste of time these meetings allowed in an otherwise impossible schedule. He had studied for hours, and if he was not ready now, he never would be. After all, for him there was more to life than tests, grades, and high scholastic rank. He preferred people to grade points. He was glad to begin the test. He smiled at the professor and took the exam from the professor's hand as he passed.

Days later, the first student awakened with the irritating tickle in the back of his throat that always signaled a severe cold. He was forced to cancel plans to attend the student government party. He was disappointed, for he viewed such parties as stepping stones to enhance his future career opportunities. He blamed his situation on the failure of the university to heat the classroom adequately. He remembered being cold during the exam and thinking even then that it was incomprehensible that a major university could not adequately maintain its buildings.

The second student experienced no cold symptoms. He frolicked happily at the survivors' party, which the first student saw as a meeting of marginal students with "room temperature intelligence quotients."

Both students were only points away from one another on their test results. Both had been influenced by various degrees of test terror. Both had experienced the impact of the most complex yet most vulnerable of human systems: the supersystem made up of the human brain and the body's immune system acting together to determine the health status of all of us.

LOSING OUR MINDS

One of the most helpful, and at the same time most destructive, events in the history of medicine has been the separation of the mind from the body. Before Descartes proposed that the mind and body were separate, it was felt that dissection and research on the human body was equivalent to cutting, even destroying, the soul itself. It was pure sacrilege even to consider cutting open or taking apart the human cadaver.

Descartes suggested that mind and body were different entities, related but separate in every way. As this position became accepted, physicians were allowed to learn about the body and its miracles by cutting, slicing, comparing, and arranging various parts in jars for the general terrorizing and, hopefully, education of medical students. Without this separation of mind and body, none of the modern breakthroughs in medicine would have been possible.

Unfortunately, we forgot to put things back together again. Physicians and researchers misunderstood the difference between brain and mind. The brain is in the head; the mind is "us." The mind is a supersystem of every part of us working together. It has been pointed out by many brain researchers that if the brain were simple enough to be understood, we would be too simple to understand it. The body, the brain, the heart—all of a human being's parts make up an inseparable whole sparked by the energy of our human spirit.

Samuel Butler summarized the negative side of the mechanistic, simplistic view of the body-mind connection. He stated, "The body is but a pair of pincers set over a bellows and a stewpan, and the whole fixed upon stilts." Some of us may look like such an apparatus, but medicine is beginning to learn the same lesson learned by physicists: in God's world, everything is one and separation is never possible without severe consequences.

A few years ago, I was asked to conduct what hospitals call "Grand Rounds." I know of few hospitals that regularly conduct humble rounds. On such rounds the "student priests" follow attentively in the footsteps of the "teaching priests" and wait anxiously for pronouncements of truth.

One eager student approached me, name badge clamped upside down, stethoscope strategically draped in his lab jacket pocket so that the earpieces were noticeable to anyone who might not know immediately his doctoral status, or who might doubt his knowledge as much as he himself did. "I really want to see a frontal lobe today, and I hope we can see a few temporals too," he said. "I saw two gallbladders yesterday, and the kidney in Room 13 was really interesting, but really, I want to get into neurology and see brains and strokes instead of all the kidneys I had on my last rotation." This was not one of Dr. Frankenstein's students examining beakers of body parts. This was a future "healer," well prepared in the separatism that characterizes much of modern medicine and easily able to describe not people, but parts. Somehow, he felt safer with the false security of a description of elements than with the ultimate mysteries of our wholeness. He had forgotten—no, most likely never knew—the history of his art, which may have pointed him toward the light responsible for the mysteries that at the same time awed, inspired, and frightened him so. Without knowledge of that history, he would listen through a seriously blocked stethoscope.

PSYCHE, SOMA, AND A SUPERSYSTEM

Francis Bacon pointed out that progress in medicine occurs "rather in circles, than in progression." Researchers on the interaction between body, brain, and immune system are rediscovering centuries-old ideas regarding the relationship of mind and body. From prehistoric times, disease has been seen as caused by evil spirits, with the will of the person becoming overwhelmed by negative influences. More than 10,000 years ago, exorcisms were used to remove the evil from the body in order to restore health. Disease was seen as coming from inside, not from outside, due to an imbalance in the person's life.

The Sumerian-Babylonian-Assyrian civilization (2500–500 B.C.) focused on the patient's self-examination, a search for internal causes of disease. The early Hebrew culture focused on disease as punishment for disobeying or in some way contradicting God's laws. In India, *Ayurveda*, one of the oldest of all health sciences, focused on the concept of the delicate balance between mind, body, behavior, and environment. Health was seen as a balance between these factors, and disease as a disruption of this balance. Although the medical science of Ayurveda has been traced back to early Vedic writings several thousand years before Christ, ancient texts claim that it goes back to the very beginnings of consciousness and life itself. According to *Ceraka*, a book which was written in about A.D. 300 and which continues to serve as a basic text for students of this approach to medicine, "The life stream carried in its own current its own supporting and protecting wisdom."

The ancient Greeks were well aware of the mind-body relationship. Socrates said, "As it is not proper to cure the eyes without the head, nor the head without the body, so neither is it proper to cure the body without the soul.'' Patients would isolate themselves within the temple to become closer to their own emotions, to search their private spirit world for a cure from within. They sought a reunification that would activate the "life force" housed within the body and the soul.

The nineteenth century widened the division of the mind-body dichotomy initiated by Descartes. New evidence in the twentieth century, however, points strongly to a reconnection of mind and body to save our wellness. Several investigators have shown a relationship between psychological functioning and disease. Some disorders documented as related to psychological factors, stress, and strain include allergic rhinitis, malignant hypertension, hyperthyroidism, paroxysmal arrhythmias, diabetes mellitus, backaches, and glaucoma. In 1968, Dr. Silverman reviewed research documenting the relationship between mind and body in each of these conditions, but it has taken more than 15 years for researchers to focus our attention more clearly and directly on psychosomatic illness. Telling someone that a disease is "all in your head" has been an accusation rather than an explanation, somehow diminishing the reality of disease as some type of psychic illusion.

As we learn more and more about the intricate relationship between mind and body, we learn that all disease is related to our wholeness. Epidemiology, the study of large numbers of people and emerging patterns of disease, also points to the importance of the psychosomatic relationship. In 1976, Dr. Thomas published results of a study of medical students who were followed for 30 years. She found that profiles of psychological tests were predictive of such sicknesses as cancer, heart disease, and high blood pressure. Dr. George Valliant conducted a similar study published in 1974 and 1977. In his study, a large population of Harvard students was followed for 30 years, and the relationship between emotional maturity and disease vulnerability was clearly shown. If history, correlation, and group studies do not point strongly enough to the mind-body connection, research in the laboratory should convince the most skeptical of the importance of continued research in this area.

Lesions, or surgical changes in the brains of animals, have shown a relationship to the development of certain disease patterns. In particular, lesions of the hypothalamus, a major control center within the brain, produce changes in the immune system. Stimulation of the immune system by injecting antigens, or challenges to that system, alters the electrical activity in specific regions of the hypothalamus. This suggests a two-way connection between the immune system and the brain. It is this two-way system, the immune system interacting with the brain and the body, that constitutes the supersystem.

Dr. Michael Fauman, psychiatrist at Sinai Hospital of Detroit, conducted a comprehensive review of the neuroimmunological literature and concluded that there is a strong suggestion that the central nervous system plays a major role in the development and function of the immune system. His review showed the same circular relationship between the brain and the immune system.

Thousands of years ago and now again, through carefully designed research, a new "old" model of disease emerges. It is a model of the possible hyperactivity or hypoactivity of the supersystem, the brain-immune system. It is a model of function, not personality—a model of style, of life strategy and response to the continued challenges (stresses) that produce the changes (strains) in our whole being. There are not disease-prone people, but rather disease-producing lifestyles. We can change our styles by first being aware of them and then consciously altering them for a better balance, running warm instead of hot, cool instead of cold.

It is a physiological fact that when you run hot, your heart accelerates, your bronchial tubes open up, your stomach relaxes, secreting no fluids, and your intestines retract. Your bladder relaxes, and your blood vessels constrict. When you run cold, your heartbeat decreases, your bronchial tubes constrict, your stomach secretes acids, and your intestines are agitated. Your bladder contracts, and your blood vessels dilate. The immune system follows suit, heating up or overheating when you run hot, and freezing up to the point of ineffectiveness when you run cold. High blood pressure, migraine headaches, heart disease, thyroid conditions, and diabetes relate to hot-running times in our lives. Low blood pressure, ulcers, ulcerative colitis, asthma, and even cancer can result from functioning too cold for too long.

It is how you are running, not who you are, that is important. It is your own yin-yang balance—a flow of your own life stream, the excess or deficiency of your life force at given times—that influences the effectiveness of your immune system.

BELIEVING AND HEALING

The brain and its as yet uncountable secretions interact profoundly with every other part of the body, forming what neurologist Dr. Barbara Brown calls the "supermind." Dr. Brown summarizes data on the mind-body relationship. "Some evidence about minds signals . . . the emergence of a human super potential." She, as do most current neurophysiologists, sees this supermind as a "complex of innate capacities of mind/brain to appreciate, organize, and control the body and brain."

If you are confused with the words "brain" and "mind," remember that the brain is the physical site where most of the body's activities originate, are moderated, and are controlled. The mind is the totality of all that makes us human.

Research at Michigan State University has shown that a single cell can be controlled by how we think. In summing up this and related research, Dr. Brown writes, "The mind alters every cell in the body."

Each of the 200 trillion cells in a person responds to the super-system, that combination of our central nervous system, hormonal system, and autonomic nervous system that affects our general physiological orientation to life. Some amazing findings from scientific literature document the impact of our thoughts on our cells and on our selves.

A serious skin disease called *congenital ichthyosiform erythroder-mia* results in a hardening and blackening of the skin. A 16-year-old boy was seen for this condition after being shunned by his teachers and friends. His skin condition had worsened, and bacterial infection had found a welcome environment in the rigid and cracked surfaces of his body. As the skin grew harder than the boy's own fingernails, blood-stained serum oozed from the slightest bend in the skin.

All major dermatology textbooks report no known cure for this terrible disease. Hypnotist Dr. Mason saw the boy and offered mental imagery suggestions to relax him and to help him learn to see his skin as becoming normal. Hypnotism is not some magic process that some-how overrides disease. It is a guided and carefully chosen process of learning to focus, remember, think, imagine, and experience ideas and events to help achieve a healthier state. It is really a systematic way of more effective thinking and believing, of taking responsibility for the supersystem. Within 5 days, the hard, damaged skin had fallen away, replaced by reddened but more normal-appearing skin. In 10 days, the skin had returned to normal. Dr. Mason's results, published in the *British Medical Journal*, were later verified by three other medical researchers.

Following the publication of these data, other physicians attempted to work on other "incurable skin disorders." Positive results for other conditions were obtained. *T cells* are special cells in our immune system that help us deal with foreign invaders or allergens. We now know that "T-cell-mediated skin response" relates to our emotions and beliefs, that the skin reacts intensely to our feelings.

Taking control of our supersystem can help us not only to treat unwanted ailments but also to achieve positive states. Five published studies of women desiring larger breasts indicate that imagining the breasts as larger results in an average increase in circumference over a 12-week period of 1¼ inches. Follow-up of these studies has indicated that over 80 percent of the reported increases remained more than 3 months later.

These changes should not surprise us. All of us know that our feelings, attitudes, and beliefs profoundly affect our body image and sexuality. We all experience strong and evident changes in our genitalia in reaction to various feelings, so it is to be expected that more long-lasting changes may be effected through the mobilization of our super-system.

In other research, a woman experiencing a severe hay fever reaction to pollen for 12 years was helped to imagine herself free of symptoms. She became completely free of her symptoms for the first time. Another research team studied the reaction of persons to the well-known "TB test." A positive Montoux reaction (a reddening and swelling of the skin at the site of the injection of a small amount of tuberculin) was produced through injections of water by suggesting that the water injection was really tuberculin. Research subjects were able to change the reaction from arm to arm, with the arm receiving water developing a reaction and the arm receiving the actual tuberculin not reacting, depending on the verbal directions given by the researchers to the participants in the study.

The impossibility of separating the mind from the body, and our profound capacity to influence our own supersystems, has been documented for decades. Cosmopolitan medicine, which continues to have essentially a mechanical, separatist approach, has been slow to accept the reunification of mind and body. Certainly breast size, asthma, allergies, skin diseases, and even blistering of the skin could not be accomplished through "the mind alone." Something more tangible must have happened. Yet studies continue to confirm the link between thought and wellness and disease, documenting that this interaction is as real as any virus under a microscope.

Imagine an impressive "wart-killing machine" operated by a well-known "wart doctor." Patients come by the dozens for treatment. Each patient places the wart-afflicted part of his or her body on this machine, and the wart doctor warns the patient not to move while the wart machine rumbles, hisses, flashes, and shoots "powerful x-rays" through the warts. The patient then withdraws the treated part, and the wart doctor paints each wart with bright-colored magic medicine, warning the patient not to touch or wash the warts until they disappear. Imagine that almost one-third of the patients coming to the wart doctor see their warts disappear during the first treatment by the wart machine. What you have imagined actually happened in the office of Dr. Bruno Block in the early 1920s. He became known as "the wart doctor" for his consistent success in ridding people of warts. Since that time, other researchers have confirmed the power of suggestion in this area.

The machine actually did nothing. No current or rays were involved. It was a machine that could have been made for a set for a Broadway play, but it represented a symbol for convincing the patient that cure could be effected. The dye was not medicine, just simple food dye. The cure came from within, not without. The wart machine was really the belief system.

One of the highest-priced models in the Michigan area was concerned about a wart that had developed on her right hand. She had gone to her dermatologist and had sought the opinions of several other doctors. They diagnosed it simply as "a wart and nothing to be worried about." Various physicians offered to cut it off, burn it off, and in other ways attack "it," without regard to "her." She was concerned about scarring from burning and about other damage that might result from various destructive approaches to "healing."

She sat in my office now because, as she put it, "I'm not so sure I'm not losing my mind." What had brought her to speak with me was the fact that her grandmother had looked at the wart and said that she was willing to "buy it off me for a quarter." The grandmother had taken a quarter from her purse, by this patient's report, and rubbed the quarter over the wart; 1 week later the wart disappeared.

I assured the patient that such a phenomenon was entirely possible according to what we know from research. The skin is simply another part of the immune system, and changes can be made by simply changing our belief system. Her fear of the doctors and her love for and childhood-based trust in her grandmother combined to change her viewpoint regarding the wart. Her mind, her belief system, and her feelings, not the quarter, made the wart disappear.

MR. T'S MAGIC BLOOD STOPPER

A round-faced, smiling little boy was waiting with his mother in the hall of the hospital emergency room area. He had cut his finger rather badly while attempting to win a bet from his younger brother that paper, indeed, could not really cut someone. He had run his finger along a cardboard box edge and promptly lost one dollar and what his mother and he felt to be approximately 2 gallons of the reddest blood in medical history. Actually, it was only a superficial cut bleeding the way that only children's cuts seem to bleed.

The boy began to panic, however, and the mother contributed to the panic by rushing him to the emergency room. A triage nurse checked him and asked him to wait because "there are very sick people needing my help. People are dying here." She was impatient and overworked; she saw the superficial cut as an annoyance and became angry. As the boy and his mother fearfully sneaked another look beneath the handkerchief clasped over the cut, they noticed that blood continued to pour from the wound. I stopped by as the boy's happy face was turning white, not from loss of blood, but from fear.

The nurse saw me standing by the boy and his mother and signaled to me. The nurse's lips moved in a sentence without sound that said, "They are a real pair; he's just got a silly cut on his finger. Tell them to go buy a bandage and go home." I handed the boy a tongue depressor on which I had quickly written in ink, "Mr. T's blood stopper." I told him to push the unmarked side just once against the wound, go to the rest room, wash the wound out very carefully, and come back. I told him that the blood would be stopped and things would be fine and that he would see only a line where the blood was before.

I went to the patient I had originally come to the emergency room to see, and by the time I was leaving I had actually forgotten what had transpired earlier. As I walked to the parking lot, a horn from a passing car drew my attention. The mother of the boy in the emergency room leaned her head out to state, "I can't believe it. You stopped that blood like it was a faucet being turned off. Thank you for everything." The boy held up the special Mr. T tongue depressor and waved his unbandaged finger happily in the air.

Time, natural clotting, and a quick change of belief had combined to change the body process. Our immune system not only includes cells but is "us." This boy had exercised control over the part of himself that is skin. A blow against Cartesian dualism had been struck by a tongue depressor and a little boy's belief.

HEART ATTACK AND THE MARX BROTHERS

Harvard physician Richard Bergland describes in detail how the brain is altered in its patterns of secretions by our thoughts and feelings. "What is significant," he writes, "is that brain secretions can be stimulated or diminished by thoughts, behaviors, feelings, and environment." A new journal, *Advances*, published by The Institute for the Advancement of Health, presents articles throughout the year that explore the relationship between the brain, the body, and the mind. The split between mind and body may be beginning to heal.

From warts and paper cuts to the life-threatening situation of a heart attack, belief is important. A man was rushed from his workplace to the emergency room, sirens wailing, lights blinking. Like the Marx Brothers jumping on a bed, people pounced on the litter transporting the man to a treatment room. A large staff of medical people worked frantically in an attempt to regulate a potentially fatal irregular heartbeat. As I watched from the distance, I could see the man's face. His eyes showed panic as he searched for someone who would look at him. Everyone worked on "his body, his heart, his circulatory system." No comfort, only an occasional yell that "you'll be okay," could be heard. All professional eyes were too busy to see his panic, to react to the appealing searching of his eyes.

I walked to the side and squeezed my way into the crew working so frantically. They hardly noticed my presence. I leaned over, stroked the man's forehead, and stated, "You are really doing well. You've got the best doctors I've ever seen, and things seem to be improving. I can't believe how hard your heart is working to regulate itself, and how strong it's looking." With these words, his heart rhythm began to return to one that was manageable by the medical team.

Once again, the treatment used by the medical team, their concern for his survival, the rapidity of their intervention, and a subtle, crucial change of belief had saved a life.

TRAINING THE TERRAIN

A new field called *psychobiology* has emerged. It is defined by physician Richard Restak as a field concerned with the mind's attempt to know itself through the study of the brain. Research in this area is leading to fascinating discoveries that underscore our potential for superwellness, for transcending the mere absence of symptoms by mobilizing our supersystem. We should remember the warning issued by Diane Hales, former editor of *The New Physician*: "The causes of our vulnerability may lie not in our stars or in the twist of fate, or in roving pathogens, but in ourselves."

Several months ago a news item in *The Los Angeles Times* reported an event that took place at Monterey Park Football Stadium. During the game several persons reported being ill with symptoms of severe food poisoning. At the first-aid station, a doctor suspected a soft-drink machine and decided to make a public announcement over the PA system to the effect that drinks from such a machine could be the cause of severe nausea and other symptoms.

Within several minutes, nauseated, pale, retching persons flocked to the first-aid station. Ambulances carried people from the stadium to local hospitals, where hundreds were kept for observation. It was later established that the soft-drink machine was not at all involved in the food-poisoning instance. When this fact was announced, symptoms began to disappear immediately. An announcement, a statement of belief, and a hypothesis about illness had caused illness not only in one person but in hundreds. So it is in our world that words, thoughts, and feelings are as powerful as any bacterium.

Dr. Lewis Thomas is aware of the revolutionary implications of the interaction between thought and wellness. He hypothesized that a form of "superintelligence" may exist in each of us that is designed to help us grow, develop, heal, and fight off disease. This superintelligence that Dr. Thomas describes is the force behind the supersystem. It is not a blind, reflexive system coping with germs and viruses, but a responsive healing and defense system directed by the subtleties of our own cognition and emotions. The biologist Claude Bernard stated that germs hover constantly about us, but they do not set in and take root unless the terrain is ripe. This terrain is cultivated by our thoughts, cognitive style, feelings, and perceptions.

I return to the two students described in the beginning of this chapter. The first student, who was so concerned about power, control, and success, became seriously ill. He developed pneumonia and had to be hospitalized. For the first time, he was forced to take time to think and feel.

He learned early on that survival in hospitals depends upon being a person and not a patient. He thought about how he got so easily upset and about how unimportant most of what he got upset about seemed to be now. A female nurse spent hours with him during the crisis period and helped his fever to break. As he returned to clearer thinking, he began to be attracted to the nurse. He took what was for him a major risk. Late one evening he shared with her his appreciation for her caring and the fact that he now cared for her as well. The nurse sat on his bed, discussing with him the possibility of a year of travel through Europe together, a total vacation from everything, the sharing of perhaps "total freedom just to be together for a while." Comfort from the nurse and the lesson learned by the student on the importance of people in his life to balance his career development had helped in the healing process.

The second student, the student who could enjoy nonsense and a complete waste of time, who particularly wanted to be around people and enjoy their company, had gone to the survivors' party with his woman friend of 3 years. He left her to go for food and drink. Next to him in the food line was an old flame with whom he had shared a passionate relationship years earlier. She seemed somehow more erotic to him now than ever before.

His supersystem went into action. His heart beat faster, his palms sweat, his stomach gurgled. He felt completely agitated as he noticed his date for the evening approaching, and in an effort to put a quick end to this spontaneous meeting, he blurted out, "I have to go now, but I would really like to see you." As the evening wore on, he thought more and more about how he would like to see the woman from his past. As the party neared its end, he noticed her leaving and she stopped by once more to say, "Please get in touch with me. I would like to show you pictures of my children and, by the way, this is my husband, Dave.'' He felt depressed, hopeless, somewhat embarrassed, and saddened by the thought that his fantasy had been so quickly erased.

For several weeks he felt strangely lonely, longing for the woman from his past. He developed severe gastritis and intestinal irritation. The development of his illness was for different reasons, at different pacing, and in different ways from that of his fellow student, but just as real. Not only how we think and feel but also how we interact and fantasize are processes of communication within the supersystem of the mind and the immune system.

Chapter Two

THE SUPERSYSTEM'S SOGGY COMPUTER

The care of tuberculosis depends more on what the patient has in his head than what he has in his chest.

SIR WILLIAM OSLER

More than a trillion cells race through the bloodstream and lymph system on search-and-destroy missions against any invaders, whether bacteria, viruses, fungi, or the body's own cells gone awry. Lymphocytes identify and proliferate so further identification and resistance can be offered against antigens or foreign bodies attacking the human system. These cells produce antibodies that reach out and destroy antigens, those threatening outsiders and misfits. The phagocytes finish off the battle and clean the battlefield of all debris. Natural killer cells act as an early-warning surveillance system against cancer cells and the spread of tumors and fight off attackers all by themselves. The more active and alert these killer cells, the more effective is the defense against cancer.

About the size of a grapefruit, the human brain weighs about as much as this book. It contains more cells than there are stars in the Milky Way. Billions of interactions take place between these cells, and the resulting electrochemical dance is the system we call our brain. Working together, these two systems make up a supersystem that responds to our awareness of our world, our theories of life. It responds to whether we are running "hot" or "cold" in our thinking and feeling at any given time. If we fail to control this powerful system, if we leave it to its own prewired, inherited patterns, we surrender control of one of the most powerful systems in the universe.

The brain is not "in charge" of the body or the immune system; it is a coordinating, cooperating part of that system. The immune system does not just respond to the brain; it affects and is affected by it. Try as we may to identify "centers" and "command posts" to explain the interaction of these systems, the magnificent oneness of human functioning cannot be denied. The brain responds as much as it controls, and it continues to develop and change in response to our thoughts and feelings and environment throughout life. The brain is never too old to learn, to adapt, to develop, and the same is true for the immunity system.

We have only two windows to our world. The brain reacts automatically to sounds, sights, and stimulation coming from all the senses. The immune system reacts to any stimulation to the body. What we feel, hear, see, or imagine stimulates the brain to respond, coordinate, and store information for the future. Every foreign particle, germ, or virus results in a reaction by the immune system. The supersystem is the interaction between these two master networks.

One study done at the Yale School of Medicine demonstrates the interaction between brain and immunity clearly. In an attempt to learn more about the high rate of mononucleosis at the West Point Military Academy, Stanislav Kasl, Alfred Evans, and James Neiderman screened all entering cadets for susceptibility to the disease, which is caused by the Epstein-Barr virus (EBV).

Those cadets whose blood samples contained evidence of an antibody to EBV had developed a defense against the disease; their immune systems had readied a resistance because of a prior confrontation with the virus. Cadets without the antibody were susceptible to the disease because their defense systems had not had earlier training for this specific invader.

At West Point, about one-fifth of susceptible cadets become infected with mononucleosis each year. Only a quarter of these cadets develop symptoms, the other three-quarters have an immune-system efficiency and effectiveness that wins the battle against EBV. Those who succumb generally tend to see their fathers as overachievers, and they state that they sorely want a military career but do poorly academically. These vulnerable cadets perceive their world in such a way that their immune systems are made ineffective. The stress of military school affects them and their supersystems differently from the "immune" cadets.

Dr. Steven F. Maier and Mark Laudenslager at the University of Colorado studied how readily T cells, the defending lymphocytes, can help fight off infections and malignancies. The most effective T cells were found in rats who perceived their world as controllable—they were given shocks that they were able to do something about. This research team found that it is not just the stress of being shocked that affects the immune system but also the perception of being unable to do anything about the stress.

The Colorado research team wondered whether other aspects of the immune system might not be responsive to "perception," the way the brain deals with our world. They studied natural killer cells, which seek out overgrowing or badly growing cells and destroy them, and found again that the issue of not being in control of administered shock results in killer cells that are less effective in their surveillance for early tumors.

So it is not just stress or life pressures that affect our immuno-efficiency, but our perceptions of our world as well. Dr. Steven Locke at Harvard University Medical School found that natural killer-cell activity is diminished, not by severe changes or stressors in the life of healthy human volunteers, but by people's interpretations of stress: whether or not they see themselves as able to deal effectively with the stress that they are experiencing. It was as if immune cells behaved as confidently and effectively as the thinker in which the cells circulated.

This is not to suggest that resignation, surrender, or denial results in a more effective immune system. Dr. Sandra Levy also studied natural killer-cell activity, and she found that women who are treated for breast cancer differ in the rate and degree of the spread of their cancer cells. Women who accept their disease, and are resigned to it, show less effective killer-cell activity than women who are more agitated. Again, perception plays the key role, not just random reflexes of cells working in isolation from the brain.

Researchers now know that cells within the immune system and within the brain itself have receptors on them that allow for interaction between the immune system and the brain. Every thought and every feeling we have alters the immune system, and every challenge to the immune system alters the way we think and feel. Remember, the key is to learn more about our subtle styles of daily living, thinking, and feeling, not to discover a type or character style.

A bright, articulate businesswoman came to my office for help with what she called her "free floating, ever-present anxiety." Her cardiologist had referred her to me because of an abnormal rhythm to her heartbeat, which she felt was due to "stress." Before using medication to restore a normal beat, the doctor had hoped that this patient could learn to see her world differently and, therefore, effect significant changes in her body system, specifically the electrochemical balances affecting her heart rhythm.

"I can't understand it. I'm in love. I'm going to get married. Now I am getting sick and having heart trouble. Why now of all times?" she said incredulously, with red face and clenched fists.

I asked how plans were proceeding for her wedding, and she responded, "Are you kidding? Both of us have so much junk to get cleared out, so much to get organized, it seems impossible."

I asked, "Why does it make so much difference right now? Who really cares about all that junk at this time anyway?"

Her anxiety, ambivalence, even uncertainty were obvious. "What difference does it make? What difference does it make?" She raised her voice and stood up. "I care, I can't stand clutter. I want organization, structure. I want it and I will have it if it kills me!"

Like a computer screen printing back green letters on command, this woman ran through her computer tape. She was being directed by her brain, not taking responsibility for her own thoughts. Her brain was programmed for order and now it demanded it. Unless an overriding or replacement program was inserted, the brain would persist in its historically determined direction; it would disrupt and deregulate the system designed to protect itself.

All disease is metaphor, and learning about our world and our strategies about dealing with it at different times in our lives is as important as any nutritional or exercise program for overall health. The "soggy computer" part of our supersystem is only beginning to be understood by scientists. Researchers at Cambridge University have spent more than 3 years utilizing several computers and teams of scientists to attempt to count the connections in the brain of a simple little worm with only 23 neurons. They are still at work.

The neurons that make up the brain are unlike any other cells in the body. They cannot reproduce themselves, and those you have from about 3 months after conception are essentially the ones you will have throughout your life. Once damaged, they cannot be repaired. Researcher and neurologist Richard Bergland calls the brain a "master gland," capable of dealing through its secretions with the most complex bodily processes.

This magnificent organ, as powerful as it is, is unable to heal itself; for that reason, it may sense its own vulnerability and maintain—at all costs—a selfishness, a dedication to survival, that can sometimes cause even more of a threat to our lives. When we fail to see our connection to the world, when we behave as our brains might have us behave, as selfish, isolated beings, we are much more likely to get sick, for we break from the system, from the flow of our world. We run hot or cold as if without a thermostat or thermometer to sense changes in our psychological temperature.

From the viewpoint of evolution, the soggy computer is relatively new. If all the history of our world were condensed and viewed as a 24-hour day, our brains occurred 5 minutes before the end of that day. Almost all human history took place in the last minute of that same day. The selfishness of the human brain is new too, for history teaches us that the blessings of our advanced brain capacities come with the price of selfishness, of alienation from the human community caused by a focus on "I" that developed along with our intelligence.

We are as much "I quotient" as we are "intelligence quotient." I will show you how important it is to change such a focus if you are to maintain and enhance your health.

WHERE IN THE WORLD ARE YOUR BRAINS?

The human brain contains the fossil memories of its past, just as a stratified landscape contains earth's past in the shape of horned type titanotheres and stalking dirk-toothed cats.
LOREN EISLEY

Place your index fingers beneath your earlobes on both sides. Right about there, and in toward the center of your head, is the part of your brain called the *brain stem*. Developed only 500 million years ago, this brain stem is referred to by some scientists as our "reptilian brain." Dr. Paul MacLean spent years studying this and other structures of the brain. He sees the brain as an archaeological site, with the brain stem being the deepest and oldest part of that psychological dig.

It is not difficult to see our mammalian ancestry in our day-to-day lives. Notice the way we posture ourselves, wrinkle our brows, stick out our tongues. Notice the way we smile or frown. Notice how our eyebrows go up in a signal of safeness to approach or as an appeal for understanding and permission to approach. Psychologist Kathlyn Hendricks states, "Our bodies are a visual representation of our life's stance."

Our brain stems have a great deal to do with how we carry ourselves. Notice how we line up behind one another and walk to the beat of a stick hitting a stretched animal carcass. Notice how we march with our heads held high, legs moving in unison. Notice how we lick our lips when we are hungry and rub our hands together when we are in a state of anticipation. Notice how we place our hands on our hips and cock our heads to one side as an expression of doubt or curiosity. Notice how we show our teeth to others, as if signaling we will not bite, and call this a smile. Notice how our "prejudice muscles" stiffen when we feel threatened. Notice how our heads go up and our trunks stiffen in an attempt to be taller than our perceived adversaries. Notice people who feel threatened, and you will see their heads dart from side to side, much like lizards on leaves in search of food or alert to predators. Notice how we cling to our personal leaves, protecting our turf, sometimes getting so mad that we could spit. This is hot behavior.

Traditional Japanese medicine focused on some of the subtle indicators of the functioning of the brain stem. George Oshawa discussed ancient Japanese medical techniques for reading some of the brain stem signs, such as "*sanpaku* eyes." There are three sides of a person's eyes that may be visible: at both sides of the iris and just beneath the iris. In Japanese, *san* means "three" and *paku* means "sides." Look at pictures of Abraham Lincoln and you will notice his *sanpaku* eyes. Lincoln was plagued by low life energy and depression throughout most of his life. He was running cold. Physician John Diamond describes the *sanpaku* eyes of such well-known people as John Kennedy and Marilyn Monroe. *Sanpaku* reveals not really the eyes, but the posture that the eyes reflect, a life orientation at a given time in our lives, how we consciously or unconsciously choose to present ourselves to our world.

A netlike series of cells called the *reticular activating system* is located slightly above the location of your fingers when you place them beneath your earlobes. This is the ON and OFF switch of the brain. About the size of your little finger, it monitors your environment constantly.

A clock ticking in a quiet room will gradually leave your awareness. The reticular activating system "hears" it, however, and will alert you to the absence of the ticking should the clock break. Something will seem amiss. Even though you do not "think" that you are aware of the change in your environment, your brain is on alert through the reticular activating system. It is possible that hot-running people have a particularly alert reticular activating system, while cold-reacting people experience a rise in the threshold of that system.

It is important to remember this vigilance function of the reticular activating system as you think about hot and cold times in your life. Your brain is always on duty unless you do something to relieve it from such vigilance. It is a mistake to understand your thoughts as related to only the higher parts of your brain. Your whole brain thinks in continued interaction with your entire body.

We know that patients under general anesthesia are capable of recalling dialogue that took place in the operating room. Researcher Henry Bennett at the University of California Medical School published in *The Journal of Anesthesia and Analgesia* the warning that patients are capable of hearing and remembering dialogue in the operating room while under anesthesia. It is hypothesized that the power of suggestion could play a major role in the way we recover from surgery and in the avoidance of complications. Hypnotic suggestion has been shown to work while a patient is under anesthesia. Bennett reports that nine of eleven patients for whom a taped message was played during deep anesthetized sleep suggesting that the patient tug at his ear did in fact tug at his ear after waking up.

Think of the implications of a surgeon angry with her or his staff, pessimistic about your recovery, and talking negatively while your brain monitors and stores this programming material. It may be wise to wear earphones during surgery, receiving encouraging words even if you have to record them yourself. Perhaps you may wish to prepare a "surgical suite" of relaxing music and statements such as "You are doing beautifully, and you are going to get well quickly and be stronger than ever before." After all, this is much better to hear on whatever level the brain hears it than the statement "This poor fool is a goner."

Another part of the brain stem is called the *thalamus*, the master file system of the brain. All incoming information is sorted here and sent to appropriate higher-level locations for processing and reacting. It is interesting that the filing and directing department of the brain is located so low in the psychoarchaeological hierarchy. It is as if our entire government were run by an impulsive, immature, hyperactive file clerk. We can deal with this clerk if we understand the level at which the clerk functions. If we are unaware of this fact, we become slaves to our more primitive, less humane impulses.

The thalamus does not read, consider, evaluate, and assess in terms of the welfare of the world. It files and directs only for the survival of the brain itself. Unless told otherwise, there is no "us" in the lower levels of the brain, only "self."

In the center of your head is another of the structures of the brain. About 300 million years ago, this part of the brain evolved as the survival center. It is the intensive care unit of the nervous system, the part of the supersystem that can get you into serious trouble or help you stay well, and it is directly implicated at hot- and cold-running times in your life. Medical students are taught to remember the functions of this part of the brain, called the *limbic system*, by remembering the so-called Four F's: fighting, fleeing, feeding, and . . . the sex act.

Body temperature, heartbeat, breathing, sweating, and the general response of the body to the world go on here. This area is named the limbic system because it resembles a cap, or "limbus," sitting on top of the brain stem. It reacts first to stress or change in our internal or external world, a type of life-stress Geiger counter.

The limbic system controls all our secretions and excretions. Until recently, we thought that the essential excretions of the body were sweat, urine, and feces. We have learned, however, that everything the supersystem does is somehow related to avoiding hot and cold running in favor of a more balanced, effective temperature.

Our tears may also serve an excretory function. Research on crying provides an insight into the interaction between the brain and the immune system. Tears elicited intentionally by the inhalation of onions contain only salt and water. Tears elicited by watching sad films contain leftovers of chemicals secreted when we are under stress, a type of washing out of the remnants of our reactions to stress. Regular crying is likely to rid the body and supersystem of our stress by-products. William Fry, in his book *Crying: The Mystery of Tears*, suggests that the more frequent and open crying socially allowed of women may enable them the opportunity to excrete their "stress waste" more readily than men, who are conditioned to block this natural cleansing system.

Psychobiologist Dr. David Goodman at the Newport Neuroscience

Center in California reports that men encouraged to weep intensively and uncontrollably experience a drop or rise in testosterone levels, depending on the prior level of hormones in their systems. Those with high levels of hormones lower these levels; those with low levels tend to raise the testosterone levels in reaction to their crying. The hormone testosterone is related to male aggressiveness and competitiveness. It is implicated in male vulnerability to stress-related diseases such as stroke and heart attack. Once again, the concept of balance emerges as the key to the supersystem.

Goodman found that men with low levels of testosterone at the start of his research program experienced as much as a 30 percent increase in testosterone following their crying. They also reported feeling more assertive and comfortable with themselves. Some of them actually grew more hair on their chests. At puberty and afterward, males experience an increase of testosterone which, when combined with social mores against the display of emotion, may result in less crying.

Perhaps men can learn to cry their hearts well.

THE BRAIN'S BRAIN

The body/mind connection is a discovery that relates to process . . . the reorganization of one helps reorganize the other.
MARILYN FERGUSON

Located in the limbic system is a tiny "brain of the brain," the *hypothalamus*. It is about the size of a pea and weighs about 4 grams, or about one-seventh of an ounce. Although it is small, it is the director of a symphony of body interactions. It directly affects the body's master gland, the pituitary gland, which secretes hormones affecting every major gland of the body. As you will learn, it is the gland directly involved when we run hot or cold. A "keeper of the flame" capable of turning our temperature up or down in reaction to our world, it reacts to how we choose to think. The hypothalamus is directly involved in our sexuality, playing a major role in our sex drive and our responsiveness to erotic stimuli.

Near the hypothalamus is the *amygdala*. Stimulation to this area produces anger, rage, hissing, and threatening behavior in animals. Just as the hair of a cat stands on end when a cat is angry or threatened, as a type of evolutionary trick to fool an enemy into thinking the cat is larger than it actually is, so the hair on the back of your neck stands on end when you are threatened or angry.

The interaction between the amygdala and the hypothalamus is important in understanding hot- and cold-supersystem functioning. Hot reactions are often characterized by hissing, raging, and the threatening posture related to the amygdala. In actuality we are most often threatening ourselves.

Also in this area of the brain, and another part of the limbic system, is the *hippocampus*, which is related to the recognition and enjoyment of novelty in the environment. Damage to this area in animals will result in docile, redundant, surrendering behavior. Cold functioning in our lives may be related to those times when this part of our brain is more active than other parts, seeking input, stimulation, involvement. It becomes apparent that even within the structure of the brain there rests a prewired hot-cold cycle reverberating in response to the environment.

An incontrovertible principle of the brain is that first and foremost it wants newness, information, and novelty. In fact, if boredom is the primary state and we "run cold" for too long, the brain may direct the body to produce novelty and change from within itself, perhaps producing extra cell growth, cell disease, and cancer.

While such thinking is speculation at this time, Dr. Augustin De La Pena, in his recent book *The Psychobiology of Cancer*, proposes that the brain will not tolerate docile, redundant, surrendering behavior by the body in which it resides. It seems to "eat" new information and may, if all else fails, entertain itself to death if it senses a stimulus starvation. Dr. De La Pena suggests, that the selfish brain will create perturbations to help entertain itself, and he even goes so far as to suggest that the area of the body chosen for perturbation is related to the lifestyle of the person. He theorizes that world conflict, war, and even the possibility of nuclear holocaust relate to the brain's desire for novelty, change, and stimulation. If Dr. De La Pena's speculations are correct, we have even more evidence of the importance of taking control of the supersystem, of providing it with stimulation we choose to feed it, rather than allowing it the autonomy of an immature young child left unattended.

Located just behind the limbic system is the part of the brain responsible for balance and coordination. Watch a belly dancer or skilled athlete to see the workings of this part of the brain in action. This three-lobe structure, the *cerebellum*, has been theorized as responsible for more than just our physical balance. Dr. James Prescott, developmental neuropsychologist at the National Institute of Child Health and Human Development, hypothesizes that gentle cuddling, rocking, swaying experiences early in life can result in the development of more loving, peaceful, less hyperactive persons. Perhaps failure to be treated gently and to get used to such movement early in life produces an overreaction to movements later in life. In effect, the cerebellum seems to be saying, "Rock me early and rock me often, or I will rock you later," causing you to overreact to daily stimulation, perhaps to overheat the supersystem.

Under the control of the brain, within the limbic system, we have centers for fear, rage, withdrawal, regression, hostility, and boredom—states that relate closely to running hot and running cold. This is also the center for intense feelings, sexual impulse, and the desire for human interaction—all of which can relate to wellness.

Our health depends not just on the higher centers of the brain, but on understanding the functioning of our "lower" brain as well.

One of the most controversial biologists since Charles Darwin, Edward O. Wilson of Harvard University states that our knowledge of self is shaped by the hypothalamus and limbic centers of our brain. He points out that to overcome our subservience to these emotional control centers of our brain requires the expenditure of time and energy, increased effort, and awareness.

Wilson discusses the concept of vegetarianism, a style of eating contrary to the meat-eating culture of our ancestors. The evolution of hunting big game for meat required higher degrees of cooperation which, in turn, led to higher development of intelligence. This accelerated the process of mental evolution. Meat eating is now built in. It is easy and effortless. Vegetarianism requires effort, self-monitoring, commitment, and reprogramming of our brains. It requires control and not response to evolutionary predisposition. The type of control and the change in internal dialogue that are necessary to transcend the limitations of our biological ancestry, our hot and cold cycles, are achieved primarily through our "higher" brains, the two sides of our neocortex.

We must next learn what we can do to assume more control over these lower levels of the human brain. Our higher brains are the center of self.

HALF A MIND TO LIVE

The only satisfactory way of existing in the modern, highly
specialized world is to live with two personalities. A Dr.
Jekyll that does the metaphysical and scientific thinking that
transacts business in the city, adds up figures, designs machines, etc. And a natural, spontaneous Mr. Hyde to do the
physical, instinctive living in the intervals of work.

ALDOUS HUXLEY
"Wordsworth in the Tropics"

The so-called higher parts of the brain are the left and right hemispheres
of the cerebral cortex. It is a mistake to consider them as separate parts,
for everything about us as humans works together. The left and right
hemispheres, however, have their own unique cognitive styles, and each
may take on more significance during hot and cold times in our lives.
We are now learning that this left-right specialization of the human brain
has profound implications for our immunity and wellness.

The left and right halves of the cortex are joined by a massive
bundle of nerves called the *corpus callosum*, containing some 200 million fibers. In spite of this complex connection, it is the left hemisphere
that seems to know it is thinking and seems to equate itself with you
as "self." It is here that a self-dialogue takes place which can alter the
entire supersystem.

There are strategies for gaining access to the right hemisphere as
well, but the programming is quite different. The language of the right
hemisphere is one of symbolism, of dreams, of ambiguity. The language
of the left hemisphere is one of linearity, rationality, and logic. Jerry
Levy at the University of California suggests that women, who tend to
enter adolescence as much as 2 to 3 years sooner than boys, experience
an earlier development of the corpus callosum and, therefore, that their
two hemispheres are joined more closely together in cooperation, developing a more whole-brain orientation to their world, perhaps a capacity to more rapid change between hot and cold reactions or less
drastic opposites.

To get some idea of the structure of these two brains, make two
fists and place your hands together at the wrists, knuckles touching
knuckles, bottom of palms touching bottom of palms. Now move your
two middle fingers. This area corresponds to the part of the brain that

represents movement of the body parts. Moving your hand slightly outward, toward the little fingers, indicates the area associated with memory. Your right hand represents visual memory, your left hand represents verbal memory. Move your little fingers to see the area associated with vision. Move your index fingers and they will correspond with the part of your brain responsible for incoming stimulation sent up from the thalamus filing system.

Now move your thumbs. They should be facing toward you, and they represent the part of the brain associated with thought, speaking, and emotional control.

Now think of your hands as covered by thick gray gloves. This will correspond to the gray matter of the brain, the *cerebral cortex*. This is a new evolutionary development, less than 100 million years old. This is the area where day-to-day thinking, and the general location of your limited sense of self, is housed. It is here where much of your self-dialogue takes place and where much can be done to regulate other areas of the brain and the supersystem—and where much of your control of the hot and cold running styles can be achieved.

The neocortex is directly related to the functioning of the immune cells. Dr. Norman Geshwind of Harvard University documented years ago that left-handed persons (who more typically experience right-hemisphere dominance) manifest more problems with their immunity systems. Recently, Dr. Gerard Renoux of the Medical School of Tours in France demonstrated that the destruction of large portions of the front of the left hemisphere of the brain (around the area of your left index finger in our two-fisted model) resulted in significantly reduced numbers of certain types of cells important for fighting disease in mice experiencing this surgery. We are beginning to learn, then, that our brains interact in complex ways with our immune systems, sending signals back and forth for the protection of our health.

Researchers have shown that certain brain chemicals discovered in their research attract special immune cells important for healing wounds and infections. There is even preliminary evidence that some immune cells can produce some of their own brain hormones.

Much has been written about gender differences and the dominance of the left or the right hemisphere. In fact, men do tend to be more localized, more specialized, in their brain functions and to have more of these functions located in the left hemisphere. This may in part explain the existence of the mathematical-genius phenomenon and the finding that this occurs more frequently in boys. Male genes may relate to the specific development of a very localized area of the brain in the left hemisphere for such a capacity.

The male's propensity to left dominance may also relate to the male tendency to value autonomy, independence, and self at the expense of relationships and intimacy. It is also true that the male tendency to more localization and specialization within higher levels of the brain makes men more vulnerable to brain damage. The female "brain generality phenomenon" has resulted in easier recuperation from brain injury and stroke for women. Other areas of the brain can take over for the injured part of the female brain in an easier fashion than in the case of the more specialized male brain.

Carol Gilligan, author of *In a Different Voice*, has suggested that parenting and learning experiences contribute to male independence and problems with intimacy and to female problems with autonomy and preference for intimacy. It is also possible that this difference is related in some way to the selfish brain theory proposed by Dr. De La Pena. If the male is more left-brained, he may tend to be more "self" oriented. Whole brains tend to be more "other" and "us" oriented, more in tune with a oneness concept underlying the principle of healthy living in our world and for our world.

Understanding the left-hemisphere–right-hemisphere issue is important in preparing to alter hot and cold systems, for the language of each hemisphere is quite different. People who can visualize very well, who can see things clearly, are usually processing things in the right hemisphere. Their comprehension takes place by seeing mental pictures. These people are *visual learners*. Those who comprehend by hearing are usually processing in the left hemisphere and are *auditory learners*. Those who cannot localize their comprehension, and who must learn by doing, are called *haptic learners*. They have to touch, to do, to experience, and to feel in order to learn.

Color sensitivity, singing, music, dance, art expression, creativity, visualization, feelings, and emotions are associated with the right-hemisphere function. The right hemisphere is more holistic, intuitive, fantasy-oriented, and timeless, while the left is more linear, logical, symbolic, sequential, verbal, and reality-oriented, emphasizing time and the abstract. ·

Utilizing these guidelines, personal programs can be established for moving from left- to right-hemisphere dominance and altering the temperature of our supersystems. I suggest that the left is closely associated with those times in our lives when we run hot and that the right may dominate at those times when we run cold.

None of us is left- or right-"brained," but we tend toward cycles of dominance. Our left hemisphere has to do with our socialization, language and movement in our world. The right hemisphere has to do with our ties to our limbic system, emotions, and body image. All of us use both hemispheres together, with different emphasis at times of challenge.

Which hemisphere seems to be dominate for you now? Take the following cognitive style test, and perhaps take it with your family as well.

Cognitive Style Test

1. Take a round cardboard tube left over from a roll of paper towels. With your eyes closed, lift the tube and hold it to one of your eyes. This will be your dominant eye, and the opposite hemisphere will likely be your hemispheric orientation.

2. Hold a pencil in your preferred hand, and write the word "brain." Stop at the end of the word and do not remove your hand or the pencil from the paper. If you are right-handed and you curled your thumb inward, with your palm up, almost writing from on top of the writing line, you are probably right-hemisphere-dominant, even though you use your right hand. If you did not curl your hand, you are most likely left-hemisphere-dominant. The reverse is true if you are left-handed. Curling your left hand at the end of the word indicates left-hemisphere dominance. No curling indicates right-hemisphere dominance.

3. Your eyes tend to gaze toward the opposite side of your brain dominance. That is, if your left hemisphere is engaged, your eyes look to the right. If your right hemisphere is engaged, your eyes will turn to the left. Under stress these movements are even more predictable. Ask someone who knows you whether they have noticed which way you tend to gaze. Look at some family pictures. You may notice that you hold your head in a way that favors a gaze to the right or left. Ask people questions regarding various

issues, and you will see whether they tend to use the right or left side of the brain to process such issues.

4. Stand straight, look forward, and raise your right arm straight out from your body. Point your thumb down, and close your fist. Have someone push against the top of your arm. Reverse the process, and test your left arm. The strongest side will be the side opposite your dominant brain hemisphere.

5. Look in the mirror and smile. Which side of your smile goes up the highest? If the right side goes up more perceptibly, you are typically left-hemisphere dominant. If the left side goes up higher, you are more likely right-hemisphere dominant.

6. Stay at the mirror and cover one-half of your face with a piece of cardboard. Which side of your face appears happiest, largest, and strongest? The side of your brain opposite the stronger side of your face will be the dominant hemisphere, or the one primarily used in your cognitive style.

7. Hold your hands as if in prayer. If you are right-handed and your left thumb is on top, you are not as totally left-hemisphere-dominant as a person who places his or her right thumb on top. The reverse posture for your thumb will seem awkward. If you are left-handed and your right thumb is on top, you are more right-hemisphere-dominant than the typical left-handed person. This may indicate some mixed dominance for both left- and right-handers who have opposite thumbs on top. Our gestures tell us much about how we are thinking. Neurological discharges generalizing throughout the brain may explain why some people gesture extensively with their hands. (Perhaps a brain with more to say than just the mouth can handle?)

8. Applaud yourself. If you are right-handed and you clap your right hand into your left, you are more likely left-hemisphere-dominant. Left-handers who applaud their left hands into their right tend to be more right-hemisphere dominant. Applauding to the center, with both hands meeting at midline, indicates a more whole-brain, mixed-hemisphere dominance.

9. Do you tend to think about the past and future more than the present? If so, you tend to be more left-hemisphere-dominant. If you tend to think more about the present, to be more spontaneous in your interaction with your world, you tend to be more right-hemisphere-oriented.

10. Without hesitation, answer the following question: Are you governed more by your heart or your head? If you responded ''head,'' you tend to be more left-hemisphere-dominant. If you responded ''heart,'' you are more right-hemisphere-dominant. If you hesitated and thought about the answer, you tend to be more left-hemisphere-dominant. If you are arguing about the validity of this question, you also are more likely to be left-hemisphere-dominant.

Look over your results and try to determine a tendency to hemisphere orientation. Remember, this is only a general indication of your learning style and may relate to your immunity style. As I will discuss later, diseases of the left hemisphere tend to be heart disease, stroke, and hypertension. Diseases of the right hemisphere are more likely to be cell disease, allergy, and bowel problems. Do not forget that failure to use a hemisphere can result in diseases associated with that hemisphere, just as overuse of a hemisphere can result in the experience of diseases of that lateralization.

The cerebral cortex and its complex divisions and folds are so complicated that our heads have had to become larger to accommodate this new and developing part of the brain, with its unique left-right characteristics. Unfolded, this part of the brain is about the size of an open newspaper sheet. The wonderful aspect of this newspaper sheet, however, is that we may write, erase, and rewrite on this sheet to influence our own destinies. We can create our own news, not just read it. There is nothing better or worse about any one cognitive style, but knowing your orientation can open up new vistas toward a wholeness that we know promotes health.

Chapter Three

THE GOLDILOCKS PRINCIPLE

As we learn more about the regions of self, where mind and
body act as one, indivisible and interdependent, we may also
understand more about the internal dynamics that can make
us ill and the balancing forces that may keep us well.

DIANE HALES
Former editor, *New Physician*

Once upon a time, Goldilocks found porridge. One bowl was too hot,
one was too cold, but one was just right.

The supersystem needs to maintain an effective temperature, to
reject elements of the world that are "other," while not overheating or
cooling off too much in the process. The immune system, in coordination
with the brain, must run effectively if we are to be healthy. Our immunity
porridge must be maintained at a physiological temperature that allows
us to protect ourselves from disease and at the same time to grow and
develop and flourish. A hyperactive or hypoactive immune system turns
on us, failing us when we need it most. When we run too hot or too
cold, we lose the miracle of the supersystem, the reverberating circuitry
of brain and immune system that protects us from disease.

There is a little gland just beneath the upper part of the breastbone,
about where the "V" in a V-neck shirt or blouse points. Everyone

thought it was a useless gland for adults, because it was always shriveled and small in the bodies that were studied at autopsy. People finally learned, however, that such specimens of the gland are very small because disease processes have weakened them. People learned that the *thymus gland* is important in something called immunity and in our ability to stay healthy. Now that people are learning more about immunity and how it relates to our thinking and feeling (and how our thinking and feeling can enhance or reduce our immunity and even the size of the thymus gland itself, as well as other glands related to immunity), they may learn to live happily ever after.

As the brain and its neurons deal with other stimulation, make sense of it, and adapt to it, so must the immune part of the supersystem make sense of the continual invasion of "other." The new field of research that examines the interaction between the brain and the immune system is called *neuroimmunomodulation*. This field attempts to determine the degree and manner in which the brain and immune system interact. The field of *psychoneuroimmunology* studies interactions between stress and change in our world and reactions of the brain and immune system to our psychological interpretation of events. This field goes further than the field of neuroimmunomodulation and speculates about thought and its relationship to wellness.

Psychoimmunology goes even further than psychoneuroimmunology. It suggests that a supersystem of interaction between the brain and immune system exists and is under our own control through modification of our internal dialogue. It suggests that understanding our supersystem style, whether or not it is hot or cold, and understanding our cognitive style can help prevent and cure illness.

To understand the immune system, remember there are two kinds of *lymphocytes* (white blood cells) that fight disease. Each relates to a different function of the immune system. The thymus gland is a crucial component of the immune system, referred to by Dr. G. J. V. Nossal, an immunologist, as a "school and factory for lymphocytes."

Thymus-derived lymphocytes, called *T cells*, are responsible for immunological reaction of the body. *B cells*, which are produced in the bone marrow and so named because they originally were identified in birds, also serve an immunological function. These cells have surface immunoglobulins that function as receptors for other stimulating substances and react rapidly to environmental and personal change.

One theory for the origins of cell disease, or cancer, was formulated by Sir MacFarland Burnet, the Australian Nobel Prize winner. He suggested that of the billions of new cells generated every day, some will go wrong. They will be broken cells, unable to control their own development. They clone, divide, and crowd out healthy cells. When the crowding becomes too excessive, there is no more room for health. One of the functions of T cells, or lymphocytes, is to recognize these abnormal cells and destroy them.

There are actually two types of immune functioning in the body. One type is called *cell-mediated immunity*; it is involved in the body's rejection of transplanted tissue or organs, infections, or poisons to the body's system. *Humoral-mediated immunity* utilizes primarily B-type cells which release specific antibodies for attacking agents or invaders called *antigens*.

B cells proliferate or divide into antibody-producing cells which are called *plasma cells*. These cells, in turn, produce specific antibodies required for very specific jobs of killing off unique agents invading the body. These are the custom-made "soldiers" of the immune system. They make the immune system capable of its own form of learning, remembering, and reacting, just as the brain learns and remembers.

As the brain seeks stimulation, perhaps the immune system seeks stimulation as well. Too much health may result in "immune lethargy." Like an army which is prepared and waiting but never called into action, an unused immune system may become obsolete, not sufficiently prepared for new types of attack. It appears that the supersystem must do what it is designed to do, or it will begin to create its own problems.

Another type of lymphocyte is referred to as a *null lymphocyte*. It is designed to attack and kill overgrowing cells, such as the type of cell that may cause cancer. This search-and-destroy surveillance, carried out by the "police force" of the immune system, may help in cancer prevention as mentioned earlier. Dr. Novera Herbert Spector of the National Institute of Neurological and Communicative Disorders and Stroke designed experiments that studied the functioning of killer cells to see whether the supersystem could be taught to produce them in higher numbers to fight off disease.

Just as Pavlov's dogs were taught to salivate to a bell, mice were taught to produce more killer cells in reaction to the strong odor of camphor. Pavlov's dogs first salivated in response to meat. The mice were given a drug called I:C, or polyinosinic-polycytidilic acid, which is known to enhance the activity of natural killer cells. Pavlov's dogs matched the bell with the meat and finally salivated to just the bell. In like manner the mice matched I:C with the odor of camphor and finally produced increased activity in the killer cells in reaction to just the camphor. Whether or not the same effect applies to the entire immune system and several other types of immunity cells remains to be studied, but it is clear that immunity efficiency can be taught. Reginald Gorczynski of the Ontario Cancer Institute states, "There is probably no measure of immunity that will not prove subject to conditioning."

Classical conditioning is the technical name given to the process of matching stimuli previously unrelated to one another so that over time other stimuli can elicit a response formerly brought about by only one of the stimuli. At the University of Rochester Medical Center, psychiatrist Robert Ader and immunologist Nicholas Cohen injected rats with cyclophosphamide, a drug that can diminish immune efficiency. At the same time these rats were given saccharine-flavored drinking water. Following the period required for learning to take place, these same rats were given only saccharine-flavored water. The effectiveness of their immune function diminished in response to simply drinking water—more evidence that the immune system learns just as the brain learns.

Such research projects raise an important question. Is it possible that the dangerous side effects of drugs used for such diseases as cancer can be reduced by alternating the administration of drugs with unwanted side effects with the administration of other, less harmful substances to patients who have been previously conditioned, whose immune systems have been taught to respond to the less toxic substances?

Newspapers are now reporting several stories regarding the transplant of organs. Dr. Gorczynski operated on mice, grafting skin from other mice to assess the immune system's response to these grafts. He then subjected the mice to grafts in which all the same operating procedures were employed but no skin was grafted. Going through the surgical procedures, the mice showed the same lymphocyte response and immune reaction as they had shown when they had actual skin grafts. Is it possible that persons receiving multiple grafts and organ transplants have immune rejection to such grafts on the basis of a learned response? If so, could the immune system be taught to accept these grafts, in effect, be retrained to help instead of hinder the transplant process?

Just how powerful the effect of learning and thought can be on the immune system is illustrated in a report in the *Journal of the American Medical Association*. In a thoroughly documented case of a 28-year-old woman from the Philippines, a serious disease called *systemic lupus erythematosus* vanished following her return to the Philippines for removal of a curse which she felt had caused her symptoms of weakness, skin rash, anemia, and disorders of the liver and lymphatic system. The hormone drug prednisone had been effective in treating this disease, but serious side effects followed the use of the drug, including problems with the thyroid gland and kidney function. When her belief system changed, without the dangerous side effects of artificial substances injected into her system, the disease vanished as the curse of illness was lifted.

There are several other components of the immune system at work to protect us from disease. The *macrophages*, or "cleanup" crew, are important for healing wounds and infections. They actually ingest, or "eat," antigens or invading foreign bodies. Under a powerful microscope they can be seen crawling to, surrounding, and destroying "other" substances. Research has documented that the mobility and effectiveness of the macrophages is negatively affected by stress and depression. These cells tend to behave as we think. If we think in a sluggish, withdrawn, surrendering, hopeless manner, they seem to follow our mental que and behave accordingly.

In addition to T cells, B cells, null or killer cells, macrophages, and the division of the immune system into cell-mediated and the more specific humoral-mediated responses, there are cells called *T helper cells* and *T suppressor cells*, specialized sets of cells that are designed to regulate the immune response. T helper cells encourage B cells to generate the specifically responding plasma cells mentioned earlier. Remember that these are important because of the specific antibodies they offer. T suppressor cells, on the other hand, inhibit such formation of specific antibodies. This illustrates the check-and-balance principle of the supersystem. Too much is as bad as too little for the supersystem. The balance is maintained in part by a ratio of T helper and T suppressor cells. Fortunately, we have more control over the balance within the supersystem than we ever imagined. In fact, imagination is one way we achieve that control, one way we control the temperature of our "health porridge."

To complete a preliminary understanding of the immune system as it has developed over the last 20 years of research, two more terms must be understood. First, the concept of *tolerance* refers to the immune system's ability to identify and eliminate only non-self or antigen substances. When the tolerance function goes wrong and the self is attacked by the immune system, the malfunction is called *autoimmune disease* or, literally, "an attack on self." This concept of tolerance is also found in the brain. When our lives are stressed beyond our coping capacity, something can go wrong with our sense of self. We engage in thinking and behaviors destructive to our own welfare. This is a form of what might be called "autocerebral disease," or self-destruction through smoking, driving without a seat belt, drinking to excess, or eating unhealthy foods. In effect, we exceed our human tolerance.

The second term related to the immune system is *specificity*. Each antigen or invader elicits a rejection response only from those immune cells designed specifically to work against that type of invader. As I have discussed, the immunoglobulins on the surface of every B cell are long, full chains of proteins and are part of a chain of uniquely fitted, specific lock-and-key apparatuses. If the key fits the lock, rejection of the invader is accomplished.

Our genes precode us for the development of this specific system and design it to do this highly specialized work. I suggest, however, that it is not disease which kills us, but our living, believing, and thinking. Our supersystems are under our control and awareness; they are not simply reflex systems.

In the time it has taken you to read this far into this book, more than 30 million new lymphocytes and 3 million new antibody molecules have been produced, refined, and designed as uniquely yours. They are as unique as your fingerprint and millions of times more complex. The number 10 multiplied by itself 28 times equals the approximate number of atoms in your body. Ninety-eight percent of these atoms are replaced annually. Over a 5-year period you develop an entirely new body with entirely new cells. In effect, you are a completely new you. We are always in-process, always developing through what physician Larry Dossey calls a "biodance," interacting between our universe and the small cells within our bodies.

To understand how our immune systems can get out of balance, consider the following relationships. If our immune systems overreact to outside, or exogenous, agents, it is likely that we will develop allergy. You may detect it in your children by noticing dark "allergic shiners" beneath their eyes or a small line on the bridge of their noses from the constant rubbing (with palm of the hand brushed against the nostrils) and sniffing of the allergic solute. If our immune systems underreact to outside agents, however, we are likely to experience severe chronic infection. You may notice this in children who experience continual colds, sore throats, and problems with their ears.

If the invasion is endogenous (from within the body), perhaps created by a bored brain or immune system attempting to entertain itself, and our immune systems overreact, internal imbalance and autoimmune disease problems may result. Our systems may malfunction by continually attacking themselves. It is speculated that if our immune systems underreact to endogenous agents, or overgrowing cells, we may be prone to cancer due to failure of our surveillance and killer-cell systems.

The same pattern is present in the brain. If our environment contains stressors to which we mentally overreact, we can become allergic to our own bodies, perhaps resulting in a clogging of the vessels to and around our hearts. If our brains underreact to outside stressors, we can develop chronic emotional disorders.

If our brains overreact to our innermost thoughts, we become consumed by our problems. We begin to distrust the world in general because we distrust ourselves. If our brains underreact to our innermost conflicts, we can lead lives of desperation. We can be trapped in redundant patterns of self-destruction, even though the persons around us who love us see our problems clearly. We are unable to see the severity of our inner turmoil, and sometimes only those who love us feel its full wrath.

THE SAM AND PAC SYSTEMS: HOT AND COLD PORRIDGE

Life without the challenges which induce stress responses
would be no life at all.

KENNETH PELLETIER

The "porridge" which can be too hot or too cold is actually a hormonal porridge. The "ingredients" are *trophic hormones*, so called because they affect other glands and parts of the body as they run through our supersystems as messengers of our interpretations of our experiences.

When we are running hot, the adrenal medulla (the inside of the little gland on top of the kidneys) secretes hormones that heat us up even further. This is called the *SAM system*—the sympathoadrenomedullary system. Research has shown that this system is responsible for the secretion of catecholamines, which can inhibit the effectiveness of the immune system.

When the SAM system continues unchecked, tissues in the body interacting with the immunity cells begin to deteriorate. The master immunity gland, the thymus, shrinks to half its size within a day or so of severe injury, sudden illness, or stress or change in our environment. Millions of lymphocytes can be destroyed or impaired.

The deactivating part of our nervous system I call the *PAC system*—the parasympathoadrenocortical system. Reactive to the parasympathetic or more settling aspect of our nervous system, the adrenal cortex (the outside of the adrenal gland) secretes cortisol, which over a period of time has a negative influence on the immune system.

It is important to remember that these systems do not operate as separately as these shorthand terms would indicate. Actually we have elements of both operating within us at all times. However, when we are running hot or running cold, either the SAM or the PAC system tends to dominate, sometimes for too long and too intensely. As Dr. Herd, who coined the term "SAM system," comments, "SAM activity is essential for normal physiological functioning . . . it is the excess of SAM . . . that predisposes to cardiovascular disease." So it is with the less studied PAC system. Without this system we would cease to exist, but when it functions to excess our immune systems can shut down.

Our task is to strike a balance. When we run hot, we have a tendency toward alarm reactions. We activate the hypothalamus to stimulate the amygdala and the brain stem, causing trophic hormones, in turn, to activate the entire SAM system. This raises the amount of catecholamines, which lowers lymphocyte production and other aspects of our immunoefficiency. When we run cold, the supersystem is in a vigilant or watchful state, rather than an alarm state, like a guard who has been too long on duty. When the PAC system dominates, cortisol moves through the system. The cold reactor may seek novelty and stimulation from without instead of from within, and the thalamus, pituitary, and hippocampus parts of the brain dominate. Corticosteroids lower levels of sex hormones, perhaps even sexual desire. Macrophages are slowed in their work. Whether we are under the control of a hair-triggered guard ready for destruction or a half-asleep guard oblivious to possible infiltration, each cycle represents a lack of balance, a failure of the Goldilocks principle.

Researchers may question this. Some will say that research has not yet clearly documented the relationship between disease and the SAM and PAC systems. I suggest, however, that whether or not we have enough proof, we have nothing to lose and everything to gain by attending to lifestyles and seeing them as directly related to our suffering and illness.

Oscar Wilde warned of the difficulty in understanding complex fields such as the field I propose, psychoimmunology. He states, "There are works which wait, and which one does not understand for a long time; the reason is that they bring answers to questions which have not yet been raised." I hope I will raise several questions throughout this book that will draw your attention to your day-to-day life orientation, for I believe that our survival depends upon such attention.

I do not know for sure that thought, emotion, and imagination can work magic, change our entire lives, and greatly enhance our immune systems through the power of controlling our supersystems, but I hope so. One of the leading researchers in the field of healing, Dr. Jeanne Achterberg, states, "The imagination should not be regarded as a panacea for all that ails the human species . . . unless, of course, we choose to believe there are no limits to consciousness and its inherent ability to alter the state of things." I confess to being a believer, and I hope this book for laypersons will serve as an early translation of some of the most important research in history.

I turn now to an examination of the hot-reaction style, the SAM-activated cycle that we all experience at various times throughout our lives. Maybe you should take a short rest before you read the following "hot" chapters. It may help you keep your own SAM system in check and encourage just a little more PAC as you read through all this hot material.

Part Two

HOT- AND COLD-RUNNING PEOPLE AND PROBLEMS

The most compelling factors of the environment, the most commonly involved in the causation of disease, are the goals that the individual sets for himself, often without regard to biological necessity.

RENÉ DUBOS

In Part Two you will learn two supersystem styles. All of us have within us both hot and cold capacities for maladjustment. As you read through this part, identify your own tendencies to run hot and cold and learn how heart and cell disease can result from running too hot or too cold for too long.

Chapter Four

HOT-RUNNING PEOPLE

Ever since I made myself naught, every day has been a vacation.

GHANDI

"I've got complete control of the entire eastern seaboard market," bragged the man next to me on the airplane. "I've built my company from the ground up, and I've got it so that I can push one computer button and see the whole picture."

Throughout the 2-hour plane ride, this successful businessman spoke of himself and the impact of his own strategies in dealing with day-to-day life. His central theory—his philosophy of life was one of self-involvement and self-centeredness. Research on "Type A" risk factors for heart diseases and other studies of the mind-body connection are becoming more specific; they seek ever more precision in the identification of risk factors to our health. I maintain that there is an equally important need for awareness of our own philosophy and life orientations that may predispose us to disease. I suspect that the major health risk is the impact of our personal values and relationships with others.

At those times in our lives when we are running hot, we are not only more hostile, competitive, and impatient, we are also guided by the central view that we, ourselves, are indeed responsible for everything, control everything, and are not only the captains of our own ship but the crew and cargo as well. Our supersystem becomes totally consumed by this self-focus. Drs. Scherewitz, Graham, and Ornish have completed a review of research studies and have highlighted the importance of self-centeredness as a key component of what I mean by *running hot*. Frequency of the use of such words as "I," "me," "my," and "mine" is correlated to cardiovascular risk. I suggest it is not only *that* we are running hot but *why* we are running hot that affects our health and that *why* is our "I-it" rather than "I-thou" lifestyles.

The following 12 questions will help you decide whether or not you are oriented toward a hot style of life at this time. This "Dirty Dozen" test will provide you with the key factors that make up the hot style of living. Once you have examined each of these items, go on to construct your own psychograph on the hot style. This psychograph will help identify specific areas within the hot style that are uniquely applicable to you. All 12 items to follow are derived from research on hot living. Stop and think about each one and, if possible, discuss each with someone you know well.

Hot Characteristics—The Dirty Dozen Test

1. Do you feel hostile much of the time, although you may stringently deny or repress this hostility to others?

    YES_____ NO_____

2. Do you think about time, trying to figure out how to get more and more out of it, viewing it as "yours"?

    YES_____ NO_____

3. Do you think competitively, comparing yourself to others, even in little things such as dress, driving, tennis, recreational activities?

    YES_____ NO_____

4. Do you think about achievement, always striving toward goals and, in the back of your mind, thinking of step-by-step success plans, sometimes only to find that the ladder you are climbing is leaning against the wrong wall?

    YES_____ NO_____

5. Do you think impatiently, rushing others in your mind, hurrying past their thoughts, focusing on your own thoughts? You may even be thinking of other things as you read this question . . . ?

YES_____ NO_____

6. Do you find your mind restless, always looking for something to think about, even when sitting quietly?

YES_____ NO_____

7. Do you think in a hyperalert fashion, with the slightest stimulation such as a phone ringing setting off a whole chain of thoughts that distract you from the event itself?

YES_____ NO_____

8. Does door slamming or dog barking cause your mind to go into high gear immediately?

YES_____ NO_____

9. Do you speak as you think, in an explosive manner with gestures accompanying each phrase? Does it appear that your gestures are a model of the way your mind is functioning?

YES_____ NO_____

10. As you respond to this item, notice three sets of muscles: your forehead, your upper back by your shoulders, and the small muscles at the junction of each of your jaws, called the *temple manipular joints*. Are any or all three of these muscles tense right now? If they are, your shoulders are slightly elevated, your jaws are clenched, a little wrinkle exists between your eyebrows over your nose, your muscles bulge slightly in front of your ears, and your breathing may be in your chest, not in your belly.

YES_____ NO_____

11. Do you spend time thinking of all the responsibilities you have, and does it seem to you that you have more responsibility than almost anybody else and that people dump on you, thereby avoiding their responsibilities?

YES_____ NO_____

12. Do you sometimes think that relationships and intimacy would be nice but that time does not allow them to be a priority? Do you think that your achievements are your form of giving of yourself? Do you seem to give every gift but the gift of yourself?

YES_____ NO_____

If you said "yes" more than six times, you're hot! More than four yeses and you're at least warming up.

Now that you know the basic characteristics of the hot reactor, you are ready to construct your own psychograph and look for those areas that apply to you. Have someone who knows you well score you on these same items.

Score yourself as follows:

1—Almost never

2—Sometimes

3—Almost always

4—Always

Competitiveness

1. When listening to a story about someone else's accomplishments, do you automatically think about how you might have done better than the person in the story?

_____

2. When someone else is praised, do you think that you have done things that deserve even more praise and that you seldom are praised enough?

_____

3. Do you usually think of ways to get the edge on others, even in small activities such as getting a slightly closer parking place or having a place closer to the front of the line?

_____

4. When playing games, do you go strictly by the rules and never give any advantage to your opponent (giving a point that really is very, very close), sometimes to the point of cheating in your favor?

_____

5. When in social discussion at dinner or at parties, are you always "on," trying to be just a little more clever, quick, accurate, or intelligent than everyone else?

_____

_____
Subtotal

Impatience

1. When standing in line, do you find yourself getting just a little angry that other people are even in front of you at all?

_____

2. Do you interrupt others when they are talking, or at least want to interrupt them because you have thought of something to say?

_____

3. When people are late for an appointment with you, do you start to think they probably are inferior or not too smart?

_____

4. Does it seem that there is never enough time in the day and that there are always a hundred things left to do? Even when you are doing one thing, are you thinking of something else you have to do?

_____

5. Do you sometimes want to rush others as they speak, perhaps by offering a little verbal encouragement to get them to talk faster—even to the point of giving hand signals to "make it quick?"

_____

_____
Subtotal

Hostility

1. Do you think of physical violence toward someone who has frustrated you, even when the frustration is minor (such as being cut out in traffic)?

   _____

2. Do you fantasize what seem to be beautiful put-downs of people long after you have had a run-in with them?

   _____

3. Do you talk in negative, harsh, aggressive terms when relating stories or events to others? Do your stories typically contain yourself as the hero gaining some advantage over someone else?

   _____

4. Do you tend to think in sarcastic terms (looking at people who have frustrated you and thinking that if Moses had seen them, he would probably have created a whole new commandment)?

   _____

5. Do you spend time thinking negatively about yourself, not qualifying for any positives (as in "Sure I work hard, but I'm such a twit when it comes to handling my money")? Do you get mad at yourself for failing to work well enough or hard enough?

   _____

   _____
   Subtotal

Once you have completed the three tests, add up the subtotals to reveal your own hot-psychographed score. (Your observer should do the same.) Using the accompanying graph, indicate your results by coloring in the outside thermometers. Are you surprised with the outcome? To review each of the categories separately (and more dramatically), multiply each of the subtotals by 3 and mark your scores on the center thermometers. (Your observer should do the same.) Sitting with someone to discuss your subscores, your total score, and comparisons between your own and the observer's score may be one of the most

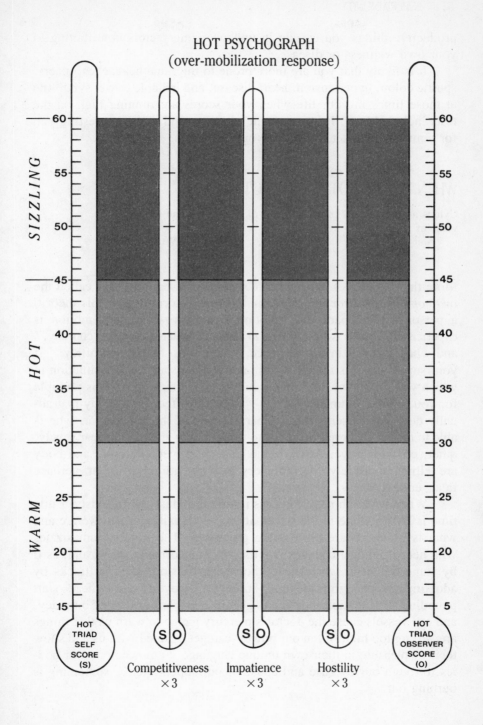

productive things you can do in understanding factors contributing to your own wellness or disease.

It is likely that you are more prone to migraine headaches, ulcers, spastic colon, hypertension, heart disease, and irritable bowel syndrome at those times in your life when your scores are running high on the tests included here. It is important to understand that I am testing you for your "mental set," not just your behaviors.

WHEN YOU'RE HOT YOU'RE HOT

Cynics are those who know the price of everything and the value of nothing.

OSCAR WILDE

More than 2 decades ago, psychologists discussed what was called the *two-component theory* of emotional arousal. According to this theory, a person feels a particular emotion based on where the emotion is experienced. That is, when you are in a church, you tend to feel "churchy," and when you are in a post office, you tend to feel "post officy." If your supersystem is in a fear and high-arousal state but the situation in which you find yourself calls for quietness and steadiness, it is possible for you to label yourself "steady" when, in effect, your body is gradually destroying itself. This is characteristic of the hot reactor, who is able to match his or her behavior to the situation and may appear steady, quiet, contemplative. At the same time, however, the mind and body are telling an entirely different story with an entirely different, perhaps fatal, ending.

When we are hot, we process information fast and furiously. Little time is left to relate to the information emotionally. Where we are and what is going on are all that are processed. The supersystem sizzles with neurochemical changes, we roast in our hormonal stew, and, as if by some universal wisdom, the body can be stopped in its tracks by adopting an "enough is enough" strategy. We overload, our heads start pounding for attention, our hearts get attacked for our lack of intimacy, and our vessels cause the doctor's mercury gauge to warn us that things are getting too high. Even our bowels can get irritated with us and show their displeasure in their own unique language. Somewhere in our bodies, through our overuse and abuse of our supersystems, something is burning out.

Dr. David Burns has written about a cognitive behavioral theory suggesting several types of thinking errors that people make. Some variations of these thinking errors also characterize the hot style. As you read each of the following thinking styles, take the time to determine whether or not they characterize you or a loved one at any given time.

"Nontweeny" Thought

I assigned one of my groups of heart patients the task of sorting a hundred art reproductions into three piles: beautiful, in between, and ugly. The five men sat down to begin work. The first few paintings were easily classified and group decision was rapid. As they progressed, however, one of the men commented, "I think this one is sort of a tweener." He explained that he meant it was in between, not beautiful or ugly, but sort of somewhere in the middle. One of the other men in the group commented, "There ain't no tweeners. It's good or it isn't." This "nontweeny" approach is hot thinking.

The world is viewed as either-or, a projection of the thinker's inner turmoil, an ON and OFF switch. People and events are never *sort of* or *kind of*, but *complete* or *total* as in "complete fool" or "total jerk." All assessment is accomplished through this inner dialogue of opposites.

To understand hot-supersystem people better, apply their all-or-none type of thinking to them. When they describe something as a "complete waste of time," put their names at the beginning of their critical sentences, and you will see how they are really thinking about themselves. "*I* am a complete waste of time. *My* life is a complete waste of time. *Everything* seems a complete waste of time" is the orientation. Of course, do not let on to them that you are doing this private test, or you, too, will be seen as a total fool.

In fact, one way for hot people to cool down is for *them* to learn to put their names in front of their all-or-none statements. Over time, they are sometimes able to gain insight into their own thinking style, perhaps even recognize the self-centeredness that underlies hot times in their lives.

The supersystem itself responds to the hot type of thinking, becoming quick on the draw and easily being set out of balance. The result can be diseases related to an impulsive type of immunity system, or one that is too quick to identify *other* as "enemy." It is a potentially fatal mistake to ignore the fact that our brains react to our thoughts and that a pattern of hot thoughts may result in brain chemistry changes signaling the immune system to behave in this same poorly controlled, overly selfish manner.

Claim Jumping

"I can't believe it. Every ride in Disneyland done twice, all in one day." This was the report of a man to his family as they were almost the last persons to leave the gates of the amusement park. The entire family had the look of survivors rather than revelers. It was clear that at least at this time, this was a hot man who was even "recreating" in a hot fashion.

If there is one type of thinking that hot-supersystem people value more than any other, it is fast thinking. They tend to offer as their highest compliment labels such as "lightning quick," "on the ball," "like a pistol," "sharp," "quick as a whip," and "a mind like a knife." Their minds quickly stake claim to ideas and viewpoints, quickly forming conclusions. Their own thinking is so fast that they seldom allow persons to finish thoughts or sentences.

Hot people have processed the "other" incoming data before it has even stopped coming in. As a result, hot people are often without complete information with which to make rational decisions. They have thought for two persons at once, staked their claim, and moved on.

You can test a hot person on this conclusion-jumping style by stopping your sentences to him or her in midstream. "I'd like to tell you that . . ." and then pause. Most likely, the hot person will complete the sentence for you and have the answer. "You want to tell me that the water heater is broken. I'll call the shop tomorrow. Next issue . . . ?" Even worse, the hot reactor may not notice that your sentences are incomplete and may finish them for you in his or her own mind, draw conclusions, and move on without having communicated at all.

To test the hot system, change your message even if the hot person is right in his conclusion. Finish it with a feeling statement, such as, "I want to tell you that . . . I really love you." You will probably get a response such as "Me too" or "Yeah, thanks" or "Why, is something wrong?" The hot person's brain is confused at what it finds as surprising, incomplete, dissonant "other" messages. It is keyed to deal with *other* as "it," not "thou," with everything and everyone rotating around a narrow definition of self.

The supersystem is keyed to offer inappropriate responses or input. The result may be a complete turnoff of the immune system by the hot reactor. The supersystem responds to this claim jumping with inappropriate, poorly functioning responses. It makes mistakes about what is other and what is self. It may get so confused it begins to see everything as other and attacks part of the body because it thinks that it, too, is other. It literally overheats, and things begin to bulge, stretch, clog up, and block, especially around the heart, as if the very heart of the hot person were being separated from the body itself.

"Musturbatory" Thought

The young husband turned to his successful executive wife, after listening to her 5-minute discourse in the therapy session. She had outlined her obligatory lifestyle and her ambitions in terms of money and status. Her husband responded, "You make us both lead a 'shouldy' life. Everything is should, should, should. What about words like 'like,' 'want,' 'wish,' and 'love to'?"

Hot-supersystem people think in a style of obligation. They are mired in a sea of *should*s, *ought to*s, and *have to*s. Applied to self, such thinking results in guilt and dissatisfaction, a form of impatience with self. When this "shouldism" is applied to others, the result tends to be anger and impatience and intolerance. All these emotional states are destructive to the immune system.

Set your watch and count how many times in a 5-minute period the words "should," "must," "ought," "have to" are used by someone you feel is thinking in the hot style. Hot-running people will use such words several times every 5 minutes, revealing an inner dialogue that is using such language at an even higher rate.

I asked one of my patients, as we walked to the hospital, what time it was. Without looking at his watch, he responded, "It should be two." Hot people not only keep time, they try to control it.

The supersystem of the hot-thinking person gets trapped in a response pattern that "right or wrong" in its responses to invasion from others causes it to continue in an obligatory, trapped overreaction. It is unable to shut off or turn down. The hot reactor can get sicker and sicker, and the immune system can respond in the same ineffective manner over and over again. Chronic illness can result. Even though an effective immune system is in place, it becomes trapped in a childlike "he or she told me to do it" style of defending against disease. This is "the devil made me do it" syndrome, and in this case the devil is the brain unchecked by rational thought.

Label Making

The hot reactor is almost always a cynic. He tends to be a "cognitive bigot," grabbing on to the slightest perceived weakness or flaw in someone and generalizing it as a character trait. People do not make mistakes in the eye of the hot reactor; they are utter "incompetents."

As I walked through the waiting room in my clinic, I noticed one of my patients counting change by lining dimes and quarters along the arm of the chair. The patient noticed my gaze and responded, "That arithmetic idiot in your parking booth shortchanged me again. He can't read tickets. He can't add or subtract. I doubt if he breathes correctly" was the evaluation of the patient. He finished with, "It's okay, he's just another one of those people ruining the American economy."

This cognitive bigotry extends not only to behaviors but to race and religion as well. Although hot-supersystem people are typically bright and articulate, they will reveal their bigotry in not so subtle ways. They will identify certain flaws with certain races, certain strengths with certain religions. They may be smart enough not to show this in public, but the partner of a hot reactor has heard such bigotry in the privacy of the home.

This labeling and arbitrary style of thought extends to the immune system as well. George Solomon of Stanford University has divided the immune system into afferent, central, and efferent components. The *afferent* function is the labeling process of the immune system; the *central* function is the organization for dealing with invasion; and the *efferent* function is the actual destruction of "other," or antigens, affecting the body. The hot reactor has serious trouble in the afferent, or labeling, function. If this function goes wrong, the whole immune system starts out wrong and could become more vulnerable to disease.

Oh-No-ism

As I sat in the hospital room of one of my patients and discussed the results of some medical tests, he suddenly sat up in the bed stating, "Oh no, I missed the news." He showed tremor, sweating, anxiety, as if a nuclear attack were imminent. This is the *oh-no-ism* characteristic of the hot style of thinking.

Hot reactors exaggerate events, making whole worlds of sandpiles. Their self-dialogue is tied to a cycle of "one day lost is a wasted week which messes up a whole month which can ruin my life." It is as if they were looking through binoculars at each event. An unmade bed can be a signal of family collapse through lack of cooperation and respect. Hot reactors go into "situation red" over a spilled soft drink, and rage that "everyone is always messing everything up around here."

When the immune system reacts to this type of thinking, it is in a type of Defcon Three situation similar to the high level of military mobilization just short of actual nuclear war. Two dangers result from this. First, just as our country is at great risk when it is in a Defcon Three nuclear war status, so our health is forever threatened when we are living on this thin edge. Second, the immune system can become fatigued by this constant state of overreadiness. Readiness states may be prolonged for years in response to this destructive thinking pattern and magnification style of processing incoming data, leaving the immune system fatigued at times of invasion.

The wife of one of my patients commented about her husband: "Harold almost never gets sick, but when he does, he almost dies. I call him Defcon because he's always on a scramble alert. The trouble is, he is scrambling our entire family." Harold has an immune system so scrambled it becomes ineffective and dangerous to itself.

POWERFUL PEOPLE AND WEAK DEFENSES

For this is the journey that men (and women) make; to find
themselves. If they fail in this, it doesn't matter much else
what they find.

JAMES A. MICHENER

When people are thinking hot, they tend to use defense systems, strategies for avoiding confrontation with central problems in their lives. The problem is that when we run the hottest, we tend to have available to us only our weakest set of defenses. When we run hot, we tend to become "power people," valuing control, frustrated in our ability to achieve it, and tending to ignore or to devalue the importance of other people in our lives. When all this is combined with the behavioral characteristics of the Type A person, the time illness, and the anger of the Type A, we have a potentially fatal combination.

Researcher George Vaillant suggests that certain types of defenses or ways in which we avoid confronting our own inner conflicts and internal dialogue are related not only to our emotional well-being but to our physical survival as well. He has found that the maturity of our defense systems and the degree to which we are in tune with our innermost wishes, feelings, and thoughts is a stronger predictor of heart disease than smoking.

In my experience, most hot-supersystem people are characterized by what Vaillant referred to as the "neurotic" defense systems. Most people who come to see a psychotherapist have problems with what used to be called "neurosis" or with "character disorder." Simply, the person who is neurotic assumes too much responsibility. The person with character disorder does not assume enough responsibility for his own life. This is described well by Scott Peck in his book *The Road Less Traveled*. While changes in psychiatric diagnoses have occurred and the term "neurosis" is no longer used, it is helpful to use this framework to understand the functioning of the immune system.

Five types of defenses are characteristic of the hot person who is thinking in a neurotic, overly responsible manner. While defenses are necessary for healthy day-to-day functioning, blindness to the overuse of such defenses can be as crippling as having no defenses at all. In effect, we all have two defense systems—the immune system and emotional defenses—and we need both to survive.

Hyperheadism

One of my patients suddenly lost one of her closest friends. She had come to therapy to deal with her grief. Her husband accompanied her, and during the session he stated, "Look, dead is dead, gone is gone. She was good when she was here, and now she is gone. Nothing accomplished by moping about it. Onward and upward." The patient turned to him and said, "You are such a hyperhead. All you have is head. Don't you have any feelings?" His response was, "Sure I have feelings. I just don't allow myself to be bothered by them like you do."

Shakespeare wrote in *Twelfth Night*: "Better a witless fool than a foolish wit." Hot reactors are foolish wits, theorizing away their hot style with high-sounding, complicated, abstract theories, supported by carefully selected and biased "research" that upholds their limited view of the world.

Hot people are able to win most arguments, not only because they tend to be smart and articulate but also because they would not be aware of losing. They are caught up in their own thoughts, and others' views are not likely to result in more than a pause for hot reactors to collect more self-oriented materials to buttress their case.

Anything that is not "intellectual" is seen by hot reactors as weak or soft. Even in medical schools, which can be factories for hot reactors, students and faculty describe "hard" courses as those dealing with numbers, data, bodies, cutting, and chemicals. "Soft" courses are those dealing with feelings, concepts, and thoughts. I will show you later that this causes trouble when you try to talk to hot doctors about diseases related to cold styles of life.

If you are lying in bed as you read this book, and are next to a partner who has already dismissed most of the information you may have shared, try again. Share this section on hyperheadism with your partner and note the response. It is likely to be similar to the report of one of my patients who referred to this material as "psychological ballyhoo designed for frustrated stay-at-homes." One hot-reacting husband told his wife, "A person would have to be crazy to go to a psychologist anyway."

The hot person's focus on head rather than heart results in the brain's disrespect for the symbolism of the heart and its associated emotions, carings, and focus on relationships. This may account for the brain's dismissal or even removal of the heart. One wife, testing the material in this book with her husband, stated, "I'm really worried about you. I think you are too much head. You are characterized by this hyperheadism." The husband's response was, "You need a lot more theory and a lot less worry. Use your head, will you. If you wear your heart on your sleeve, someone will always wipe his nose on it."

Deep-Sixing

Hot reactors have very little access to their own underlying emotions and events in earlier life that may affect their present living. In spite of the fact that they may have had severe problems in childhood and life crises that have taken a toll obvious to others around them, hot reactors are both unwilling and unable to examine with others these developmental setbacks. Instead, they are functioning under a curse of living and reliving the same pain and distresses that affected them earlier in life. As Shakespeare wrote, "Past is prologue." To hot reactors, "The play's the thing."

I have yet to see a hot-reacting person in my office who is not able, with support and encouragement, to describe childhood events that were extremely painful and related to present difficulties in life. The wife of a man in treatment for hypertension stated, "It's like talking to a wall when I talk to him. Actually, it's worse, because this wall is crumbling and it's falling on myself, on him, and on our children." When I talked to this man about his background and, through the use of imagery, traced difficulties he had experienced with an abusive father, he responded to me, "I've just deep-sixed that stuff, buried it down there deep, no sense dealing with that. What's gone is gone."

The combination of hyperheadism and "deep-sixing" affects the immune system by leaving it victim to, instead of interacting with, the brain. Hot people are stuck in a mode of reaction that will never be as effective as it can be, for hot reactors must first acknowledge the obstacles to efficient functioning of the supersystem. They must look to the past as well as to the present. This past has become a type of historical "other," constantly aggravating the immune system, resulting in sometimes subtle but often chronic hypertension and bowel disease.

Dog Kicking

The "neurotic" style of feeling totally responsible and overwhelmed at hot times in our lives can result in a tendency to express feelings and thoughts in the wrong places. Hot reactors tend to blame the kitchen sink, the car, and the notorious *them* for any problems that occur. Hot reactors seem to have an innate sense that those who love them are safe targets for dumping the frustrations that would be better dealt with in the setting in which the frustrations occurred. Families of hot reactors sometimes dread their return home, knowing that they or even a family pet may catch the wrath of the hot reactors' day. One such reactor told me, "That's nonsense. I do not bring my problems home. I go right upstairs, undress, throw up, and then join my family."

The immune system that "displaces" is likely to attack the wrong other as well. It may unsuccessfully attempt to protect a weakened and vulnerable self by attacking a part of the body that should not be attacked. It may become distracted and allow the hot-running heart to be closed off from the brain, symbolically maintaining the distance between thought and feeling, an "MH" (or maladaptive hyperarousal) before an "MI" (or myocardial infarction).

Na-Na-ism

We all remember our almost universal tendency to deal with conflicts during childhood through a rhythmic "na-na-na-na-na." It is not unusual to notice groups of children issuing na-nas to one another for an entire afternoon. The hot reactor uses this same infantile defense.

The hot person tends to be more than ready to avoid acknowledging his hot style through sarcastic "opposite" reactions, sometimes called by therapists a *reaction formation*. If a spouse asks the hot reactor to calm down, he or she may respond by saying, "Great, I'll sleep for three years and buy a mantra. Maybe that will make you happy."

One of my hot-reacting patients responded to his wife's plea for moments of quietness together with "Quiet! You want quiet? I'll leave for a couple of years and you can have all the quiet you want." He had missed the appeal for closeness, denied his feelings of frustration and fear, blamed himself for not achieving this closeness, and sarcastically attacked and embarrassed his wife. As if sticking out his tongue and issuing the na-na-ism of childhood, he had avoided confrontation of the intimacy issue at hand.

The immune system that responds to such reaction formation can cause severe infection by its "sarcastic" response to the smallest cut, pneumonia from the slightest cold, or severe hypertension from the simplest stress of daily life. It is as if the immune system were without direction, reacting in the same sarcastic overreaction style of the brain. In effect, it fools around with our health as the brain has fooled around with our feelings and crucial issues of relationships. This reaction, sometimes called a *defense through the opposite*, can develop an immune style that reacts entirely inappropriately to challenges.

Cradle Diving

"Why don't you just dive right into your cradle? That's where you seem to belong." This was a statement from a wife who had become frustrated with the tantrums of her husband. His recent tantrum had resulted in a chair being thrown through the television screen because he disagreed with the commentator. Fortunately, the regression and immaturity of the hot reactor is not always as drastic as chair throwing, but hot-running times can produce temper tantrums worse than any children's tantrums which we may feel precipitated some of our own. Persons who live with hot reactors have noted that the hotness can escalate the smallest crisis, the smallest event, to a major crisis within the family setting. Comedian Bill Cosby has said "Being a parent can destroy the last vestiges of maturity and intelligence in anyone." We all have difficulties with our maturity levels from time to time. The hot reactor is capable of diving to the depths of immaturity.

Tantrums of the immune system can ravage the body. Regressing to childlike immature behaviors can signal the immune system to do the same, to overreact or to sulk, to disrupt everything just because of some small "something" in the system.

MENTAL MELTDOWN

Drs. Meyer Friedman and Ray Rosenman publicized their research on Type A behavior patterns in 1974. Decades before this work, Walter Cannon described the fight or flight response, illustrating the impact of emotions on our bodies. In 1920, Wilhelm Raab discussed the dangers of elevated levels of cortisol and adrenaline, the cold and hot porridge of the supersystem. In 1956, Dr. Hans Selye made the word "stress" a household word. He illustrated the effect of catecholamines, or stress-type hormones, on our bodies. Dr. Robert Eliot at the University of Nebraska recently described what he called "the hot reactor" as a person characterized by rapid and significant rises in blood pressure and other physiological measures when confronted with situations as seemingly innocuous as being asked to perform quick mental arithmetic. All this work has done much to clarify the type of damage we can do to ourselves and others by allowing our bodies to get out of control. I maintain that it is our internal philosophy, our style of dealing with day-to-day life, that predisposes us to all the behaviors described by the above researchers.

Whether we consider Friedman and Rosenman's Type A's with their hurriedness, agitation, and anger, Dr. Eliot's hot reactors with the physiological response identified in his research, Cannon's and Selye's work on the stress hormones, or Dr. McClellan's power people with their frustrated need for control and alienation from others, I suggest that the important point is whether or not we are able to transcend the self-centered philosophy underlying all the above findings. If our supersystems are instructed by us, even unconsciously, to maintain and enhance the self at all costs, these costs might be much more severe than we ever imagined.

The answer to meaningful change rests with understanding how we take charge of our brains and our supersystems. Joggers still die of heart attacks, some of the most well-known practitioners of meditation are not physically well, and many heavy smokers never get lung cancer. Beyond genetics, which we cannot change (at least yet), are our thoughts, our orientation to life. They are under our control. When we run hot, we run selfishly; we experience high levels of tension, feeling charged up, defensive, overmobilized, and ready to act. Our bodies and immune systems function in the same way. Hot-running people feel that something must be done, when sometimes the answer may be that nothing should be done, that time should be taken to find not only self but the relationship between self and the world in which we live.

It is important to remember that I am focusing here on thinking and internal dialogue, not just the outside behaviors measured through the Type A characteristics. While millions of dollars are being spent on wellness programs throughout the United States, we have tended to "McDonaldize" the wellness movement, seeking quick behavior modification solutions to our "quickness diseases." Wherever there is gold, there will be counterfeiters, profiteers making quick money off of hurry illness.

When we are only self-involved and self-defensive, the stage is set for a potentially fatal meltdown. Hot-running people are caught in thinking errors compounded by crippled and immature defense systems, and they become victims instead of masters of their supersystems. They view their entire world as a threat to their control. They are in a constant state of being threatened by actual or imagined challenges. This threat "orientation" is manifested through the behavioral signs in Type A and even Type B behavior. However relaxed or agitated our outside appearance may be, threat exists when we burn on the inside for the enhancement and maintenance of self, when we lose control.

When we are running hot and perceive a threat to self, an alarm reaction kicks in, and hot people fall victim to time illness. They feel there is not enough time to deal with all the events in their lives, and they become alarmed, feeling they must do something fast. For several years this has been known as the *fight or flight* response.

Stimulation goes to the hypothalamus and to the lower parts of the brain, causing chemicals to be secreted to the adrenal medulla. This is an activation of the *SAM* system—the sympathoadreno medullary system. This causes a rise in adrenaline and the sex hormones. Arteries constrict, blood pressure goes up, and free fatty acids increase in the blood. The brain becomes overly controlled by the newest part of the brain, the neomammalian brain, or cortex. The left hemisphere in its rational, intellectualized dimensions is overly influential. Spiegel and Spiegel, at New York University, have identified this type of thinking as the *Apollonian* style, named after the god Apollo, with implications of order, structure, and control. The system "hypercoagulaters."

Running hot is defending immaturely, being driven yet frustrated by the need for power, feeling alienated from others, living in a state of alarm, being driven by time, and sometimes frantically attempting to protect a narrow but precious view of self. As all mammals experience in this state of frustration, a prewired reflex occurs. When threatened, mammals become territorial, agitated, and aggressive. Thinking has caused a reflex which, in turn, causes more thinking and an ever-heating spiral results.

In ancient eastern writings, the term *yang* implied an aggressive, demanding orientation to life, focusing on progress, the immediate, consciousness, the now at all costs—a form of egocentrism at the expense of "ecocentrism."

I return now to the man who had reported his complete control of the eastern seaboard market. As we approached our destination and prepared to land, the man turned to me and stated, "If you don't mind, I'll be stepping over you. I need to get off quick. The last time I flew into Detroit, some fool stood there and let half the plane get off before him. I swear he waited for every last person. Man, I stood behind him; I tell you, I could have died." How right he was.

The following chart summarizes the factors contributing to those times when we are running hot. Trace through each of these factors as a review of the hot supersystem. As you identify each factor, think of times in your life when you ran hot and use the suggestions in Part Three to help cool down. You can cook or cool your own emotional porridge. Unlike Goldilocks, you do not have to choose from available porridges. You can make your own.

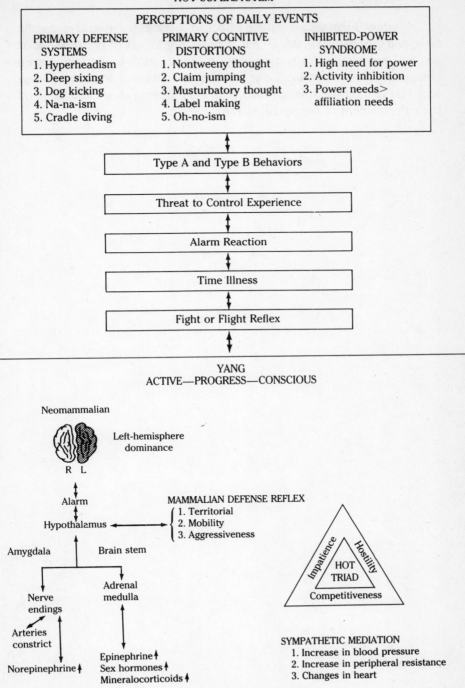

HOT SUPERSYSTEM

PERCEPTIONS OF DAILY EVENTS

PRIMARY DEFENSE SYSTEMS	PRIMARY COGNITIVE DISTORTIONS	INHIBITED-POWER SYNDROME
1. Hyperheadism	1. Nontweeny thought	1. High need for power
2. Deep sixing	2. Claim jumping	2. Activity inhibition
3. Dog kicking	3. Musturbatory thought	3. Power needs> affiliation needs
4. Na-na-ism	4. Label making	
5. Cradle diving	5. Oh-no-ism	

Type A and Type B Behaviors

Threat to Control Experience

Alarm Reaction

Time Illness

Fight or Flight Reflex

YANG
ACTIVE—PROGRESS—CONSCIOUS

Neomammalian

Left-hemisphere dominance

R L

Alarm

Hypothalamus

MAMMALIAN DEFENSE REFLEX
1. Territorial
2. Mobility
3. Aggressiveness

Amygdala   Brain stem

Adrenal medulla

Nerve endings

Impatience Hostility HOT TRIAD Competitiveness

Arteries constrict

Norepinephrine ↑

Epinephrine ↑
Sex hormones ↑
Mineralocorticoids ↑

SYMPATHETIC MEDIATION
1. Increase in blood pressure
2. Increase in peripheral resistance
3. Changes in heart

Chapter Five discusses the effect of overheated porridge on the heart and circulatory system. One of the major killers of our time, heart disease, has elicited in some people a hot reaction to avoiding, even conquering, this crippler. I suggest that the answers to heart disease may rest less on the soles of the latest-style jogging shoes and more on the enhancement of our spiritual soul.

Chapter Five

ON CHEATING OUR HEARTS

We see things as we are, not as they are.
LEO ROSTEN

Imagine a typical professional football stadium, full of cheering fans on a Sunday afternoon. Think of a thousand of these stadiums filled to capacity, and that is the number of people who will die this year of diseases related to the heart and circulatory system. More people die in our country of diseases related to the heart than of any other illness, yet the cause of heart disease has remained a mystery.

Cigarette smoking, high blood pressure, elevated serum cholesterol, diet, genetic considerations, diabetes, and other factors cannot explain the dramatic increase of coronary heart disease during the first 60 years of the twentieth century. Changes in these factors do not fully account for the recently reported decline in deaths related to heart disease. To further confuse matters, the same factors that we associate with heart disease in this country cause entirely different diseases in other countries. Why do our hearts cheat us so? Or is it that we have cheated our hearts in ways we do not fully understand?

The idea that we can think ourselves sick is not new, but it is neglected as a factor by a cosmopolitan medicine that almost totally ignores our beliefs in favor of a mechanistic view of illness and wellness.

In about A.D. 30, Cejus said, "Fear and anger and any other state of the mind may often be apt to excite the pulse." Seventeen hundred years later, the physician J. P. Hunter observed, "My life is at the mercy of any rascal who chooses to put me in a passion." William Osler, a famous physician, thought that diseases of the heart were related to "the high pressure at which men live, and the habit of working the machine to its capacity."

Cardiologists Friedman and Rosenman suggest that Type A persons are aggressive and attempt to do more and more in less and less time. This is contrasted with the Type B orientation, which is a more relaxed, less time-driven style of life. Type A behavior is not a personality trait, but a set of behaviors characteristic of people as they relate to different challenges in their daily lives. People are not Type A, but behave in a Type A fashion. What provokes a Type A reaction in one person may not produce that same reaction in another person because it is our internal dialogue, our life perspective, that I suggest is the major factor in any disease process.

Current research is extending and building upon the work of Friedman and Rosenman. Dr. Robert Eliot at the University of Nebraska has suggested that heart disease is related to a physiological reaction style of individuals who, when under stress, experience a hot reaction. Describing his own heart attack, which occurred when he failed to cope well with the stress of a busy lecture schedule, Dr. Eliot comments, "My brain cried out for rest, but my body wasn't listening." The result was a heart attack experienced while Dr. Eliot lectured on the topic of heart disease.

Norman Cousins, in his book *The Healing Heart*, reports much the same occurrence. A busy lecture schedule from which he unsuccessfully attempted to extricate himself led him to excessive stress reaction, time illness, and a sense of being trapped by professional commitments. Unable to free himself in order to rest, Cousins reports that his heart took care of this need for rest by "attacking him." The heart attack demanded that his body take an almost fatal rest.

Both Cousins and Eliot knew better than to let their lives get out of their own control. Both men are knowledgeable about rules of wellness, yet they both experienced their own heart disease. They were both unable at a given time in their lives to manage the brain-body conflict. They could not alter their thinking and behavior sufficiently to prevent their own illness, because at that time in their lives they had not really altered their philosophy and perspective. Neither man made the facts he knew a part of his inner life, his "self."

You have scored yourself on the hot-supersystem test, and by now you have a pretty good idea of your own tendency to run hot. I will now focus on the internal dialogue, the psychological set of the hot reactor who is so prone to heart disease. It is not Type A behavior that kills, but the type of thought the brain insists upon that leads the supersystem to fail us. The heart becomes "other," not "self"; it is ignored or rejected by the body and is cut off from everything else. We psychologically clamp off the supply lines to our own hearts. Even if we know better, our brains continue their hot patterns unchecked. Participators and observers of the development of our own heart disease, our brains stand by, accessories in the commitment of a major health crime, watching as fibrin "cocoons" clog our system.

What is significant, then, is not whether you are Type A or Type B in your behavior. You may appear hurried, speak in a rapid, explosive manner, and be agitated, always on the move, trying to do more and more in less and less time. These behaviors are only external markers, indicators of what your brain is telling the rest of your body to do. The internal dialogue, the ways in which you talk to yourself, results in these behaviors. Changing behavior can help, but external change without internal change only stresses the system further.

When overheating of the supersystem occurs, significant biochemical changes take place. Since the early 1960s researchers have shown that cholesterol in the blood increases in response to the way we think about external changes or stressors. The cholesterol level of accountants increases almost one-fifth at tax preparation time. The increase begins with the anticipation of the coming season, months before the actual tax season and accompanying behavioral changes occur. One study showed that the way in which the body reacts to breakfast, the way it processes the food, is more damaging to the heart if we think about life in hot ways. Researchers can measure hurry easier than they can measure worry, but it is the internal worry that kills us. Subjects have to tell scientists that they are worried, but sometimes the brain will not allow itself to be "turned in to the authorities." Changing behaviors accomplishes little if we do not change how we think.

I have discussed the fact that the alarm reaction, the activation of the SAM syndrome of the hot reactor, affects the inside of the adrenal gland, or the adrenal medulla, to increase the production of catecholamines. This negatively affects the tissues which produce our immunity to disease. The hot reactor is forever seeking more and more information, more and more stimulation, more and more novelty, more and more accomplishments, as if the brain is saying, "Self, self, self, enhance, enhance, enhance." Simply trying to force the hot reactor to relax is not likely to help. It is possible that even worse diseases may result if our attempts are focused on behavioral change without altering internal dialogue, without changing the actual programming process of the brain. There is no research on what happens to "cured" Type A's, who may not be cured from the inside out. Perhaps the brain will cause different types of disease once we catch it as a conspirator in the destruction of the circulatory system. Perhaps it will just keep on causing other problems until we tell it what we want from life.

Researchers have found increases in ACTH, adrenocorticotropic hormone, in the blood of hot thinkers. This is also associated, in elevated levels, with damage to the circulatory system. It results in the buildup of plaque in the supply line to the heart. Whenever the SAM system overreacts, the heart is vulnerable. It is as if the brain were saying, "I don't need this feeling stuff; just pump me the supplies I need to work faster."

This theory of heart disease suggests a focus on the thoughts, internal dialogue, belief systems, and internal feelings that may be the crucial variables in the diseases of hot reactors. These include not only heart disease but ulcers, spastic colon, hypertension, and irritable bowel syndrome. All these have in common an agitation and disruption of tissue. The Goldilocks rule is violated, and things are not "just right."

In the case of heart disease, we become allergic to our own hearts. We reject the heart by clogging all the arteries around it. The result may be a more gradual cutting than is removal by scalpel, but the effect is the same. The heart has been cheated of the positive chemistry that comes with the thoughts and feelings of joy, celebration, love, faith, and laughter. It is cheated of the will to lead life. Instead, life leads us.

Certainly, if negative emotions can debilitate the immune system, positive emotions should be able to enhance the supersystem. We know that no two emotions can be experienced at exactly the same time. It would be difficult to be aggressive and peaceful simultaneously.

HEART DISEASES

We have no indication where precisely psyche leaves off,
and only reflexes and neurophysiological events remain.
                                    LUDWIG VON BERTALANFFY

I have noticed certain patterns of internal dialogue in the heart patients
with whom I have worked. To best understand the interaction between
the internal dialogue and the neurophysiology of the overheating of the
immune system, we begin with a 10-item test, which takes us deeper
into the hot person's mind.

Heart Cheater's Test

To best understand the possibility of psychological "heartectomy,"
please respond to the following questions using this scale:

> 4—Almost always
>
> 3—Sometimes
>
> 2—Seldom
>
> 1—Almost never

1. Are you the victim of the "little things mean a lot" phenomenon?
   Do people and events in day-to-day life take a great deal of your
   thinking time? Can small events sometimes send you into hours of
   reconsideration, private anger, and impatience? Do others say that
   you "get on something and just don't let it go"?

   Score_____

2. Do you notice that people seem to approach you cautiously or avoid
   you because they know that in spite of what you say, you are
   thinking critically and impatiently about them? When you talk to
   people, are you at the same time thinking, "I can't imagine how
   you survive when you are so incompetent"? Do your thoughts
   favor events, goals, places, and things, rather than people, relationships, and feelings?

   Score_____

3. Do you find yourself going over and over the same daily events in your mind? Does it seem that these repetitious thoughts are circling faster and faster in what I call the *thought carousel effect*, spinning around and around on the same issues and accelerating with each spin?

Score_____

4. Do you find yourself thinking about how everything happens to you, and how if you don't watch out and think faster or more clearly than everyone else, bad things will happen to you? Do you think that in spite of your efforts, you seem to get the short end of the stick? Do you spend time thinking about how to overcome this "short stickedness" of life?

Score_____

5. Do you think that you have been hurt by others' lack of appreciation for what you have done for them? Do you feel you have gone through much and made many sacrifices only to be unappreciated? Does this hurt feeling lead you into thinking that you will stop doing things for others because you find that the more you do, the more they expect and the less they appreciate? Does this type of thinking apply to colleagues, friends, and family?

Score_____

6. Do you think that time is accelerating faster and faster? Do weekends blur into other weekends, months into months, holidays into holidays? Do you think that there is a constant march of your life, that you seem to be throwing away the wrapping paper minutes after you went shopping for the gift? Do you think, and sometimes even say out loud, that there is never enough time in the day?

Score_____

7. Are you thinking about how you can get more and more out of less and less or how you can do several things at once? Do you become angered and uncomfortable about wasting too much time thinking and not spending enough time doing? Do you try to prevent any wasted motion when walking through rooms by picking something up and transporting it to another room in an attempt to save time and effort? One hot-reacting patient said. "There is no sense

doing one thing at a time when you can do six. I can't go through a room without picking something up to transport it. I do this while I am thinking and planning my next move. Of course, sometimes this results in not being able to find those things I transport because I get busy on something else." Does this type of thinking apply to you?

Score_____

8. Have you read about or heard about Type A and Type B behaviors but thought to yourself, "Sure, I'm a Type A, but only for now"? Do you think, "I am not as Type A as other people think, and I'll be Type B anyway some day"? Or do you think that you are "really a latent Type B" or that you are "a Type A and proud of it," because "Type A's shall inherit the earth"? If everyone is telling you that you are Type A, do you think that you are the only one who really knows what you are, and do you tend to disregard these multiple reports?

Score_____

9. Do you think fast and find yourself mentally frustrated by the slow, plodding thinking of others? Do you think in staccato fashion, thought following thought following thought, rather than focusing on one thought for a period of time?

Score_____

10. Are you typically mentally alert? Are you on the watch for any challenge to your turf? Are you mentally in the alarm mode, ready to process, deal, dispense, and complete thoughts at the hint of any new data?

Score_____

If you have scored over 20 points on this test, you are strongly leaning toward the heart rejection syndrome we have discussed. Over 30 points, and psychosurgery is already in process. But cheer up. I will be offering some new ways to alter your internal dialogue so that your brain can direct the supersystem toward wellness. First, let's look at the characteristic that corresponds to each question of the test so that you may understand more fully the internal dialogue related to the items you have just scored.

1. Hassles

Some years ago researchers developed scales to measure the impact of major life events and the stress they cause in people's lives as related to their development of disease. This scale was devised by Drs. Holmes and Rahe, and forms of this test commonly appear in popular magazines. The test is still used in many research programs throughout the United States.

Holmes and Rahe hypothesized that it was indeed possible to die of a broken heart and that the body would respond most negatively to major life events, such as assuming a mortgage, becoming divorced, experiencing a loss in the family, or making a job change. Positive events such as marriage or buying a new car could also cause stress and strain reactions, and were also on their test.

More current research has suggested that although major events such as loss of a loved one can relate to serious illness, it may be the little things that really "get to us." Fifteen years ago I designed a program, which I still direct, called the "Problems of Daily Living Clinic" at Sinai Hospital of Detroit. Over the years of operation of this clinic, I have noted that although there is no disagreement that major events can take a significant toll on one's wellness, it is the day-to-day hassles, the smaller problems, that build up and actually nibble away at the individual. It is not stress or change that damages us, but the way in which we interpret such change. Perhaps we rally our strength at major events, and perhaps we are forced to think more clearly and consider the influences of others. In reaction to the little hassles, however, our brains take charge of us and we react in a patterned, automatic fashion.

A balance between hassles in day-to-day life and what researcher Dr. Richard Lazarus calls *uplifts* in day-to day life seems to be important to our wellness. He states, "Stress resides neither in the situation nor in the person; it depends on a transaction between the two." When we run hot, we lose the balance between the aggravations of daily living that cause us to feel ineffective and helpless and the uplifts that can help us feel competent and successful in our coping.

The work by Dr. Lazarus and others indicates clearly that what we perceive as hassles or uplifts depends again on our life orientation. The hot-running person sees any delays to his or her self-oriented goals to be hassles. A red light is either a chance to pause and rest or a barrier to our progress. It is truly up to us.

If we have expended our energies and adaptive strengths on daily hassles, we have less strength available for dealing with the day-to-day stress of outside agents that affect the immune system. It is a fact that most of us spend much more time being sick with little illnesses such as colds, bowel upset, and flu than we do with major illnesses. The immune system seems somehow more ready to deal with major crises than with the constant bombardment of daily irritants from the environment.

Hot patients tell me that they are aggravated by people who slow down for yellow lights or who get in their way. People in bank lines who seem to always pick the one day that the hot reactor has to be there are aggravating. People who move their shopping carts in front of the hot reactor's at a newly opened checkout lane, even though the hot person has been waiting much longer, can cause minor irritation or major disruption. Of course, there is always the major aggravation for the hot reactor of confronting the people in the ''10 items or less line'' who have 11 items in their carts.

In response to these daily hassles of our thinking and immune systems, our blood chemistry gets trained and acclimated to overreact. We get addicted to the rush of excitement and stimulation that comes with the hormones and chemicals released in this alarm state. If we are hassled to alarm almost every day of our lives, we may need to search for more and more information, getting hotter and hotter as we get older and older. The Goldilocks phenomenon is disrupted, and a poisonous dose of chemicals gradually begins to remove the heart from our own being.

2. Isolation

Hostile, competitive, impatient people are not fun to be around. We tend to pull away from them. We can never seem to make them happy or to live up to their high levels of expectation. We cannot compete with their time-management and time-dominance approach to life. We feel that we are forever disappointing them through our own inefficiencies and time wastefulness.

If it is true that hot reactors are like burners on a stove from which we pull our hands after just a few trials, it is possible that the isolation of hot reactors causes their supersystems to isolate their own hearts psychoimmunologically. Their brains, in search of more and more information and enhancement of self, are willing not only to sacrifice friendship and intimacy for the sake of self-oriented goals but also to sacrifice their own bodies as well. Hot reactors ultimately end up alone and heartless.

A study done at Ohio University illustrates the isolation hypothesis of heart disease. In 1980, Dr. Nerem and his colleagues fed rabbits a diet high in fats and cholesterol to assess the impact of such a diet on arteries and the possibility that such a diet was responsible for atherosclerosis. All the rabbits received this diet, which was almost guaranteed to produce blockage of the vessels around the heart. Most of the rabbits did indeed evidence clogged arteries at the end of the study. One group of rabbits, however, showed 60 percent less *hypercholesterolemia*, or buildup of chemicals associated with clogging of the arteries. Dr. Nerem and his colleagues initially viewed this set of findings as coincidence, but the study was repeated to assess and understand more about this unique group of rabbits with healthy hearts. Multiple repetitions led to the same surprising finding. The reason for the lower incidence of blockage was that the rabbits in the group having significantly less arterial damage had been stroked, petted, and cared for by one particularly caring lab assistant. The other rabbits did not receive this preferential treatment of warmth and support. Touching and relating to the rabbits had innoculated the rabbits against heart disease. The hot reactor is caged with the unstroked rabbits, isolated from the prophylaxis of tender touch.

I suggest that the isolation of the hot reactor is as significant as any other factor in the development of heart disease. I will return to the importance of touch and closeness later. As a hint regarding the important relationship of touch and intimacy and heart disease, consider the fact that more than half the patients suffering heart attacks report problems in their sexual lives prior to their attacks. Whether some disease process had begun to take its toll on sexual function or sexual problems had taken their toll on the heart, there is evidence of a strong relationship between caring, intimacy, and isolation in cardiovascular illness.

It is not comfortable to touch someone who is hot and getting hotter, and a vicious, destructive cycle of avoiding the hot reactor perpetuates itself. Too busy to touch and care, hot reactors find themselves increasingly unaware of the absence of these factors from their lives. This emotional blindness may cost them their lives.

One of my heart patients asked me whether his sex life would be satisfactory after his recuperation from his heart attack. I responded affirmatively and encouragingly. He looked most relieved and responded, "Thank God, because my sex life has been terrible for ten years before this heart attack."

3. The Broken Record

Hot reactors are isolated and hassled, thinking autistically and ruminating about each of life's little hassles and the world plot to obstruct their own individual brand of efficiency. They spend much of their time thinking about the redundant patterns of their lives. They think to themselves about the constant recurrence of the ineptitudes and inefficiencies of those around them. Their favorite word seems to be "they": "They do this, they do that, and now look what they've done." The endless circle of preparing the taxes, sending in the taxes, getting audited, and preparing the taxes is a continual burden seemingly suffered only by the hot reactors themselves. Indeed, each new tax law seems aimed specifically at hot reactors.

No matter how planned or organized, hot reactors seem trapped in the same problems in their own minds. Their Apollonian style of thinking, as identified by Dr. Siegel, is rational, controlled, and restricted, the making of lists and checking them thrice.

I have discussed the left-hemisphere orientation of hot reactors. There is a tendency to attempt to use this hemisphere to make quick decisions over and over again. Hot reactors think to themselves, "If I've told that person once, I've told him a thousand times." The reason for their frustration may be that they think these things a thousand times but never truly communicate their thoughts to others. This is because communication takes time, a slower pace of living, a receptivity instead of the more typical emphasis on sending, on telling rather than sharing.

This redundancy shows itself as hot reactors talk to themselves, making it almost impossible to get a word in edgewise. They seem to be on a roll, and to be rolling over anybody else. The brain functions as if it were a computer connected to a word processor, turning out more and more words in a fast-copy mode.

Because of this redundancy pattern, hot reactors intellectually mistake their own redundancy of thought for correct thought. It seems to them that they have heard something so often that it must be true. They forget that where they have heard this material before was in their own thoughts. They have become legends in their own minds, mistaking validity for self-repetition.

Redundancy is characteristic of all of us, but hot people overdo it as they overdo everything else. They may brag about their 20 years of experience and fail to realize that it is not actually 20 years of experience they have had, but 20 years of the same mistakes made over and over again. They are gradually experiencing a hardening of the attitudes along with their hardening of the arteries.

4. The Victim Dictum

Hot reactors obey the *law of unequal dispersal*. It seems to them that if something hits the fan, it tends to distribute itself all over them. As they drive down the freeway thinking three things at once and planning strategically for the next lane change, some fool always pulls slowly in front of them and disrupts their strategy of quick travel. It is as if that person left home to lie in wait just to aggravate hot reactors. Hot people seem forever burdened by others who are running in a different time zone and may refer to these others as spaced-out or "airheads." If there is one thing that hot reactors cannot stand, it is space, air, and nothingness in a life of filling everything up quickly.

Following a group meeting of six of my heart patients, the elevator from the clinic became stuck. Swearwords were uttered almost in harmony, and an immediate story-telling session began. Many of the patients talked at once; there were few listeners in this mandatory group meeting caused by the stuck elevator. In each story, each person was a victim. "This always happens to me because some fool doesn't do the proper maintenance and doesn't do his job." "This always happens when I have something more important to do." Of course, hot reactors seem unaware that they always have something important to do or that everything they do is important. Ask hot reactors how many times in one day they have done something unimportant, and they will typically respond that they had little time for such foolishness. If they do report doing something unimportant, it was usually "caused" by some person not behaving appropriately and frustrating their life strategy. Hot reactors suffer from a type of problem paranoia, feeling that somewhere, somehow, a plan has been issued to frustrate their efficiency.

The group on the elevator suddenly became quiet after several minutes of mutual story telling. It was difficult to keep telling stories with all tellers and no listeners. One of the patients asked, "Wait a minute. Is this a test of our patience, some type of experiment?" The whole group chimed in with the same type of questions about some secret experiment being conducted. The six patients apparently thought they were being victimized by an ever-lurking researcher eager once again to test their "Type A personality."

5. Silent Sadness

Listen carefully to the speech of hot reactors. Type A or not, explosive or rapid or not, there is an underlying sadness and despair in their message. It is as if "It is all for nothing." It seems that they are running faster and faster and becoming more lost. They are leading lives, as pointed out by Robert Louis Stevenson, that one moment of reflection would lead them to disown. Unfortunately, they do not have enough moments or enough reflections. Their houses are burning and they are smart enough to know it, but their addiction to continuing activity and thought traps them even though they are choking from the smoke.

One of my heart patients came to my office, slammed down into his chair, and looked out the window. "I waited twenty minutes for my wife at that damn restaurant. This was our lunch day together and she forgot it. She is so damned disorganized." I asked if he felt bad or if he felt stood up. He shot back angrily, "Stood up, hell. It's just that people cannot get organized and get their lives together." I questioned further: "But don't you feel sad that you missed a chance for lunch with her, that you had to sit alone, and that she forgot you?" He responded, "Hell no, I just felt mad." This time, however, as he responded, his eyes moistened and he looked away. "Are you crying?" I asked. He began to sob. "You'd think she at least could have come for lunch. It's just our one day." He reached for a tissue on the table near his chair. The patient from a prior session had emptied the tissue box. The hot-reacting patient picked up the box and threw it against the wall.

"You have to make somebody responsible for tissues here." He then added, "Let's get on with therapy. We haven't got too much time today due to my wife's screwing everything up." This story not only demonstrates the style of hot reactors but the fact that hot reactors try to experience even their pain quickly.

6. Future Thinking

Our perception of time is a major factor in our wellness or illness. Hot reactors do not live in the now. There is only what was and what will be.

Another patient grew impatient during his therapy session. "How many more sessions will it take before I will become significantly more relaxed? I read this Type A stuff and I would like to be a little more Type B-ish in time for the slow season at work."

This style of perception not only shows how hot reactors think about time but also a common use of the Type A theory that is made by heart patients. They seem to love quick labels, and Type A seems very effective for them. It prevents them from the necessity of having to explain in more detail their feelings and orientation to life. They take great comfort in using a letter code. They seem to feel that finding the right program at the right time and on the right day can make them "B-ized."

Vacations are potentially deadly to hot reactors, because they are never truly *in* vacation, but tend to be *on* them or *doing* them. While in the cart during a golf game, they think about the future and plan a business move before the next hole.

Lying in the sun at the pool, one man turned to his wife to ask, "What are the plans for tomorrow?" The patient's wife responded, "No plans. We will just sit here and enjoy the sun." Her husband stood up, grabbed his beach blanket and a folder of papers, and said, "I didn't spend $5000 to come here and do nothing." Even at this time of rest, the brain demanded action.

The left-hemisphere dominance of hot reactors is implicated in this type of thinking about time. "Time is money and money is time" is a philosophy of hot reactors. They seem to be always vested in capital gains of the future. They fail to experience things now, always thinking of what things will be like later. Ask hot reactors to describe things in the present, and they will have difficulty. Ask about what happened before and what is going to go on in the future, and they will be at their best. Baba Ram Das has stated, "Be here now." The philosophy of hot reactors is "get ready for later."

7. Cramming in Time

Hot reactors try to squeeze as much into a given block of time, activity, or conversation as possible. They can look you in the eye, apparently listening, and be thinking of several things at once. You may note that their gazes change as you talk to them. They may look up to the right, indicating engagement of the left hemisphere, a sign that they are rationalizing, plotting, and planning, not really receiving your message.

An interesting phenomenon related to thinking more and more in less and less time is the fact that hot reactors squeeze dreaming together with thinking and control. Dr. Steven LaBerg reports a collection of research supporting the occurrence of what are called *lucid dreams*. These are dreams that take place while the dreamer thinks and observes the dream. The dreamer is able to deal with the dream as if she or he were awake, manipulating its contents and theme. Hot reactors are such monitors of their own thinking and such "squeezers" that they seem unable to allow themselves the luxury of a dream that guides them. They value only reality and tend to bring their dreams into that arena of their lives.

Psychiatrist Havilock Ellis once stated, "Dreams are real as long as they last. Can more be said for living?" Hot reactors, by squeezing thoughts into their dreams and accelerating the patterns of their lives, rob themselves of the escapism provided by dreams. They are trapped in the reality of thought, a reality created by a brain striving to protect and enhance self when, in effect, it is destroying the entire supersystem.

One of my hot-reacting patients stated, "Tonight I am going to dream about my new summer home. Then I think I'll wake up around 6 A.M. I don't have to use an alarm clock, you know, because I can set my own mind to wake up at will at 6 A.M." I have noted this same phenomenon in several hot reactors. They not only control their dreams, but they are able to control bodily functions such as waking, defecating, even eating.

One of my patients bragged, "I don't let myself get hungry until I have accomplished a good day's work." Another "squeezer" reported to me, "Even when I make love, I can think of several things at once. When I jog, I take along a tape recorder and earphones to listen to medical tapes so I can stay current in my medical practice. I am even alert to my pulse when I jog."

The wife of one of my heart patients stated that she had awakened several nights during the last month to find her husband had left the bed and locked himself in the bathroom. This pattern persisted for several evenings. One night she decided to discover for herself the meaning of these late-night escapades. She waited until he left the bed at approximately 3 A.M. She heard the bathroom door close and lock. She walked to the door, placed her ear against it, and heard a tape player describing trends in the stock market and real estate. She discovered that her husband would wake in the middle of the night to squeeze another hour of learning into his life.

This squeezing pattern will be explored further when I discuss the relaxation response that can work for some heart patients. An important warning is that during the relaxation response heart patients can actually be thinking more about obligations and life strategies. There is some evidence that blood pressure actually rises for these persons even though they are attempting to relax.

It is possible that this squeezing style of thinking relates to a squeezing style within the immune system. Vessels around the heart may themselves become squeezed, failing in their role as supply lines. Cardiologists point out that there is a syndrome of angina related to spasms of the arteries around the heart. These arteries may be completely clear and healthy in every other regard, but they are in effect squeezing the heart to death.

8. Cynicism

Current research in cardiology indicates that cynicism may be one of the most significant predictors of heart disease. It seems possible that those who expect the worst of this world may end up leaving it much sooner. Hot-running people assume a protectionist posture, expecting trouble.

One of my patients went to his front door to greet a delivery person with a large package. The card read, "I have always loved you." The patient sent the delivery person away, refusing to sign for and accept the package. Although his wife waited several days for him to comment on the gift she had sent him, he gave no indication of having received this expensive token of her caring for him. When she finally summoned her courage to ask about the gift, her husband responded, "You sent it? I thought some wise guy at the office was trying to be funny. I sent it back. I'm sure they will take it off our charge card."

When I asked him about his thought patterns, he theorized in hot fashion, "I always expect the worst, and I am never disappointed. If I expect the best, I am almost always disappointed. Look for rain and maybe a little sun will shine." He concluded his reaction by stating, "Cynicism is one of the most healthy and safe ways of leading one's life."

It is important to understand that this cynicism is applied not only to the world of the hot reactor but to the hot reactor too. The immune system overreacts, because even self is distrusted. The self becomes a focus for attack. The hot reactor is so insecure with himself or herself that the hostile, impatient, competitive pattern develops into a strategy of avoiding failure rather than achieving success. The philosophical answer to the patient with a cynical philosophy might be, "Expect the worst, and sooner or later you will receive it. Expect the best and you can alter your immune system and your own lifestyle." We have seen several examples of negative feelings producing negative health states. Positive expectations and thoughts can, then, be expected to produce healthier lives.

A new research project will help illustrate this point. Patients with good health indicators on all the modern body system measures were asked to personally rate their own health on a scale of *excellent, good, fair*, or *poor*. Patients with poor health indicators on objective measures, such as blood pressure instruments and blood tests, were also asked to rate themselves on this scale. Try this yourself. As you read this sentence, consider your health and your experience of your own wellness: It is *excellent, good, fair*, or *poor*?

Regardless of the objective measures of health, the patients' own perceptions of their health were more predictive of mortality than the objective measures. Our health attitude is crucial to our survival. In fact, researchers concluded that only age is a better predictor of mortality than attitude toward one's own health. In this study, and perhaps in our lives, perception was everything.

Whether ill people have some innate mechanism that signals them regarding illness or whether their attitude negatively or positively affects their health cannot be clearly demonstrated at this time. It is reasonable to speculate, however, that negative emotions, thoughts, and self-talk can negatively affect our health and that positive emotions will positively affect our health. In the same study, patients with very poor objective measures of their health, including blood pressure, blood tests, and other measures, were able to override these negative measures because of their positive attitude toward their health. The cynical brain puts the heart in jeopardy; the hopeful brain frees the body for wellness.

9. Relaxation or Agitation?

With all the talk about Type A and Type B behaviors, the so-called A people may place themselves in jeopardy through what has been called the *relaxation response*. Discussed in some detail by Dr. Herbert Benson of Harvard, this is a response innate to the human body. It is achieved in a quiet place by relaxing the muscles throughout the body and breathing slowly. The mind is freed of distracting thoughts. Significant changes in body chemistry and blood pressure can be accomplished. Cholesterol levels are lowered significantly by this technique. *The American Journal of Psychiatry*, January 1985, contains an article supporting the importance of meditation as one form of relaxation response. It is clear that we can achieve control not only of our bodies but of our brains.

Researchers have long understood that Type B is not all that it is cracked up to be. Indeed, the original researchers are often misunderstood, for they never suggested that Type B behavior is a goal or cure strategy for Type A. Cardiologist Robert Eliot states, "Plenty of old and crabby Type A's have seen their Type B friends and colleagues die of heart attacks." We know that about 70 percent of men and 50 percent of women in the United States could qualify as Type A by the Friedman and Rosenman standards. Only a small fraction of these Type A's and another fraction of the Type B's become sick. Is B the answer if B means relaxation?

Recently we have learned that a paradoxical effect is present in relaxation. For several years physicians and health care workers have been asking their patients to sit, relax, even meditate, or at least settle down, for about 20 minutes twice a day. For some people, probably those who are already relaxed anyway and who have mastered their internal dialogue, this can be a very effective technique. For other people, however, and hot reactors in particular, disruptive thoughts are given free reign to agitate the body during such relaxation. Sometimes the relaxed state itself is so shocking to hot reactors that blood pressure goes up instead of down. Cholesterol levels can go up instead of down during the relaxation attempts of people who are unable to recognize relaxation, mistaking it for a signal to act. Relaxation, then, may not be the answer for all hot reactors. Moving one letter ahead in the alphabet may not solve the heart disease problem.

10. Thoughtless Thinking

Hot reactors are more positive than pensive. They have little time for process, only for results. There is no hesitation for hot reactors. They know right from wrong, good from bad, a good deal from a bad deal, as soon as they see it. You may recall the sergeant on the popular TV series *Hill Street Blues* who used to warn his officers, "Let's be careful out there." The new sergeant now warns, "Let's do it to them before they do it to us.'' Ironically, this alarmed, threatening stance is characteristic of hot reactors, but they end up doing it to themselves much more than they do it to anyone else.

One hot reactor, following his lecture at a business meeting, was asked, ''Do you really think you are right?'' The lecturer responded, ''I don't think—I know!'' The questioner sarcastically turned away and murmured, ''I don't think he knows either.''

To hot reactors, the person who hesitates is not only lost—but stupid. The early thinker gets the money worm. Hot reactors are on full-volume thought and highly respect fast, self-assured thinking. They may even listen to music and sports events on television at a loud volume, for those who think loud and fast tend to acclimate to everything loud and fast. One of my patients plays music at fast speed because he ''can listen to an entire symphony in half the time of other people.''

We are talking about hyperthought, not just hyperbehavior. Try this experiment to understand this principle. Following the reading of these instructions, put this book aside and sit straight and comfortably in your chair near a clock. Notice the time and then close your eyes. Be perfectly still and try to think of nothing at all. Clear your mind, but try by sense or instinct to guess approximately when 1 minute has elapsed. Now put the book down and try the test.

If you are a hot thinker, you will note that thoughts kept floating in and out during the experiment. You will also note that you guessed early on the minute or felt that time was dragging and that a minute's time was exceedingly long. I have tried this with hot reactors, and some will insist, ''You slowed the clock down'' or ''I must have misread it at my first gaze.''

These 10 internal dialogues are responsible for altering the brain and the immune system. The supersystem becomes a risk instead of an aid to the hot reactor. If you suspect that you are a hot reactor or that someone you love is suffering from this type of thinking, the worst mistake you could make would be to lecture yourself or your loved one on the urgency of change. Make sure you continue reading this book, and do not jump to the conclusion that you are a hot reactor without first understanding the cold-reactor style. We all function hot and cold in differing degrees at different times in our lives. Knowing how, when, and why we run hot and cold is the first step to health. You cannot be aware of your hot cycles without first understanding cold cycles.

In Part Three I'll tell you how to cool off. No matter how hot you are running right now, though, do not skip to the solutions in Part Three until you have read about cold reactions and cold disease.

Chapter Six

COLD-RUNNING PEOPLE

There is now incontrovertible evidence that mankind has just entered upon the greatest period of change the world has ever known. The ills from which we are suffering have had their seat in the very foundation of human thought.

PIERRE TEILHARD DE CHARDIN

The patient held the button down on the remote-control device controlling the television suspended from the ceiling above her hospital bed. She ran through every channel more than twice. It sounded as if a machine gun were being discharged within the room as the channels rattled by. "These networks ought to be shot. TV stinks and they are all controlled by the news media and the liberal press anyway. We are probably doomed by these left-wingers." She tossed the remote control to the patient chair beside her bed. The physician leaned closer and said, "But Charlotte, we have to discuss these results. I have just told you that your growth is malignant."

She looked toward her metal file held against the doctor's chest and said, "I guess I am in a bit of a mess, aren't I?" This overreaction to the trivial and underreaction to a potential life-threatening situation is characteristic of the cold reactor.

The hot reactor, by contrast, tends to overreact to any significant event. A memo announcing cutbacks at one of my patient's companies resulted in a phone call from the patient to my office. He stated, "Looks like it's poverty for me." He anticipated the worst, even though he had worked years to establish his position and was a valued employee. This same man tended to mock, even defy, recommendations regarding his health. When advised to make efforts to lower his cholesterol through dietary management, he responded, "Cholesterol, schlesterol, I like high scores in everything, even my cholesterol count."

Two people, with two entirely different reactions to events in their lives. The pattern of the cold reactor is one of defeatism and a sense of inadequacy, being passive in the face of life's challenges. While the hot reactor feels totally responsible for everything, the cold reactor feels victim to his life situation.

THE PERSONAL FREEZE

Perhaps the course of cancer can in part be altered by changing the emotions associated with depression, helplessness, and failure to cope.

SANDRA LEVY

As hot reactors melt down, cold reactors begin to freeze. Hot reactors were characterized as having the inhibited-power syndrome or being power people. Cold reactors are powerless people. They experience emotional isolation. They are overly conscientious, attempting to do everything just right, never fully understanding that such strategy is doomed to failure. They experience a high ambivalence toward themselves and others, wanting closeness yet fearing it. Desiring to be loved yet feeling unworthy, cold reactors are distanced from their inner pain by their cold-thinking, impenetrable, intellectual defense system. This inhibited-emotion syndrome results in what could be called the *Type C behaviors*. Not agitated or relaxed, not Type A or B, the Type C pattern is one of stoicism: still, apparently contemplative, but, in fact, ruminating and persevering with despair. They sense a loss of control. Less threatened than defeated, they are in the vigilance stance. As spectators helplessly watching their houses burn, wall after wall crumbles for cold reactors, and they are vigilant only for more destruction, rather than in the state of alarm of the hot reaction.

Rather than having an urgent sense of time, cold reactors feel timeless, as if suspended, victims of emotional cryogenics. They are flowing, not fighting, experiencing what has been called the *general adaptation syndrome*. A lack of novelty, newness, and growth results in a neurohormonal pattern stimulating the adrenal cortex (the outside of the gland on top of the kidneys). Cortisol rises, sex hormones deplete. The *PAC* system, or the parasympathoadrenocortical sequence, has rendered them neurochemically stagnant. The only activity is the ultimate destruction of their own health.

Spiegel and Spiegel have called the type of thinking characteristic of cold reactors a *Dionysian style*, named for the god Dionysus, who represented lack of control and structure. Neurologically, cold reactors are controlled more by the paleomammalian brain level, not utilizing the higher levels of the brain to think their way out of their entrapment. Their right-hemisphere dominance results in a pattern of negative emotions. Rather than being a strength, the right-hemisphere dominance becomes a liability, with fantasies and dreams becoming a part of negativism rather than hope. Without the rationality of the left hemisphere, we run "down" when we run cold.

While hot reactors find themselves trapped in the mammalian defense reflex, cold reactors find themselves trapped in the mammalian depression reflex. Just as cavemen and cavewomen became territorial, mobile, and aggressive when under attack, another strategy was to withdraw, to become passive and conservative, to fool predators into thinking that their prey was not worth chasing or was perhaps dead. Remember, this is a reflex to a way of thinking, not a hopelessly irreversible condition.

I call this mammalian reflex the *Livingstone response* after David Livingstone, the Scottish missionary famous for the "Dr. Livingstone, I presume" story. He was once attacked by a lion and came close to death. Twenty years later he was still haunted by the episode and wrote:

> The lion caught my shoulder as he sprang, and we both came to the ground below together. Growling horribly close to my ear, he shook me as a terrier does a rat. The shock produced a stupor similar to that which seems to be felt by a mouse after the first shake of a cat. It caused a sort of dreaminess in which there was no sense of pain or feeling of terror, though I was quite conscious of all that was happening.

The cold reaction is associated with this type of response. In the case of Dr. Livingstone, this mammalian reflex was adaptive, but just as the mammalian reflex of the hot reactor has outlived most of its usefulness in our modern society, so has the Livingstone response become a liability, except at times in some of the most severe life-threatening situations. Cold reactors fail to respond, typically functioning within the framework of anticipated failure.

One of my cold-reacting patients, following the loss of her husband, withdrew from her friends. She spent most of her day straightening closets, straightening drawers, attempting to organize her life. The result was more clutter and disorganization, with piles of materials and papers left throughout the house. Her children requested that she visit her physician regularly, but she resisted this, stating, "What will be, will be." She saved everything, every bit of furniture and clothing. Such a depression reflex may have been adaptive millions of years ago, as was the mammalian defense reflex. It may have led to the herd response of attempting to protect the withdrawn and the passive. In our modern-day society, however, such a reaction goes largely ignored, and the mammal is left by the wayside as the herd proceeds.

To test yourself as to whether or not you are in a cold sequence at this time, respond "yes" or "no" to the following 12 questions.

Cold Cognition Test

1. Do you sometimes strongly desire closeness, but feel that you have never had it, even in your childhood?

    YES_____ NO_____

2. Do you find yourself checking and rechecking work for fear of mistakes or inadequacy?

    YES_____ NO_____

3. Do you find yourself being "morbid" in your sense of humor or thinking of fatal illnesses, disasters, or loss?

    YES_____ NO_____

4. Do you find yourself ambivalent, not really enjoying activity, just simply taking part and going through the motions?

    YES_____ NO_____

5. Do you find yourself constricted in your emotions, unable to feel or think openly with elation or vigor? Are you sometimes laughing or crying but not actually experiencing either emotion as you do it?

YES_____ NO_____

6. Do you think in a rigid, conventional fashion, having difficulty breaking away from mental sets that you have established for years? Do you seem to be suffering from hardening of the attitudes more than hardening of the arteries?

YES_____ NO_____

7. Do you tend to be self-blaming and self-depreciating, feeling that you give of yourself continually and others take more and more?

YES_____ NO_____

8. Do you feel helpless and unable to organize attempts to help yourself get rid of a situation you find destructive to you?

YES_____ NO_____

9. Do you feel hopeless and, in spite of any changes you may make, that the quality of your life will never improve?

YES_____ NO_____

10. Do you find yourself being compliant, going along easily with doctors, teachers, and others in your environment? Do you yield to status and professionalism and even to friends who represent their own viewpoints and needs? Do you seem to always be the listener and the one lectured, rather than the lecturer?

YES_____ NO_____

11. Are you overwhelmed by any type of loss, even saddened by the end of a party or a brief activity or a visit from a friend? Do you find yourself reliving in your mind losses you have experienced intimately, even years after they occurred?

YES_____ NO_____

12. Do you have problems with individuation or a fear of being alone? Do you feel that your life is dependent upon one person or that your lack of one person is holding up any future development or hope for intimacy in your later years?

YES_____ NO_____

If you responded to six or more of these items affirmatively, there is a chance that you are thinking in the cold style. Four or more yeses, and you may be cooling down. I have used the Hot and Cold Cognition tests 5 years. People often say that they score high on both tests. Remember, both types of thinking are not mutually exclusive. It is possible to score high on both tests; such a situation may indicate a highly complex disruption of the immune system, perhaps a time of major life transition.

Even though our medical establishment seems to act as if we can get only one disease at a time, it is more typical that people experience more than one disease. Medical diagnosis is a singular-type diagnosis and sometimes fails to note the complexity of the patient. A man took his dog to the veterinarian, to be checked for fleas. The veterinarian, following the exam of the dog, stated, ''Your dog has worms.'' The man said, ''How can that be? I was sure he had fleas.'' The veterinarian responded, ''You know it's possible to have worms and fleas at the same time.'' To understand your wellness or illness, it is important to look for trends or characteristics, not a singular category or label, to look for an orientation now, not a lifelong label.

Diseases related to this cold type of thinking are infection, allergy, and the autoimmune diseases including rheumatoid arthritis, diabetes, lupus, multiple sclerosis, and, most particularly, cell disease. It may be that a person's failure to grow will be compensated for, metaphorically, by the body's spontaneous disruption of growth and restriction of movement.

As a further check on your status in the cold supersystem, take the following Cold Reactor Test. Score yourself, and have an observer rate you, as follows:

1—Almost never

2—Sometimes

3—Almost always

4—Always

Defeatism

1. When there are rumors that someone is going to receive a major break, good news, or a promotion, do you automatically assume that it will not be you?

_____

2. Do your fantasies of the ideal life result in thoughts of by how far you have missed such a life because you "just can't seem to do it" or "nothing good ever happens to me or my family"?

_____

3. When you have difficulty on a task, do you think "that's just like me to mess it up"?

_____

4. When you're out with friends, do you feel as though everyone looks at and admires them and ignores you?

_____

5. When you look at yourself in the mirror, do you look for flaws, imperfections, and strategies for cover-up?

_____

Subtotal

Inadequacy

1. Do you have private thoughts that sound like "That does it, I've had it, so what, and who cares"? Do you have only "last straws," seldom "first straws"?

_____

2. When playing games, do you reach a point in most games where you feel yourself losing and then give in? Does that point seem to come much sooner than it does for others with whom you interact?

_____

3. When a crisis occurs, is your first thought "Who can solve it?" rather than "I can solve it"?

———

4. Do you find yourself thinking that the whole world is going down the drain and no one cares anyway, so why should you? Do you use the pronoun "they" a lot, such as "they say," "they never do," and "they are all crooks"?

———

5. Do you find yourself thinking of your same flaws over and over again, no matter what the issue?

———

———

Subtotal

Passivity

1. When criticized, do you think "That is not fair, but it's no use explaining"?

———

2. Do you find yourself thinking of things you could have said or would have said but failed to say because you were not spontaneous enough? Having missed what you considered to be the best time to speak out, do you find yourself receiving even more harassment due to your hesitation?

———

3. When in an argument, however minor, do you think of ways to get out of it quickly, even to the point of distorting your own point of view?

———

4. When thinking about future plans, do you tend to think in terms of obligations rather than enjoyment?

———

5. Does your thinking include a "peace at any price" philosophy, almost an "it's not worth it" orientation?

_____

_____

Subtotal

Now place yourself on the cold psychograph (page 96). Add up your subtotals, and have an observer do the same. Color in the outside thermometers to see an aggregate score of your emotional and thinking "temperature." To focus on the subcategories, multiply each of the subtotals by 3 and mark your score on the center thermometers. Your observer can also mark the appropriate areas and you can discuss patterns, similarities, and differences among the categories.

COLD THOUGHTS

Five characteristic thinking patterns of the cold reactor follow. Check yourself against these thinking styles, modified once again from the work by David Burns on cognitive approaches to depression.

Smearing

Cold reactors tend to take one small bit of information from the pallet of life and paint the whole world a different color. Events in their lives tend to smear into one another. One of my patients stated, "It's like somebody had dipped their fingers in black paint and smeared it across my canvas." For this patient and other cold reactors, a rainy day is another bad day in a bad year in a bad life. The immune system slows down, almost as if it were a team whose coach has given up in the first few minutes of the game. Rather than fight or flee as the hot reactor does, the cold reactor flows helplessly.

Thought Straining

Cold reactors receive very little positive information from their environment. Everything is colored dark by the filter through which these elements must pass. Compliments, good news, or anything positive is

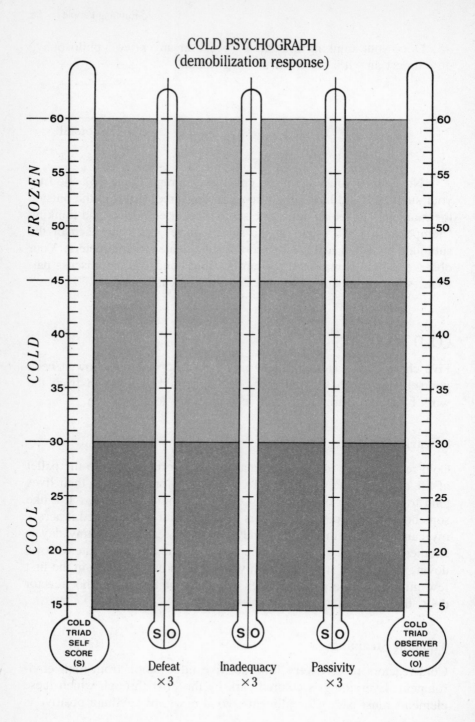

filtered away with only the negative seeping through. So it is with the immune system which allows "negative cells" free run of the body.

Negativity

Cold reactors are difficult to compliment. The statement that they are looking trimmer may be met with "But I need to lose 20 more pounds." So even if the filter is fooled, cold reactors will disqualify a positive. They may hear it, but they negate it. This puts cold reactors at great risk in terms of immune efficiency. I believe positive emotions can promote wellness to the same degree that negative emotions can interfere with health. The cold reactor's style of negative thinking produces an immune system that is impaired, sluggish, and ineffective, not allowing positives and changing any positives that sneak through to negatives, rendering the cold reactor vulnerable to chronic disease.

Minimizing

Cold reactors look through the binoculars of life from the wrong end. They minimize any positive event or positive characteristic. A promotion at work may be reported as "an easy thing to get at the stupid place where I am." They seem to believe that anything they can do cannot be worth doing, that anything with which they have success cannot be significant. Groucho Marx is quoted as saying that he did not want to join any group with standards low enough to let him in. So it is with cold reactors who seem to be on the margin of life and seem even more insecure when allowed to enter. At such times they grow suspicious, suspecting charity or pity, suffering from the Groucho Marx syndrome.

The Atlas Trap

The cold reactor tends to take burdens of family and, indeed, the world upon his or her own shoulders and psyche. Unlike the hot reactor, who takes responsibility for everything, the cold reactor feels burdened but, at the same time, ineffective and hopeless. While the hot reactor is challenged, the cold reactor is threatened. Problem children become the failure of the mother who has fallen short in her maternal role. Problems among staff become a cold supervisor's personal failure. The immune system, too, seems to sense this failure and becomes sluggish, inadequate, and less vigilant.

Unlike the self-centeredness of hot reactors, cold reactors assume the self-orientation of victims. They have a broad definition of self, not the narrow definition of hot reactors. This generalized self is vulnerable, insecure, and inadequate. The cold reactor is not so much self-involved as self-defeated, a fertile terrain for the invasion of the yin diseases, the empty diseases of metabolic disruption and unchecked cell growth or even the misdirected attack of the immune system upon itself.

Both hot and cold styles victimize the person trapped in these cycles. Cold reactors are more *aware* of the victim orientation.

POWERLESS PEOPLE AND STRONG DEFENSES

I believe the idea of a right to health should be replaced by the idea of an individual moral obligation to preserve one's health—a public duty if you will.

JOHN KNOWLES

Cold reactors often present themselves with a syndrome referred to in psychiatry as a *character disorder*, a view that the world has dealt them a handful of unfair cards. Through their hopelessness, helplessness, and sense of despair, they end up hurting others as much as or more than themselves, for those who love or relate to cold reactors feel that they, too, have failed and are responsible for what they clearly perceive as a sadness and despair in their loved ones. The five defense systems equated with the character disorder are immature defenses. They are strong only in their solidification and impenetrability, much as a stubborn child is unresponsive to discipline or control.

Echoing

Unable to see things as being under their own control, cold reactors tend to cast things to the wind and curse outwardly at problems that originated from within. Negatives seem to come from out there and everywhere. The world, not just people, seems to have failed them. Cold reactors are hurt less by feelings that someone has done something to them and more by the fact that the world or the life system has failed to allow them to take part in the joys of living.

The world of cold reactors becomes a soap opera. They are forever the observers, not the actors. As the images of joy, happiness, and productivity fade, the brain begins to generate its own amusement, possibly by creating the reality of physical illness.

Arctic Isolation

Cold reactors feel totally alone, withdrawn. While they may not actually be close to acting on their own suicidal thoughts and sense of nothingness, these thoughts are very real, and the immune system's failure may be helping cold reactors commit slow suicide. This is an isolation through withdrawal, not overactivity and distraction.

It seems easier for cold reactors to defend against the inner pain and loneliness by becoming even more lonely, for to take control of the brain by more rational thinking is a much more difficult task. Much as a child standing along the wall in a kindergarten class waiting to be invited into the game, the cold reactor waits in vain, for ultimately playing the game depends upon the player.

The Dr. Welby Dilemma

Marcus Welby, that kindly TV physician, was capable of treating any and all diseases through kindness, caring, and concern. As unrealistic as the image of this television character was, cold reactors long for such attention and concern. They create their own diseases for treatment in this television drama. A mark on the hand may be seen immediately as melanoma. A headache may be a sign of a brain tumor. The immune system may mistake this fear of disease for hope of disease and allow or, indeed, cause the dreaded disease to develop.

This hypochondriasis in search of Marcus Welby only serves to isolate cold reactors even more from others. We are threatened by their focus on disease and impatient with their continual concern for survival.

Crumbling

Cold reactors are unable to acknowledge problems that they experience, much like hot reactors. However, while hot reactors repress and hold things deeply within themselves, and are unable to acknowledge their own distress, cold reactors can only temporarily hold things back. When confronted with their own difficulties, they crumble quickly. Denial, however human, can exact a terrible price on our health, and cold

reactors have a weak denial defense that serves them poorly. Hot reactors' denial is firmly entrenched.

Cold reactors' denial is puzzling to those who relate to them.
Complaining of symptoms, diseases, and weaknesses, they meet offers
of help from other people with a cavalier or stoic denial. One mother
told her daughter as she visited the hospital, "I know this is life-threatening, but I don't want you to be concerned." The daughter responded,
"Mother, you are not even taking the medicine they are asking you to
take." The mother responded with sadness and hopelessness, "Look,
it's God's will. What happens, happens." Impatiently, the daughter
responded, "Then don't complain to me about it." Caring had turned
to anger in this daughter, stemming from her helplessness and worry
for the mother she loved.

An immune system directed by denial orientation is likely to mis-
label and misidentify agents invading the body. Recognition, not denial,
is the cornerstone of immune efficiency. The three phases of the immune
system described earlier from Solomon's work at Stanford (see p. 56)
are all vulnerable to the irrational thinking of the cold reactor. While
the hot reactor is primarily affected on the afferent level, the labeling
and identification processes of the immune system, the cold reactor is
more affected on the efferent level, the actual execution of the invading
agents. Too slow, too fatigued, too defeated to act, the defense system
surrenders.

Quiet Noise

Psychologists and psychiatrists use the term "passive-aggressive" to
refer to people who are actually hostile or aggressive through their
passivity, surrender, and inactivity. So it is with the cold reactor who
surrenders and causes others to be impatient or threatened. The husband
of a cold-reacting patient complained, "Why won't she just speak up?
She is so passive, she drives me crazy. I don't want to even visit her
any more." Failure to love yourself can deeply anger those who love
you, and the more they love and respect you, the more they may yield
to your opinion that you are not worth loving. If your immune system
becomes convinced that you are not worth caring for, it may resign its
role as protector and convert to slayer.

No one causes his heart disease or cancer. No one *makes* himself
or herself sick. Instead, we fail to understand our potential. You are

COLD SUPERSYSTEM

PERCEPTIONS OF DAILY EVENTS

Primary defense systems
1. Echoing
2. Arctic isolation
3. The Dr. Welby dilemma
4. Crumbling
5. Quiet noise

Primary cognitive distortion
1. Smearing
2. Thought straining
3. Negativity
4. Minimizing
5. The Atlas trap

Inhibited emotion syndrome
1. Emotional isolation
2. Overly conscientious
3. High ambivalence toward self and others

Type C Behaviors

Loss of Control

Vigilance Reaction

Timelessness

General Adaptation Syndrome

Flowing

YIN
REACTIVE—REGRESS—UNCONSCIOUS

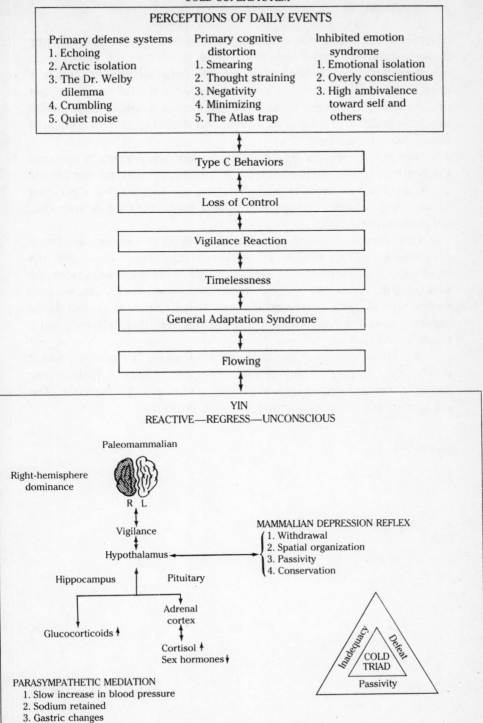

Paleomammalian

Right-hemisphere dominance

R   L

Vigilance

Hypothalamus

MAMMALIAN DEPRESSION REFLEX
1. Withdrawal
2. Spatial organization
3. Passivity
4. Conservation

Hippocampus   Pituitary

Glucocorticoids ↑

Adrenal cortex

Cortisol ↑
Sex hormones ↓

PARASYMPATHETIC MEDIATION
1. Slow increase in blood pressure
2. Sodium retained
3. Gastric changes

Inadequacy   Defeat
COLD TRIAD
Passivity

healthier at the end of this sixth chapter than you were at the beginning if the material presented here and if your test scores are viewed as a recommitment and challenge to wellness, personal growth, and new hope, because of your ability to recognize hot and cold phases in your life. As Hippocrates encouraged: "A wise person should consider health to be the greatest of human blessings, and should learn how to benefit from illness by thinking."

The preceding chart summarizes the key components of the cold reaction. As you did for the hot style, trace through each step as a review of the cold supersystem. Remember, you are looking for a personal trend, a way of thinking and feeling at a particular time in your life, not a personality trait.

One example of the impact of cold reactions on the immune system is the process of cell disease. While there is no direct evidence that any emotion causes cancer, it is clear that life orientation influences the supersystem. When that system is made cold, slow, inattentive, we may be less able to purge ourselves of overgrowing cells or to correct the as yet immeasurable disruptions in the supersystem that may eventually result in cell disease.

We know less about this cold process than the hot process, which is why this chapter is shorter than the "hot" chapter. Perhaps our society's hot pace rewards hot running and overlooks the cold. The changes of cold running are none-the-less profound.

Chapter Seven

UNDERGROWING PEOPLE AND OVERGROWING CELLS: DISEASES OF THE CELL

Well, I don't get angry, okay? I mean I have a terrible weakness. I can't express anger. That is one of the problems I have. I grow a tumor instead.

WOODY ALLEN
Manhattan

LOSS AND THE LONELY LYMPHOCYTE

She looked as if she were drained of all life energy. She had come to my office on a bitterly cold winter morning for help adjusting to a diagnosis of breast cancer. She sat beside me, looking at water drops hitting the cement sill outside my office window.

After several minutes of silently staring at the drops, she began to speak without diverting her attention from the water. "They are so much like my life, you know," she said, without an external show of emotion. "It seems to take forever for just one drop to work free from that large icicle way up on top of your window. Ever so slowly, just one drop will break loose, then fall quickly, break, and disappear. It really is like the days of my life.''

This woman is typical of the hundreds of male and female patients who have come to my office after having been told by a physician that they are cancer victims. They not only seem frightened and despairing regarding the diagnosis but also have a history of disappointment and relate life stories with symbolism of expectations that never worked out. It is as if the need for personal growth somehow mysteriously translated itself to the metaphor of overgrowing cells.

A person who experiences an overgrowth of cells engages in a dialogue of defeat, inadequacy, and passivity. Their cold orientation to life may be thawed only by the burning of disease.

One example from current research illustrates this issue clearly. Bereaved spouses, and most particularly widowers, are significantly more vulnerable to disease than the unbereaved. We know that lymphocyte responsiveness—the effectiveness of one part of the immune system that is designed to fight disease by maintaining the internal balance and preventing over production of cells—becomes sluggish in a person who has lost a spouse. When we sample lymphocytes for the lab and stimulate them with something called *mitogens*, which have the capacity to cause lymphocytes to reproduce rapidly, the lymphocytes of the bereaved reproduce at a significantly lower rate than those of individuals who have not lost significant persons in their lives. A direct relationship between thought, feeling, and immunity has been demonstrated.

We also know that some lymphocytes have tiny receptors on their surface designed for the reception of various secretions from the brain so that they may respond to the brain's signals. It is possible that the severe reduction in incoming information to the brain—the information of intimacy, closeness, sensuality, sexuality, day-to-day interactions, and even the predictable presence of another human body—is the food which an overstarving brain is deprived of by loss. Caring only for itself, the brain signals the body cells to develop more rapidly than normal or in ways that are unusually challenging to the immune system, as if the brain were attempting to entertain itself, to find new company, to keep itself busy. The lymphocytes, in turn, have been rendered less effective by chemical changes interfering with the response at receptor sites, and cell disease is initiated. Unless you take control of your brain, unless you give it something more constructive to do than playing dangerous games with your body, the brain will continue its deadly self-stimulation at those times when you are running cold.

While speculative, this theory of cell disease does not violate anything we know about the supersystem. This is the *surveillance theory* of cancer. It suggests that we overproduce cancer cells daily and that our immune system is designed to seek out these cells and destroy them before they crowd out our healthy cells. If undergrowing people have overgrowing cells and underactive supersystems, it would seem that they may be vulnerable to this disease.

Our concern about this process is heightened when we recognize that the number of bereaved persons in the United States is staggering. Returning to our football stadium reference point, it would take more than 1500 college football stadiums to hold all the people who lose spouses by death in one year. Almost one out of every four persons will develop some form of cancer in his lifetime. If even a small percentage of cell disease is related to the processes hypothesized here, it is important to understand the interaction of our supersystems with our thoughts and feelings, our perceptions of our world, and the fact that we can speak to ourselves in a more healthy language, even at times of crisis and loss.

CELL CHEATER'S TEST

Over and over again, the recent lives of cancer patients are linked to loss and life change.

DENNIS T. JAFFE

Before describing the concept of cell disease and its relationship to our thinking process, we begin with another test. You have completed the Heart Cheater's Test and learned that it is not agitated, aggressive patterns of the Type A syndrome that cause heart disease, but a pattern of thinking that misdirects the supersystem, resulting in a clogging of supply lines to the heart. So it is with the case of the cold reactor, who is more vulnerable to cell disease. It is not the slow, withdrawn, more pensive behavior that relates to a proclivity to cancer, but a cluster of internal dialogues revealed in the following test, which probes deeper into the cold psyche.

Respond to the following 10 questions using the scale below:

4—Almost always

3—Sometimes

2—Seldom

1—Almost never

1. Do you suffer from the "little red hen" syndrome? You may remember the children's story in which a little red hen had to do everything herself. Do you think that you will have to carry the load, to mobilize more and more energy because no one can or will help you?

_____

2. Are you extremely conscientious, checking and rechecking everything you do? Does the slightest criticism cause you to reassess your total approach to life?

_____

3. Does it seem that nothing you might do will help your present situation? Do you think in a helpless fashion, self-talk being primarily about how ineffective everyone is in this cruel world of ours?

_____

4. Do you think there is a "they" set of people who are selfish, hurried, impatient, insensitive, irresponsible, and noted for their lack of caring? As you read about hot reactions, does it seem that the they in your life are very often hot reactors (hostile, impatient, competitive) and you are more the cold reactor by contrast (defeated, inadequate, passive)?

_____

5. Are you conventional in your thinking, seeing things in black and white, right and wrong, and wondering why others cannot see the truth according to you? Does it seem to you that everything would be very clear if only people would take the time to talk, share, and listen to you?

_____

6. Do you think a lot about intimacy, closeness, family, and sharing and think how few of these things there are in your own life? Do you think to yourself that "my family is gradually growing further and further apart, and I am becoming more and more alone?"

_____

7. Do you think that any good news is only an exception, a drop in the bucket compared to the bad news and bad luck you have experienced? Do you think that it is best to minimize the impact of good news so that you have more practice dealing with the bad which seems more frequent in your life?

8. Do you think that time seems to drag by, sometimes actually standing still? Do you feel like an observer on the shore near the river of time? Does it seem that everyone else is short of time when you have plenty of time you would be willing to share?

_____

9. Do you think that there is little hope for you or, even, the entire world? Do you think that every time you get your hopes up, everything else tends to fall on top of them?

_____

10. Do you think that you may as well comply with people at work and at home, including doctors and therapists? Does it seem that you have little choice anyway, because the system cares little about you or any individual, and there is no use in fighting that system? Do you think that professional people are busy, consumed in their own life systems, so that you may as well follow their instructions and not take their time with questions and your need to talk and share?

_____

If you scored any more than 20 points on this test, you may have a tendency to cheat yourself. You may be vulnerable to a pattern of self-undergrowth, and the cycle of the cold supersystem may result. Check back on your psychographs. Look at the subtests and your observer scores. Look for a pattern to your self-talk, and you may note a disease fingerprint, a tendency toward vulnerability to the cold diseases.

BORED LIVES AND EXCITED CELLS

We have learned that the body possesses a complex machinery
of checks and balances. These are remarkably effective in
adjusting ourselves to virtually anything that can happen to
us in life. But often this machinery does not work perfectly.

HANS SELYE

Some surprising and controversial findings are beginning to accumulate
about cancer. We know that people with a hypothyroid, or underactive
thyroid condition, are more likely to have cancer than those with hyperactive thyroids. We know that the condition of low cholesterol and
low blood pressure, which is typically seen as a sign of health, is more
typically present in patients who develop cancer than those with higher
levels of cholesterol and higher blood pressures. We know that being
thrust into a concentration camp in World War II tended to decrease
the stress diseases being experienced by the victims, such as heart
disease, diabetes, and high blood pressure. Certainly there was an increase in infectious diseases and other trauma from this unimaginably
inhuman experience, but a change in types of disease was recorded.

We know that during wartime the incidence of diabetes significantly
lowers. We know that injecting a live tuberculin vaccine called *BCG*
into a patient with a tumor can sometimes result in a shrinking of the
tumor, actually reducing the impact of one disease by giving the supersystem another disease to grapple with. We know that cancer does
not exist in any organism that does not have a brain.

What does this set of seemingly unrelated findings mean? I propose
the theory that cell disease is a disease of brain deprivation, of a type
of boredom with life. Is it a coincidence that the incidence of cancer
increases with age, when such life circumstances as retirement or even
preparing for retirement are in process? While one cause never explains
any disease process, and aging is a most complex phenomenon, I suggest
that emotional state and self-talk are as important as precoded genetic
changes related to aging for explaining disease vulnerability.

Most theories of aging are related to equally contested and as yet
unproven theories. Such ideas include the following hypotheses:

•   A predetermined and self-limiting number of breaths and heartbeats
    are assigned to you for life

- The idea that "noise" levels increase within the body until these bodily disruptions can no longer be tolerated

- Correlations with the lifeline in the palm of your hand

- Newton's law of entropy, suggesting that all systems become more and more disorganized with time, eventually resulting in death

- Heiflick's theory that the number of cell reproductions is limited and gradually runs out, with the result being aging

- Genetic approaches suggesting that repair by a body chemical called *DNA* becomes more inefficient as we age

- The error theory, suggesting that the more cells divide, the more likely is the possibility for error in "transcription"

- The "free radical theory," suggesting that certain cellular changes result in a graying of our hair and a weakening of our tissues

- The theory referred to as *lipofuscin* accumulation, or the idea that waste products build up, resulting in the formation of age spots and the reduction of elasticity of our skin

All these are only some of the speculations about aging. None of these theories deals with self-talk and emotion and the possibility that boredom, lack of incoming stimulation, and isolation for the person who is aging may relate to cellular and immunity changes. These theories ignore the brain's compensatory effort to challenge itself if the world fails to continue to be a challenge to the developing person. If age causes us to give up and if our brains are never ready to give up, we have, in effect, left the soggy computer *on* with no new programs coming in. I suggest that aging is not synonymous with disease and that the illnesses which come with our later years are related to our eviction from our own systems.

When I suggested these ideas 4 years ago at a meeting of oncology nurses in California, one nurse rose from the audience to say, "I understand your theory, but you know, children get cancer too." Of course she was right. The age group of about 3 to 14 years is particularly vulnerable to some types of cancer.

Cancer researcher and theorist Augusta De La Pena clearly traces the development of his theories of cancer to evolutionary theory and the development of the nervous system. He suggests not only that underload of the brain may result in perturbation of body systems to create additional information flow for the brain but also that excessive overload—as perhaps could happen in an overly stressed, challenged, emotional, overwhelmed, or despairing child—may result in a protective shutdown of the information system. In compensatory overreaction to the shutdown, the brain attempts to reestablish the information flow, and overstimulation of cells can result, in effect, turning up the heat too quickly after a shutdown of the furnace.

To accept these theories without continued and replicated research would be foolish. To interpret these theories as some sort of patient blame, causing those already hurt to criticize themselves or their families or diminish their own value, would be destructive to the healing process. However, to ignore the role of self-talk and interaction of the supersystem with self-talk is to take an exclusively mechanical approach to understanding cancer. Cancer is no more a disease of cells than a traffic jam is a disease of cars. Each of us is a supersystem and each of us functions as a whole. Any disruption of the whole can result in illness.

Other findings lend support to the theory that the cold reactor's defeated, inadequate, passive style of internal dialogue results in an overgrowth of cells and an underkill of the overgrowing cells by the supersystem. People with severe intellectual impairments that reduce the capacity of the brain are virtually free of cancer. Is it possible that their "brain appetite" is reduced, therefore resulting in a lower level of requirement by their brains for new and challenging information and thus a less compensatory effort by their brains?

We also know that people report, and we can sometimes document, that long periods of superior health exist prior to diagnosis of cancer. We know that it typically takes several years for a tumor to be noted or diagnosed accurately. Is it simply a coincidence of time until diagnosis, or does the state of superior health result in boredom for the brain, leading to its compensatory overstimulation of the body?

All of us seem to require an optimal state of information flow, suited to our own brains and the efficiency of our immune systems. Is it possible that when this state does not exist, the flow of life energy is disrupted, with cell-growth problems the end result?

In my discussion of hot reactions, I hypothesized that relaxation may not be the strategy of choice for some of these people. Even though their information-flow demand is high, perhaps the problem rests with their tendency to seek information, the food of our brains, from the external world. This world is not under our control, and we are, to some extent, victims of it. Our brains continue to insist that we are separate from that world, from our universe. Perhaps we have failed to recognize that we can control information flow, that we can generate from inside, from the spirit and from the soul, and achieve a change of focus.

Simply having hot reactors slow down may result only in the development of different forms of disease unless we alter their self-dialogue. Perhaps the houses of the hot reactors are burning down while they rush through their neighborhoods in search of the source of the smoke that is actually emanating from their own internal fires. Perhaps hot reactors are overheating as the system of the race car overheats, not shifting into a different gear as the engine requires. Perhaps cold reactors have stopped running, causing their own cars to develop internal overstimulation in an attempt to restart the system. Driving too fast and too recklessly is no more dangerous than the stagnation of not driving at all.

Our failure to recognize that we generate and do not just respond to information causes an information-flow crisis. All healing comes from within and is related to the interaction among all of us. Our selfishness may kill us all if we do not learn that it is not looking in or out that matters, but realizing that there is no in or out; there just *is*, and what *is* depends upon our perceptions and theory of our lives. We must learn that imagery is everything. We create our world, or it will be created for us. We will be effects if we are not effectors, victims instead of masters of our own destiny.

Studies have shown that B cells, which produce antibodies, and particularly those T cells that destroy and transform cells, are sometimes diminished in number and effectiveness when we run cold, when we are depressed, defeated, isolated, or in a state of grieving or despair.

Studies have also shown that special T cells, called *T helper cells* (T-4), which amplify the immune system, and *T suppressor cells* (T-8), which control and inhibit the immune response, are also affected by running cold. An effective immune response requires a balance between the T-4 and T-8 cells, but Dr. Richard Krueger and his colleagues have found that T helper cells decrease in number while the inhibiting T suppressor cells remain unchanged in those people identified as depressed. In other words, the cells that encourage the immune system diminish, and those that hold it in check continue their job in cold-running people. Dr. Sandra Levy has reviewed several studies suggesting that survival from cancer is related not only to tumor biology but also to the person's psychological response to disease. While her review and integration of the data are not applied to the development of disease per se, but to surviving the disease, her findings indicate that a relationship exists between how we feel and our coping mechanisms against cancer.

"Cancer" is actually a general term for a complex set of various cell diseases, and most studies show only relationships, not direct causation between emotion and this set of diseases. It is wrong to suggest that any emotional state causes cell disease. It is equally wrong to continue to approach cancer as a mechanical malfunction unrelated to the person as a whole. Research to date is clear in its documentation that it is not possible to separate the biology of the cell from the psychology of the person, either in the development or course of the disease.

In the medical literature, there are several documented instances of what are called *spontaneous remissions* from cancer. Drs. Eric Pepper and Kenneth Pelletier collected over 400 such cases and constructed a bibliography, listing the sources and backgrounds of such occurrences. There are no doubt hundreds of other such cases that have not found their way into print. Spontaneous remission, one of those magic terms used by the medical profession, may be translated to "all of a sudden this disease went away and we have no idea why, and we didn't seem to do anything to make it go away based on our treatment."

Drs. Elmer and Alyce Green examined the 400 cases in spontaneous remission and found only one factor common to each case. That factor is the factor stressed throughout this book. All these people had changed their attitude prior to the remission and, in some way, had found hope and become more positive in their approach to the disease.

It puzzles me that physicians sometimes forget that the bombardment of the system with deadly chemicals against cancer is also related to how we feel and that spontaneous remissions occur during these treatment regimens as well. Studies on the successes of radiation and chemotherapy seldom include reports on changes in the belief systems and attitudes of the patients receiving the treatment. It seems equally plausible that people's belief systems change when an encouraging, trusted doctor, in this case serving in the role of shaman or healer, administers a magic elixir in the form of strong chemicals or buzzing machines that alter not only cell biology but personal psychology.

I definitely do not suggest that we ignore modern medical practices, for they can certainly save lives. Failure to benefit from the continuing gains in medical research is to ignore one of the most profound strengths of our civilization. To dismiss them would reveal the blindness similar to that shown by those who dismiss the importance of attitudes and feelings as related to disease.

FIGHTING, FLEEING, FLOWING, AND BEING

Realize the presence of health and the fact of harmonious
being, until the body corresponds with the normal conditions
of health and harmony.

MARY BAKER EDDY

Some researchers have suggested that there is in fact a Type C super-system. This is a supersystem dictated by the thinking pattern typified by loss of control. We learned earlier that cold reactors are in a state of vigilance, an observer state rather than a more active seeking state. They do not fight or flee, they flow, as if passively floating on the river of time—drowning within it alongside hot reactors, going down without a fight while the hot reactors thrash ineffectively.

Fighting, fleeing, and flowing may not be the desirable states to enhance our own health. Perhaps the movement-oriented strategies of fighting, fleeing, and flowing should be replaced by just *being*. "Sit down and be quiet" was the advice of our parents. It may still be an effective health strategy.

The vigilance or observer style of life of the cold reactor results in a chain of events through the hypothalamus, or the brain of our brains, through the pituitary and hippocampus. Remember that the hippocampus of the brain stem is involved in processing and dealing with novelty in the environment. A lack of novelty for the brain may result in the brain seeking a cell novelty. Working through the adrenal cortex, or the outside of the adrenal gland, this produces an increase in the cortisol hormone and an accompanying reduction of sex hormones. The super-system is turned down instead of up as in the hot reactor. Not only cell disease but infection, allergy, and the autoimmune diseases including rheumatoid arthritis, diabetes, and multiple sclerosis can result.

The significance of changes in the sex hormones is related to the cold-supersystem style. Sexuality is profoundly related to our internal dialogue and our state of wellness. Fulfilling sexuality is one of the most fulfilling states of being, for it involves not only self-enhancement but the enhancement of another and the merging with "other."

Abraham Maslow wrote of the psychology of being, the idea that longing for the past or hopefully awaiting the future was less healthy than living for now. We no longer have to learn to fight, to flee, to flow. Our task is to learn who we are now, not what we were or can be. Rabbi Hillel has pointed out, "If I am not for myself, who will be for me? If I am only for myself, what am I? If not now—when?"

If we are fighting, fleeing, or flowing, we are going *past* people, not living with them. The wellness of hot and cold reactors depends upon developing their ability to interact with others, the universal whole. As E. M. Forster wrote, "Only connect! Personal relations are the important thing forever and ever."

The cold reactor talks more of feelings than of events, more of frustrated impulses for caring and closeness than of accomplishments and gains. This reveals a right-hemisphere brain orientation.

When we look carefully at Leonardo da Vinci's *Mona Lisa*, her puzzling smile is related to the fact that only the left side of her face is smiling. Researchers have found that we seem to express emotion on the left side much more often than we do on the right side, and the right hemisphere is controlling that side of the face. One researcher, Dr. Davidson, has shown that the left hemisphere may be related to more positive emotions and the right more negative ones, such as anger. The cold reactor with a right-hemisphere dominance may be experiencing a great deal of anger turned inward, with the result being depression and a lowered efficiency of the immune system.

FREEZING OUT

When something doesn't go my way, I let go of my idea of how it should be, trusting that my mind doesn't know the larger picture.

ELIZABETH RIVERS

I now return to our Cell Cheater's Test to discuss in more detail the importance of the internal dialogue of the cold supersystem. You may wish to check back on your scores on the Cell Cheater's Test as we discuss each of the numbered characteristics corresponding to the quiz. Better yet, talk about some of your scores with someone else as you read the following examples of cold thinking.

1. "I'll Do It Myself"

The first characteristic of the cold reactor is the thought pattern of *aloneness*. The thinking seems to be that a bird in the hand is better than one overhead. That is, if I do it and think it myself, I am less likely to get "messed on" by someone else.

A patient in one of my groups of people with cancer discussed the fact that he had been amazed at the lack of skill shown by hospital staff in making his bed. This orientation of little things mean a lot is typical of cold thinking. He was a former marine who bragged, with some substantiation, that he could bounce a quarter off the tightly wrapped sheets on his bed and felt that the only things capable of being bounced off his staff-made hospital bed were the blankets continually disappearing during the night due to what he saw as "carelessly undisciplined bed making."

He had attempted to teach the staff a better way to make beds, but he was sent on his morning walk as thanks for his unsolicited directions. As he walked the halls, he thought, "This is typical. I have to do things myself. Everybody just rushes through things. I pay all this money, and then I will have to sneak and remake my bed myself." In the discussion group, each member was experiencing cell disease. The members shook their heads in apparent understanding of the fact that he had not only spent hours a day thinking about this relatively minor incident in his life but also learned to remake his bed during the night and then awaken early to unmake it so the hospital staff would find the bed made in the style they had expected. This exmarine in addition to making his bed was thinking and becoming sicker in it. Those people who think they have to do it themselves, who are little red hens, typically end up doing it not only themselves but to themselves.

It is an interesting metaphor that the cold reactor thinks in the "I'll have to do it myself" system of thought, for this may in fact be what the brain is attempting to do. Lacking incoming information, it adopts a strategy of "I'll have to do it myself and create my own stimulation through disrupting the body of which I am a part. I guess I'll have to do it all myself."

2. Conscientiousness

The cold reactors' philosophy of never letting anyone down translates to a thought process of monitoring their behavior continually. Their thinking is full of examples of others or circumstances letting them down, and by contrast, they think, "I would never do that to anyone else. Perhaps my overcompensation will teach them by example." The strategy fails them, however, as people in their environment do not seem to learn by their example. These people only seem to take more and more advantage of cold reactors and see their behavior not as example, but rather as a gesture of giving.

Cold reactors seem to be thinking in a checking fashion. They check and recheck so frequently for details that they seem distracted, aloof, and distant to those around them. Although desiring closeness and intimacy, they can appear withdrawn. They spend so much time thinking and rethinking that they miss opportunities to act, detect, or respond to overtures from others around them.

One of my patients calls this "garbage truck" thinking. He complained that it was predictable that each day he would miss the neighborhood garbage truck. Forgetting until the last minute to take out trash and noticing the back of the garbage truck vanishing quickly down the street as he ran from the house with garbage can in hand, he always seemed just a minute too late. No matter how conscientious in terms of preparing garbage, setting the can in a noticeable place, he was unable to beat the crew of the garbage truck, who seemed to him destined to win the race to the dump. A strategy developed within this patient that is characteristic of cell disease patients, one of "next time I'll be more than ready"—and that is just the trouble. They become *more* than ready, thereby rendering themselves ineffective, observers of their own failures. They prepare so much that they miss their chance. Like children getting ready to jump from a diving board and frustrating everyone as they warm up for what seems like an infinity, cold reactors spend more time getting ready than actually jumping in. By contrast, hot reactors seem always ready and jump in to a sometimes empty swimming pool.

I was walking through the hall in the oncology unit several years ago. It was almost 4 A.M. as I looked into the room of a patient I had talked with a few days before. I noticed the bed was empty. I walked into the room and saw her sitting in the bathroom on a chair she had taken from beside her bed. Considering the fact that all hospital patient chairs are made of the heaviest metals in the universe and are typically held in place by their own form of hospital gravity, this was an extraordinary feat for anyone, and much more so for a very sick and weakened woman. I asked her if anything was wrong. She sat writing in her chair under the light over the medicine cabinet. Without looking up, she responded, "I forgot to check my menu preference for tomorrow's meal. They want it on the door before you go to bed. I forgot completely and woke up in the middle of the night. Thank God I remembered."

I joked that she never ate the food anyway, complaining constantly about it, and that her family continually smuggled in other food (and, by the way, much more healthy food). She responded, "I know, but they want this on the door. I don't want to disappoint that cute little nurse who comes around to collect them."

3. Helplessness

The man looked down at the typical plastic-red raspberry jello on his hospital food tray. He gently prodded it with a spoon. As if addressing a young child, he stated, "Listen jello, I don't know why you are shaking so; I wouldn't think of eating you. You seem more helpless than I am." Through the humor of this patient came the truth of the helpless type of thinking of the cold reactor. There is an acclimation to this style of thinking so that it permeates almost every daily activity.

"It's no use," said one patient. "It's in the cards and I have been dealt a rotten hand." Oncology nurses typically report that their seriously ill cancer patients never seem to have one major problem but a series of problems. Impaired children, impaired parents, insensitive colleagues or administrators at their places of work, unfair or even ridiculous policies affecting them even during their stay in the hospital, and other frustrations combine to contribute to the victim syndrome of cancer.

A patient was sent to me for help with her decision about whether she should receive chemotherapy for her cancer or "play the odds" and allow the disease to take its course. Chemotherapy can exact a terrible toll on the body, for it is designed essentially to attack any cells that grow rapidly, cells that include the lining of the stomach and the cells for hair growth. Nausea and hair loss are frequent side effects of some forms of chemotherapy. In this woman's case, the chemotherapy would be particularly ravaging, with uncertain payoff in the opinion of the oncologist working with this patient. The decision was left to the patient. Her oncologist had unknowingly overrestricted her choices of therapy, forcing her to assume an either/or no-win position.

Her response was, "I guess it doesn't matter. What choice do I have? Take the chemotherapy and suffer greatly and probably die anyway, or don't take the chemotherapy and die certainly." She did not see that she had several other options. It was not chemotherapy or nothing, but chemotherapy and several other choices, including her own controlled experiment, with versions of chemotherapy modified in co-operation with her oncologist, and the use of less tested, more radical, nontraditional approaches to the treatment of cancer. Major lifestyle changes, dietary approaches, and the use of meditation and imagery were other alternatives that could be combined with or replace her chemotherapy. This patient viewed herself only as a victim, a research subject in a battery of cruel life experiments. She did not see herself as a partner with a healing team mobilized to promote her own wellness.

The hot reactor is a victim too, but a combative, grappling victim looking for alternatives, fighting to the last breath on the stretcher in the emergency room following a heart attack. The cold reactor is a helpless victim, helplessly and hopelessly succumbing to the futile at-tempts of the brain to stimulate itself. This difference in internal dialogue and perception of the world may account for significantly different disease states and recuperative strengths.

A paradox is often noted in the crisis of hot or cold reaction. While the hot reactor may be grappling on the stretcher in the emergency room, a strange calm seems to set in when the realization of vulnerability and the possibility of death becomes clear. This same calm is also noted in the cold reactor. The same pain that so immobilized the cancer patient seems to be ignored for a brief moment of calm toward the end. Research has referred to this response as *stress-induced analgesia*. Gravely injured soldiers and athletes injured in the midst of competition often report a total absence of pain in spite of the severity of damage to their bodies. It is as if "being" is a natural state sought by the mind's and body's interactive wisdom, a state that can save both the hot- and cold-running person in his or her daily living much as it protects both hot- and cold-running people in times of crisis.

Perhaps we should learn from this *end reflex* that to experience pain and disease is to be human and that the hope is not for survival but for the enjoyment of living, for living all aspects of humanness.

4. "They Did It to Me"

A 7-year-old girl in the oncology unit at our Children's Hospital attended a Christmas party. Santa Claus took her on his lap and asked, "What do you want to be when you grow up?" She responded, "Santa, it's not when, but if I grow up. And if I do, I just want to be a 'they.' " Santa was obviously saddened and felt foolish at asking his question.

Embarrassed, he quickly attempted to cheer up the atmosphere, ignored her correction as to "if or when," and asked, "They who?" "Just they," she responded. "They do everything. They are out there free, and they don't have sickness, and they are free of everything, and they can do everything."

This cold-reacting child felt ambivalent and distant from others, isolated from the world processes. *They* seem out there, distant, almost unreachable, and so it almost always is with the cold reactor.

In spite of this syndrome, it is also a characteristic of the thinking of cold reactors that they have one extremely close person upon whom they become dependent and about whom they think a great deal. This makes them excessively vulnerable, for all their eggs are placed in one basket, with one close friend and everyone else as "they."

The cancer industry of research, politics, and industrial policies continues to talk about cancer with a punitive ring, with a lethalness that frightens at its mere mention. Even Webster's defines cancer as a "source of evil." Recent polls have shown that cancer is more dreaded than heart disease, stroke, crime, earthquake, or nuclear war. It was, in fact, in all these polls, the most dreaded thing that could happen to anyone. And more than anything else, it was a thing, not a process.

This is incorrect. Disease is process. People are "cancer-ing"— they do not have cancer. In some ways their bodies are "too alive." Until we learn that things don't happen to us, but that things just are, and that we can interpret, process, and deal with things ourselves, we will forever be bound by our view of our world from a victim perspective. As long as we speak of cancer instead of cell disease, cancer victims instead of patients, and accept diagnoses as verdicts, the helpless, hopeless thinking style of the person with cell disease will be perpetuated and hopes of rallying the supersystem will be severely reduced. If negative emotions and self-talk disrupt the supersystem's efficiency and make us vulnerable to disease, mobilizing positive emotions and more rational internal thinking can encourage the brain in its healing role.

5. Conventionality

Cold reactors tend to be conservative and conventional in their thought processes. They think in terms of ultimate, static truths. Their conventionality, however, is uniquely their own and at times not even logical. One of my patients recently only half-joked, "When I turn sixty, I will have to go to Florida." I asked if he had family there, and he responded,

"No, I have to go to Florida. All people over sixty go to Florida. It's the law." As he laughed at his own joke, he failed to see that his life was indeed run by a set of cold conventions rather than adaptive self-choice.

The conventionality of cold reactors may appear to be nonsense to other people, but it is firmly embraced by the cold reactors themselves. This right-hemisphere style of thinking is often noticed in people with learning disabilities, who generate their own systems of fair play and rules of life. The brain, however, is designed for a magnificent efficiency and rationality in its total. A brain functioning beneath that capacity can be expected to cause trouble in the supersystem.

One male patient had recently had a *laryngectomy*, or removal of his voice box, and had not learned to use the apparatus designed to allow him to speak. He was continually frustrated by the hospital staff and policies within the hospital, but he could not voice his discontent. As I visited him one day, I noticed tears flowing down his cheeks as he lay in frustration over the violation of his conventionality. I asked him to prepare a list, writing on a pad I had left for him, of the rules that he considered to be in existence in the hospital at this time and that he found so frustrating. His list follows:

1. The other line of patients waiting for x-ray always moves faster than mine.

2. In order to get more pain medication, I have to prove I don't really need it.

3. I will only drop things off my hospital tray when I am trapped between the tray and the back of my bed.

4. When in doubt, nurses mumble. When they are in trouble, nurses delegate to someone else.

5. The more uncertain a doctor is, the more certain he will act. The more certain he will act, the shorter time he will spend with me for fear that I will ask more questions.

6. Anything good is against hospital rules.

7. No one in the entire hospital has ever seen a case quite like mine.

8. If an intern or resident fools around with my IV long enough, he will always screw it up.

9. My portable IV bag stand will always be hung on the wrong side of my bed, opposite the bathroom, particularly just after I have had an enema.

10. Celibacy is not hereditary, but hospitals seem to think so.

In spite of the humorous tone to this list, the humor was not the intent of the patient. He had prepared this list with a sense of despair, and was impatient with me as I chuckled at the list. He had attempted to be sarcastic and to point out the ridiculous nature of hospital life. For this patient and other cold reactors, the universality of the rules of fairness never seems to change, the world does not change, and the pattern of frustration continues.

6. Ambivalence

Cold reactors, just like their counterpart the hot reactors, have trouble thinking constructively about their relationships. Hot reactors are isolated by their hostility, impatience, and competitiveness. Cold reactors find people totally dependent upon them, taking their concern, their self-ingratiating nature for granted. Thoughts of being alone, even when in a group of friends or relatives, are typical. Their internal dialogue is one of ambivalence, wanting to relate intimately but fearing the risk of separation that always accompanies closeness. "The closer I get, the more I am afraid I'll be alone again," reported one patient.

The hot reactor is unaware of the importance of relationships, focusing on events, happenings, and things, fitting intimacy into an already hectic schedule, almost quantifying interactions. The cold reactor focuses on relationships but fears letdown or isolation.

I visited one of my patients and had to work my way through a crowd of relatives who were squeezed into the small hospital room. The room had a feeling of a social event. I noticed, however, that I had no trouble at all talking to my patient, for she was being totally ignored. People were talking about her, her condition, her family, the hospital, but no one was talking directly with her, holding her hand, or offering her comfort or intimacy.

I asked the patient how she was enjoying all this attention, and she responded, "It seems more like a funeral, doesn't it? I am lying here, they all come in, they give me some flowers, and they talk about me." I asked why she did not reach out or take part, and she responded, "It's okay, really. They have their own lives and I don't want to drag them down. I just enjoy them being here."

I asked one of the patient's daughters to join me in the hall outside the patient's room. I asked if perhaps the family couldn't involve her mother in the discussions, as she may be feeling a little overwhelmed at this time by all her visitors. The daughter responded by sharing, "No one wants to talk to her too long. She just complains and feels sorry for herself and wants you to hold her hand and stroke her cheek. Everything she says is an implied criticism of us. We love her and she ought to know that. Can't she tell? We are all here most of the time." The paradox of cold reactors is seen in this daughter's own frustration. The needs for intimacy are high in cold reactors and those who love them, yet the style of interaction resulting from the thinking of cold reactors alienates everyone.

Certainly the daughter's feelings are understandable. Cold reactors often engender a feeling of guilt and distance because of their own tendency to give so much, yet be so needful. Those relating to a cold reactor feel as if they fall short. One wonders about the inheritability of cancer and whether or not our familial patterns are equally responsible for what we see as an hereditary factor in cancer. Is it possible that families are cell disease producers, just as hot reactors can be heart disease carriers? Is it possible that family communication systems create an atmosphere, a climate, for the overgrowth of cells, a carcinogenic environment as dangerous as any contaminated environment?

7. The Gray Filter Syndrome

The cold reactor seems to have a dark gray filter through which all incoming information must pass. Good is okay, not too good is terrible, terrible is a hopeless disaster for the cold reactor. Unlike the hot reactor who is more typically cynical and processes all information suspiciously, the cold reactor personalizes occurrences to such a degree that no information can make it unimpaired through self-talk gloom. Taking everything very seriously, a cold reactor may be deeply hurt by a joke or casual comment.

A nurse walked up to a cancer patient and placed her hand on the patient's shoulder. "Your color looks much better today," she offered.

"Yes," responded the patient; "It is probably due to the additional medications that have totally upset my bowels. Besides that, you are looking at me in a dark corner and can't see how I really look." The nurse had run head on into the filter of the cold reactor.

People attempting to relate to the cold reactor often find themselves frustrated as if presenting an argument in court, trying to convince the cold reactor to cheer up, move on, and be more optimistic. Unfortunately, the verdict is predetermined. The self-accused is judge and jury.

8. How Time Drags By

The cold reactor thinks about time in years, even decades, while the hot reactor thinks in milliseconds. The cold reactor tells stories of generations and serves as a type of familial historian, while the hot reactor, if having the time to tell a story at all, talks of the next minute or of saving time and brags about how many things were done at once.

Some years ago, a hospital instituted a policy that calendars with large, tear-off numbers for the days and months be placed in each room, so patients would not be isolated from the flow of the "real world." Heart patients and other hot reactors tore the days off with regularity—sometimes ahead of time. Cold reactors seldom tore the days off, telling time by shift changes and different workers on staff in various shifts. They were alert to interactions in people, not concrete measures. For them, it seemed to take forever for time to pass.

I have discussed the boredom factor as related to cell disease. The failure of rhythm, of a sense of pulse of life, leaves the cold reactor alone and waiting forever for something to happen. Both hot and cold reactors are vulnerable to diseases of rhythm, with the hot reactor's accelerating beat and the cold reactor's dragging beat setting the rhythm for lives that are offbeat. The immune system then, too, becomes desynchronized and "disautonomitized"—Hans Selye's word for the disruption of the supersystem that results.

One of my patients recently shared her dream that everything in her body had slowed down. She reported feeling her blood flowing "as if it was an effort for my heart to move it, almost like it was circulating mud." For the cold reactor, dreams are not in the lucid style, discussed earlier, of the hot reactor who can almost observe and control the dream itself. Instead the cold reactor *is* the dream, totally immersed within it, unable to differentiate, at times, dream from reality, nightmare from fear, daydream from hopeless thinking.

9. Hopelessness

As a graduate student, I accompanied a well-known oncologist on his rounds. He was to share the results of a biopsy with one of his patients, and four of us stayed back by the door as our teacher approached the bed. Standing with a metal chart over his heart and looking down at the patient, he pronounced, "The results were as I expected. I am afraid it's worse than we thought. I am afraid there is no hope."

I looked at the patient in horror, startled that she seemed unmoved by this news and the style with which it was presented. She responded, "That's what I thought. It's okay doctor; I understand." Even at this stressful time of her life, the patient was offering comfort and support to her doctor. Of course the situation no doubt dictated the nature of the response: one pronouncer standing above the bed, an audience, and one victim. Nonetheless, this patient, as many cold reactors, seemed to think in a hopeless internal dialogue, reassuring the doctor and assuring herself of more sickness.

Of course there is always hope. Tests that count cells do not count out hope, but the cold doctor had spoken in the cold style of this patient. The fact is that the brain interacts with the body, and the doctor interacts with the patient. It is all one system. Sick patients make sick doctors, and sick doctors make even sicker patients. The same can be true for wellness and hope.

One research study illustrated that women who had received good news regarding a breast biopsy had more problems with body image and more personal distress than those who had received bad news and required a mastectomy. The surprising contradiction was explained by the fact that women receiving the good news no longer needed their denial, no longer needed to maintain a defense system, and, therefore, allowed their emotions free reign. Those women experiencing the bad news clung to a denial system and only slowly allowed their emotions to overtake them. It is important that physicians and patients alike are aware of how defense systems are employed and understand the unique styles of hot and cold defenses as part of the healing process.

There is abundant research to indicate that those patients who feel hope have a better prognosis for the same disease process than those patients who do not. Yet the cold reactor thinks, "My life has little hope, so my disease must have little hope." I sometimes wish that my patients had more "dis-ease," or discomfort with the disease, and did not just cling to the illness or accept it as fate. I wish that they would mobilize and direct their hope more effectively to coping strategies and would show less acceptance of medical pronouncements.

10. Overcompliance

Working almost 20 years in hospitals and consulting to various homes for the ill and aged, I have never ceased to be amazed by the fact that we all comply so easily with our assigned roles as patients. The cultural, almost religious right of hospitalization demands a role from the patient. The medical model, our cosmopolitan medicine, has become dogma, and the cold reactor too easily fits into dogmatic systems.

After you finish reading this sentence, close your eyes and imagine a perfect place for healing, for recovering from any disease. Did the place resemble a typical hospital? Or did your imaginary healing place include sun, light, humor, laughter, music, fresh air, warm people, warm colors, patient involvement, joy? Compliance in the medical system is dangerous to your health. Women with *metastatic*, or spreading, cancer of the breast have much longer life expectancies if they are not compliant, are more truculent, attention-demanding, and self-responsible. Even if the hospital staff may see these characteristics as cause for psychiatric referral, they may be the only defense against being "hospitalized." To be hospitalized means to be assigned a role, to be a victim and a recipient, not an active partner for cure. It is a cultural right, including being stripped, bathed, punctured, irrigated, poked, repoked, harassed, pronounced, and, if you are appropriately responsive, eventually wheeled out and released.

Over 80 percent of patients who visit a hospital will get better or worse no matter what the hospital does. Approximately 10 percent of the patients, however, may get worse due to what may be viewed as bad luck, errors, or other risks to survival. Such bad luck tends to happen to those people who are more compliant in hospitals. The 10 percent that may get better in hospitals are the 10 percent who take self-responsibility for healing, who quarterback their own team for healing.

Cold reactors think in a compliant fashion in almost all social circumstances. They tend to go along, thinking that they have little power or choice anyway. "What can one person do?" is the thought, or, "If I complain or question, they may not like me." One of my younger cancer patients was a boy of 12 with leukemia. He told me,

HOT AND COLD IMMUNE SYSTEMS

HOT	*COLD*
Anxiety ↔ depression	Depression ↔ anxiety
Left-hemisphere cognitive style	Right-hemisphere cognitive style
"SAM" system	"PAC" system
Maladaptive hyperarousal syndrome (MHS)	Learned helplessness syndrome (LHS)
Alarm reaction	Vigilance reaction
Fight/flee	Flow
"Owl" style of time	Lark style of time
Apparent "extroversion"—but power oriented	Apparent "introversion"—but "people oriented"
Lack of "r.e.s.t." (restricted environmental stimulation time)	Lack of "R.E.S.T." (really exciting stimulation time)
Hypothalamus ↔ amygdala ↔ pituitary	Hypothalamus ↔ hippocampus ↔ pituitary
Adrenal medulla	Adrenal cortex
Catecholamines (epinephrine, norepinephrine)	Corticosteroids (cortisol)
Irritation of supersystem	Decapacitates supersystem
Reduction of B cells due to sudden increase of T-suppressor cells. Tolerance problem with own system. Tissue irritation.	Slowing of macrophages—Suppression of surveillance function, reduction of number and effectiveness of killer cells. Specificity problem.
Ulcers, spastic colon, irritable bowel syndrome, hypertension, heart disease.	Allergies, arthritis, infections. diabetes, multiple sclerosis, lupus. cancer.

"I am trying to be very very good, because this is the day they decide how much chemotherapy I might need." Even when we are ill, and perhaps because we are ill, we seek approval at all costs, as if our good behavior may change our prognosis. The cold reactor seeks approval and thinks about it at the cost of wellness.

The preceding chart on the hot and cold immune systems summarizes some of the aspects of both supersystem styles. Remember, we all have both hot and cold sequences to our immunity.

ON THE MELTING OF ICICLES

Back home the healing has continued. I am learning to release my anger. I don't hold back any more. My children and I yell at each other openly when I feel like it, and we have never been so close. When I go on walks, I often yell to the roar of the ocean . . . yell out my strength, rage, laughter, joy, whatever comes. I feel a part of the whole world, at home in it. I am learning more and more deeply what a precious gift this cancer has been, teaching me how to live.

ELIZABETH RIVERS

Let's return to the woman looking out my office window at the dripping icicles. Her eyes still on the icicle, she watched as the light from the sun turned the corner of my office building. Drops were falling more rapidly, and the icicle was gradually disappearing. She commented, "There it goes. It will be a race between the drops falling or the icicle breaking off and falling down first."

I decided to try an experiment that previews some of the strategies I will be discussing in terms of enhancing our wellness. I asked the patient to rise, go to the window, and place her hand on the cold glass near where the icicle hung. She said, "This is weird; my hand is freezing." Remembering how compliant the cold reactor is, I knew her hand would remain in spite of her discomfort. The icicle broke free and shattered, almost like tiny glass tears scattering on the window sill. "Did I do that or did the sun do that?" she asked, finally looking at me. "Yes," I responded. She returned to her chair and, as she sat down, leaned toward me. "What do you mean, yes? Was it me or the sun?" I asked her and I ask you, "What is the difference. The icicle melted."

In Part Three I'll discuss strategies to mobilize the miracles of the supersystem, to cool down, warm up, and find new ways of living in a more healthy style with the supersystem.

Part Three

TAKING CONTROL
OF THE
SUPERSYSTEM

I ask those who urge me to take medications to wait at least until
I have regained enough strength and health to enable me to stand
the effort and the risk.

MONTAIGNE

This section describes strategies for being the master rather than the
victim, participant rather than respondent to the supersystem. I will
describe cooling down the hot system and warming the cool system. I
will give suggestions for boosting the supersystem, preparing it for times
of anticipated challenge. I will conclude with an example of the confrontation between the supersystem and the most terrifying disease of
the century, AIDS.

Chapter Eight

COOLING DOWN

IT'S HOW YOU *A-R-E* THAT MATTERS

If you hear that a mountain has moved, believe; but if you
hear that a man has changed his character, believe it not.

MOSLEM PROVERB

The surgeon takes his scalpel in hand and looks at the other physicians
standing around the patient. They are preparing for the first cut in a
major surgery. Just as a barber sharpens the razor on a strap, the surgeon
smiles as he scrapes the scalpel on the sole of his shoe several times.
He then uses the same scalpel to make the large incision into the abdomen
of the patient. This is exactly what took place hundreds of years ago.
Defiant and mocking of the theory that tiny invisible germs could cause
disease or infection, surgeons would engage in such acts to show their
disrespect and disdain for any idea suggesting that something invisible
could be responsible for illness.

Years ago, in the bedroom of a farmhouse a country doctor begins
the delivery of a baby. No one, including the doctor, has washed his
hands prior to the procedure, and the mother dies from an illness called
puerperal fever. Certainly, it was believed, tiny invisible germs did not
exist on the skin, and washing the hands was not viewed as necessary.
The reality of the existence of these germs was confirmed through

thousands of needless deaths of mothers and their babies, each death preventable by a more open mind on the part of health care professionals, by a respect for a new way of viewing disease—a respect for germ theory.

Much of the information I have reviewed so far in this book continues to be viewed with the same disregard, even disdain, as the germ theory was years ago. The mechanical orientation of our society and our medical model makes it difficult for some of us to accept the fact that thoughts and feelings can cause or cure disease. J. J. Ingelfinger, the former editor of the *New England Journal of Medicine*, agrees, as I pointed out earlier, that when we get sick, 80 percent of us get better or worse without physician intervention. In slightly over 10 percent of the cases, medical intervention may be dramatically successful (such as removal of kidney stones, repairing of bones, and the use of antibiotics). However, he concludes with the statement: "In the final nine percent, give or take a point or two, a doctor may diagnose or treat inadequately or he may just have bad luck. Whatever the reason, the patient winds up with iatrogenic (physician caused) problems, so that the balance of accounts ends up marginally on the positive side of zero." We improve those odds considerably when we move beyond the limits of the present medical model, the dogma of cosmopolitan medicine, to realize that immunity is not something you have, but something that you are and do. I will show you in the following chapters that you can take control of your supersystem and actually talk to it and tell it what to do and what not to do.

I pointed out earlier that the B-A-FITER system can promote wellness and healing. Our *b*eliefs, *a*ttitudes, *f*eelings, *i*mages, *t*houghts, *e*xperiences, and *r*emembrances are the keys that start the program for health. To prevent "dys-ease," or damage to the body system, and improve our condition from "dis-ease," or feedback that the supersystem needs adjusting, we must pay attention to how and what we think: We must make our imagery work for us by providing mental images that are guidelines for constructive work by the supersystem.

So it really is how we *A-R E*—our *a*ttention to the supersystem, a *r*elaxed and constructive imagery, and an adoption of constructive *e*motional and thinking states—that determines the degree to which we control our supersystems.

Cosmopolitan medicine has encouraged us to be more concerned about contamination, to prevent illness, and at all costs to fight off attacks upon our health, almost as if enough effort and enough money could cure the world. Instead of focusing our attention on our bodies, learning from our diseases, mobilizing a positive and relaxed imagery in favor of health, and attending carefully and positively to our emotional states, we have developed what Dr. Warren Bennis calls the "Wallenda Factor."

Carl Wallenda, the great tightrope artist, daringly and confidently performed feats of skill hundreds of feet above certain death. He reported that he never thought of falling, only of walking and succeeding at almost impossible tasks. Focusing on the nature of his tasks, he was relaxed, seeing himself successful in all his efforts. His emotions were characterized by happiness, joy, and pride in his work. However, after his family had a serious fall in Detroit, Michigan, Mr. Wallenda changed his theory of life and of his occupation. He began to think about falling, about preventing failure, about mistakes that could happen. He adopted a preventive, negativistic strategy to his trade. Months later, he fell to his death.

Our thinking can predispose us to illness or it can free us for a new wellness. Certainly, circumstances, bad luck, and technical factors contributed to the tragedy of Mr. Wallenda's death. Equally important, however, were his beliefs and his feelings, and it is here that I will place my emphasis for control of the supersystem. A phrase has been adopted from cancer therapists Carl and Stephanie Matthews Simonton by surgeon Dr. Bernard Siegel: "In the absence of certainty, there is nothing wrong with hope."

MEETING YOUR SELF-SHAMAN

Man is the only animal that laughs and weeps, for he is the only animal that is struck with the difference between what things are, and what they ought to be.

WILLIAM HAZLITT

If the invasion comes from our inner space, from the selfishness of our brains and our genes, which are unaware of our fit with the rest of the world, then our wellness can also come from what Dr. Steven Locke calls "the healer within." To experience this view of wellness, sit back comfortably in your chair, uncross your legs if they have been crossed during your reading, breathe from your belly (not from your chest), relax, and allow the following paragraphs to lead you through an experience that will help you discover the identity of the self-shaman on you.

Imagine that you are sitting comfortably in front of a warm, crackling campfire. You are in the middle of a large, safe, and beautiful woods and can notice the dark shadows of tall pine trees against a night sky, glowing by the light of a full moon. You have never felt more relaxed than at this moment, as you feel the warmth of the fire on your face, chest, abdomen, and legs.

As you sit relaxed, you notice through the quivering light of the campfire that a figure is present, sitting across from you. At first it is difficult to detect the figure, to see it clearly, but as you relax more, the figure comes more into view. As you look eye to eye with the person sitting on the other side of the fire, you recognize that the person is you. This "you," however, is the perfect you. This is the all-wise, relaxed, totally healthy, nonstressed potential within yourself. It is a manifestation of your very soul. For the first time in your life you are now able to address your ultimate perfection, the wisest and healthiest part of self.

As you look at this perfect you, describe the person in your mind's eye. How is he or she dressed? How does the person sit? How are the hands placed? How do the eyes look, the facial features and expression? What life attitude do you detect in the eyes of this perfect you?

As you contemplate this perfect you, imagine the one question, more than any other, that you would like to ask this person. Think for a moment, and at the end of this sentence close your eyes, pause, and ask the question. Then open your eyes and begin reading once again.

If you are at all like other persons who have tried this imagery opportunity, it is likely that your question would be "How did you get that way?" You would wonder at the perfection, relaxation, self-satisfaction, and comfort of this perfect you. You would ask how you managed to accomplish such a perfect state. It is perhaps the ultimate irony that we have within us the complete capacity to achieve states of wellness beyond our present imagination, yet when confronted with the imagery opportunity, we often seem puzzled as to how we ourselves are capable of accomplishing in the imaginary scene a perfection that eludes us in our day-to-day living.

Now that you have experienced what I call the "self-shaman opportunity," read the following instructions and then set this book down and go through this exercise in more detail.

1. Find a very quiet private place, and guarantee yourself 15 minutes of separateness from everything that distracts you in your daily life.

2. Make sure the temperature and total surroundings are comfortable to you.

3. Place this book in front of you as a symbol of the campfire, and sit comfortably on the floor in front of the book as if sitting in the imaginary forest described above.

4. Breathe in deeply through your nose so that your abdomen expands; exhale through your mouth. Feel the warmth of the fire, and smell the smoke coming from this fire.

5. Note that the temperature of the forest is comfortable. Close your eyes as you imagine the trees, the fire, and the total setting of this imaginary forest.

6. With your eyes closed, once again create the image of the wise person from within yourself. Generating that image, open your eyes and slowly ask the following questions out loud, asking each question as if you were actually talking to the wise you sitting on the other side of the fire.

- "How do I look to you, wise person? What is your first impression of me?"
- "Do I seem healthy to you?"
- "What do you see as my strongest point as a person now?"
- "What do you see as a point of vulnerability for me, an area that I need to improve as soon as possible?"

- "Do I seem to you, wise person, to be a hot or cold reactor?"

- "What is the biggest mistake I have made in my life to this point?"

- "What do you see as my most significant personal accomplishment?"

- "What is the most important thing in my life as you view me, wise person?"

- "If I were to become ill, what type of illness would most likely overtake me?"

- "Most important, wise person, how far from your wellness state am I now, and what can I do after I leave this campfire to come one step closer to your state of wellness?

Now that you have orally asked your wise person these questions, it may be helpful to write down the answers you came up with. More important than the answers, however, is the process itself. Taking time to look within for healing is a most significant step in moving toward thriving.

To help with the above process, I ask each of my patients to draw his or her self-shaman. In spite of the fact that most of my patients complain about their lack of artistic ability, they are able to sketch the shaman, and concretizing the image seems helpful to them. One of my patients has his sketch taped to his mirror, but he stated at a recent session that in the morning "sometimes I put my bath towel over the picture because I feel too guilty about what I am doing to myself to start the day."

COOLING HOT SUPERSYSTEMS

Having completed your visit with your self-shaman, you can use this technique to learn how to convert hot systems to warm and cold systems to cool, to learn how to accomplish the "Goldilocks just-right" balance.

You know that running hot, overactivation of the SAM system, is related to a set of diseases including headaches, ulcers, spastic colon, hypertension, irritable bowel syndrome, and particularly heart disease. These are all diseases of irritability, a supersystem cooking various body systems. The danger in knowing this, however, is that the hot reactor may become hostile toward himself for doing this to his own body. He may become impatient, attempting "quick" remediation by turning to the latest fad of exercise, diet, or meditation. The hot-supersystem person may also become competitive with self, trying harder and harder not to try so hard. This only results in overheating an already hot system. The purpose of the campfire assignment is to develop a comfortable, nonaccusatory relationship with self, not a critical self predestined to failure.

To cool down hot-running times, we must work toward a warm triad consisting of tolerance, patience, and caring. No one will argue against the fact that these three states are healthier than hostility, impatience, and competitiveness, but making the transition is the problem.

Transition is a process of reversal. It is a process of accurately diagnosing your own hot or cold style at a given time in your life and focusing upon the style's characteristics, understanding them, and reversing them in a constructive orientation toward self, rather than attempting to avoid confrontation of these characteristics. You will recall that the hot reactor is assessed by means of 12 yes or no questions and a psychograph, which measures hostility, competitiveness, and impatience. Combining the 12 yes or no answers with the 15 hot-triad items provides 27 items that will serve as a guide for our "reversal" of the hot cycle. Added to these 27 items will be the 5 cognitive distortions and the 5 defense styles identified earlier as characteristic of hot reaction. These will be used as starting points for our reversal exercise.

The discussion of moving the hot system to the warm system concludes with three implementation suggestions, or three techniques for facilitating the reversal process. Thus 40 concrete steps are presented that you can take now, not simply to survive, but to utilize what may have been a deficient hot system to promote a warm and healthy system. So, you see, being a hot reactor has actually provided you with an opportunity for a level of wellness that may not have been possible if you were not a hot reactor. Congratulate yourself for providing yourself with this opportunity as you begin the 40 steps that follow.

Note: It will be helpful to you in attempting this reversal exercise if you have someone with whom you can discuss the process. One caution, however: If you do have someone who will help you with the reversal process, point out to this person that you will not require her or his support. You are enlisting the person's help for change and for learning, not for support of your hot style. Contrary to popular psychology, support is not always helpful. The hot reactor is typically supported by his or her spouse, allowing the hot reaction to spread to the entire family. To stop this contagion factor, the partner of the hot reactor must set limits and not allow the hot reactor to contaminate the entire household.

READJUSTING THE PSYCHOSTAT—COOLING THE HOT REACTOR

NONTWEENY THOUGHT

Hot reactor

Thinks in terms of completes and opposites.

Reversal

I will remember that all things are conditional, somewhere in between.

Warm self-talk

I am neither a completely successful accountant or businessperson nor a completely failing accountant or businessperson. I will sound like Popeye: "I y'am what I y'am what I y'am."

Daily living example

At tomorrow's business meeting I will say to myself, "I am probably neither the worst nor the best accountant here and never will be either one. It doesn't matter anyway if I'm best or worst in comparison to anyone else. What matters is that I am doing my best for me and my health at this time."

CLAIM JUMPING

Hot reactor

Makes conclusive decisions about life on the basis of limited and self-biased information.

Reversal

I will realize that hesitating and delaying judgment are always better than rapid judgment. I will give myself time to think and never respond without hesitating first. He or she who never hesitates will end up lost. I may "eject" without the threat of a real crash.

Warm self-talk	There are no clear conclusions in life. Everything is in-process. The faster I go, the more wrong I'll be.
Daily living example	I will make no decisions today. I will jot down details and intentionally give myself an 8-hour period before finalizing any decision. I will do this as an experiment to prove to myself that hesitation and delay are constructive, not signs of weakness.

MUSTURBATORY THOUGHT

Hot reactor	Thinks in terms of "I have to, I must, I am obligated to. . . ."
Reversal	I will try to understand that we choose our own lifestyles. We establish our own sets of obligations. All life is choice. Most "have to's" are self-imposed.
Warm self-talk	I will plan today in terms of what I would like to do, not what I have to do. I will give myself opportunities to act on impulse rather than a set of long-established rules and self-expectations.
Daily living example	This morning I will write down all the "musts" and "shoulds" that await me for the day. Beside each one I will write down a "want." I will not allow myself to engage in any of the "shoulds" or "musts" unless I pay myself back by engaging in one of the "wants."

LABEL MAKING

Hot reactor	Achieves premature closure on issues by providing quick, biased, and prejudicial labels.
Reversal	I will remember that people and events are not describable by singular labels. They are understandable only in terms of my interaction with them over time. I will understand that through such interaction I will learn that all things change and that all

people and things have negative and positive characteristics.

Warm self-talk

Today I will watch my vocabulary, even when I talk to myself. I will use no labels regarding any person. I will use people's names instead of their job descriptions. If I should make a mistake and use a label, I will be sure to apply that label to myself instead of to some event or other person, for all the stress I experience comes from self and labels are a way of avoiding this fact.

Daily living example

I will talk today to some people I work with or live with and ask them what labels they think I have used to describe them. Since they will probably be able to provide answers, maybe even lists, I will apologize to them for using the labels and relate to these persons based on the opposite of the label I may have used (if I see them as lazy, I will now relate to them as people like all others, capable of a range of behaviors from lazy to energetic). I will not be able to accomplish this task completely, but the different perspective will help.

OH-NO-ISM

Hot reactor

Exaggerates events. Engages in the "total disaster" level of thinking.

Reversal

I will remember that things are probably never as good or as bad as I tend to think they are. They will always be somewhere in between.

Warm self-talk

Today I will listen to other people and notice their magnifications of events. I will attempt to put these magnifications in the *ANBD* (*a*in't *no* *b*ig *d*eal) context.

Daily living example

I will utilize my tendency to magnify as a cue to minimize. When I feel the oh-no phenomenon, I will sit down and take five deep breaths. This will teach my body to alter its readings of my reactions so that it will translate my tendency from oh-no-ism to oh-good-ism or a chance to relax. I will remember that the SAM syndrome is activated by my oh-no-ing.

HYPERHEADISM

Hot reactor

Tends to explain things away, utilizing intellectual-sounding theories of life.

Reversal

I will try to understand that intellect is not superior to feelings and that my feelings are more likely more important to my health than is my intellect. I will remember that my brain tends to be very selfish and not to realize its place with others in my world.

Warm self-talk

I will try today to talk about feelings, particularly my own feelings, and to be sensitive to other people's feelings. I will listen particularly for feelings of business colleagues and allow these feelings to enter my day-to-day business orientation. I will view feelings as valid.

Daily living example

On every coffee break, lunch break, and opportunity to pause during the day, I will keep a notepad nearby to write down feelings I am having at those times. Focus, rather than distraction, will characterize my break times, and I will focus on my feelings rather than required future tasks or lists of obligations.

DEEP-SIXING

Hot reactor

Tends to avoid confrontation with his or her own emotions from the past. Tends to avoid confrontation of prior setbacks and to avoid personal history.

Reversal

I must be aware of my past experiences and their relevance to my life now.

Warm self-talk	I will take the time to sit down and write three major conflicts that seem unresolved in my life at this time. If I need help, I will consult my self-shaman, who may have the answers more clearly in mind than I do.
Daily living example	In any conflict I experience during this week in my work or family, I will sit down and write one paragraph about how that conflict relates to my earlier life. Even though I may be tempted to deny this fact, I will work hard on establishing some connection to the past and will consult my world's greatest expert or some loved one if I need help in this regard. If I continually draw blanks, I may consider consulting a member of the clergy or a professional therapist for help.

DOG KICKING

Hot reactor	Tends to see problems in others rather than in self and to express frustrations in inappropriate places and toward innocent persons.
Reversal	I will take self-responsibility, considering myself responsible for my health, my family, my work, and most important, my own well-being and ability to thrive. I will express my feelings immediately and not store them for expression later.
Warm self-talk	I will try to use the word "I" today, using the word "you" only as the object of the verb, not as the subject. "I like you," "I love you," "I would like to," "I feel," rather than "you don't," "they don't," "the world doesn't."
Daily living example	Even though it is difficult and I may feel afraid, I will share my feelings with spontaneity and immediacy, even if I feel somewhat threatened today. If I have trouble with my boss, I will share my concerns at

that time and with that boss, rather than telling my problems to someone else. I will talk to those persons with whom I am involved, rather than engaging in frustrated discussion of what I should have said to someone. This does not mean I will explode, but that I will share feelings, not store them up. This storing is called "gunnysacking," carrying loads of problems slung over my shoulder, with a swing of that sack possibly hitting me straight in the heart.

NA-NA-ISM

Hot reactor

Tends to react the opposite from what she or he feels or really thinks as a way of avoiding conflict and discomfort.

Reversal

I will talk directly and spontaneously about my feelings and thoughts, and not attempt manipulation, indirectness, or subtle message giving. I will give rather than feel "heat."

Warm self-talk

I will avoid sarcasm and my tendency to "show people" by mocking, sulking, or leaving traces and signs that I hope they will read, thus avoiding the necessity to share myself. I will talk, not just demonstrate.

Daily living example

There is nothing wrong with being hot, it's always being hot that can kill me. If I am hot at a staff meeting, I will say that I am hot. I will not pretend that I am cool while I sizzle inside.

CRADLE DIVING

Hot reactor

Tends to behave and think in infantile fashion, acting childish while sometimes accusing other people of this same behavior.

Reversal

I will realize that I am a developing person and that childish, selfish, tantrumlike thinking is destructive to me and my family if it is chronic. I will remember that some of this behavior is necessary for my own survival.

Warm self-talk

I will make a conscious effort today to be mature and to show a caring for others. I will allow myself to regress sometimes through the use of humor and play.

Daily living example

I will make sure I have time today to regress and dive into my own "cradle." I will play, giggle, laugh, and cry at least once today, and will also sit down and be quiet at least once. Youthful characteristics are probably our species' health characteristics.

HOSTILITY

Hot reactor

Sometimes engages in repressed hostility, denied but apparent to others.

Reversal

I realize that I am hostile sometimes, and I will try to replace this hostility with tolerance and acceptance whenever I can.

Warm self-talk

I will think today about the strengths of persons, not their weaknesses. I will remember that negatives make for sickness, that my supersystem acts the way I feel.

Daily living example

I will actively seek out a chance to help some stranger today. If I notice a car in trouble, I will offer help. I will give someone the advantage in traffic.

THINKING ABOUT TIME

Hot reactor

Tends to be consumed by hours and minutes.

Reversal

I will think about people, events, and feelings, not hours and time.

Warm self-talk

I will get more out of my day by realizing that my day is a personal event, not a linear clock-measured event. I will leave earlier so that I am not rushed, and I will avoid setting deadlines. I might even sit in the office at the end of the workday instead of racing to my car at quitting time.

Daily living example   I will go to work one day without my watch and attempt to avoid all timepieces throughout the day. I will learn from this that I am able to function without the continually rotating black hands of the death monitor on my wrist dictating my life.

COMPETITION

Hot reactor   Engages in comparative thinking, one-up-manship.

Reversal   I will do what I think is constructive for myself and my family, and I will not be consumed by comparisons with others.

Warm self-talk   I will assess my day's work by how I feel and how I behave, not by comparison to my own or others' achievements in the past.

Daily living example   I will intentionally lose a game of tennis, golf or bridge and enjoy the humor of this loss, perhaps seeing who could lose the worst in a game with a friend.

STRIVING

Hot reactor   Thinks about achievement and goals.

Reversal   I will think in terms of now and the present, engaging in successful activities for the moment, not fitting them into a major life plan.

Warm self-talk   I am doing a good job now, and "now" determines my health. There truly is no before or after, only now.

Daily living example   I will try to spend one day without thinking of a life goal, my pension plan, future retirement, or promotions. I will think only of each phone call, activity, or household event.

IMPATIENCE

Hot reactor	Rushes others and self.
Reversal	I will realize that my impatience only accelerates my whole body, causing me illness. Most things that block my activities are not within my control anyway.
Warm self-talk	I am glad that I am in this traffic jam today because that means I am not in the accident that may be causing it.
Daily living example	I will walk to the longest line in the bank intentionally so that I have to wait. During that waiting period I will take time to practice my deep breathing, relax, and see this as a unique opportunity rather than a frustration.

RESTLESS THINKING

Hot reactor	Tends to be agitated, searching, thinking, always mentally "on."
Reversal	I will calm myself, slow myself, and rest myself, sometimes allowing myself not to think at all. I will sit and contemplate nothing.
Warm self-talk	I will enjoy just sitting in my office sometimes, enjoy the comfort of my desk chair, and stare out into space if I want to. If I am home, I will simply sit down, perhaps across from the campfire, and talk with my self-shaman.
Daily living example	I will realize that feeling agitated is a signal for me to engage in the "settling response." I will sit with my hands palm up on my thighs, lower my shoulders, lower my head, close my eyes, and try to guess how long a minute might be, as a resting game to interfere with my agitation. If I guessed too short, I will play again.

HYPERALERTNESS

Hot reactor	Exhibits hypervigilance, set for the alarm reaction.
Reversal	I will attempt to relax my muscles and turn off my vigilance mode. If I do experience vigilance, I will aim it at my inside feelings, not outside events.
Warm self-talk	I think I will let that phone ring three times before I pick it up. If my child calls for me, I will pause before immediately responding.
Daily living experience	I will observe others during the day and learn by watching them how hyperalert our world has become. I will look for their quick starts, quick body movements, immediate reaching for the phone, and twisting of their wrists to read their watches.

HIGH-GEAR FUNCTIONING

Hot reactor	Always runs on high speed, like a car with a stuck accelerator.
Reversal	I will realize that I have many speeds, from fast to slow to neutral. I won't use all my speeds during the day, but I will particularly try to be neutral at given times.
Warm self-talk	I think I will intentionally take the long way home from work today.
Daily living experience	If I sense that I am running on high gear, I will stand up in my office and run at a pace that reflects the gear speed I am feeling. I will attempt to slow down my running in an attempt to downshift.

EXPLOSIVE THINKING

Hot reactor	Thinks in spurts, accompanied by explosive speech and gesturing.

Reversal	I will slow my thinking patterns and allow myself to pursue a given thought without darting from one thought to another today.
Warm self-talk	Today I will focus on only one issue. My issue for the day will be . . .
Daily living example	I will put my hands in my pockets and avoid any gesturing as I speak today. I will pause between each sentence.

TENSE TRIAD OF MUSCLES

Hot reactor	Tenses forehead, shoulders, and jaw.
Reversal	I will relax the key muscles in the tense triad. When I think they are relaxed, I will relax them even more.
Warm self-talk	I will tell myself all day to lower my shoulders, smooth my forehead, part my lips gently, take a deep breath utilizing my abdomen, and let all my muscles relax as much as possible during the day, keeping my forehead cool and hands warm.
Daily living example	At work or at home I will utilize each ring of the phone as a signal to relax the muscles in my forehead. Through practice this will become a learned response in my body.

HYPERRESPONSIBILITY

Hot reactor	Experiences a pronounced sense of responsibility, the "why me?" syndrome.
Reversal	I realize that all of us, including my family, have responsibilities. I will never have to carry the entire load, I could never carry the entire load, and no one wants me to. People like to help me, and helping me is good for their health. I do them a favor by letting them do something for me.
Warm self-talk	I will spend time on my responsibilities to myself as well as to others, particularly to my body and its wellness.

Daily living example

I will attempt today to give one major responsibility that I feel I carry to someone else for the rest of the week. Even though this seems impossible, I will make an effort to do this and to see that people are happy to share my responsibilities. Sometimes if I will just ask for help, I will get it.

ALIENATION

Hot reactor

Tends to devaluate relationships, exhibits independence instead of interdependence.

Reversal

I will realize that relationships are important to my wellness and survival and to the quality of my life. They are not a distraction or a supplement; they are life itself. I will realize that my immune system must deal with "other," not as an invasion but as my total hope for health. The more people I like, the more immune cells I might have.

Warm self-talk

I will think about people, love, and "other," not just tasks, work, and accomplishments.

Daily living example

I will make sure today that I shake hands with everyone I work with and hug everyone in my family at least twice. I will send a single flower to everyone in my office. Although people will think I may be crazy, I will realize that in spite of everything else, this is a significant movement toward health for me and those around me.

DISTRACTIBILITY

Hot reactor

Thinks about self while listening to others.

Reversal

I will focus totally on someone else as she or he talks.

Warm self-talk

I will make an intentional effort today to listen to people who talk to me.

Daily living example

I will repeat whatever anyone says to me before I respond to it. I will repeat it with feeling, not just like a robot.

BEING CHALLENGED BY PERCEIVED PRAISE

Hot reactor	Competes with any praise or reward received by others.
Reversal	I will see praise to others as praise to myself, because I am part of a whole system. I will not see myself as separate from everything else.
Warm self-talk	I will realize that praise given to anyone is good for the whole world and that it eventually comes back to me.
Daily living example	I will praise as many people as possible today. I will say as many positive things as I can, and I will notice immediately the change in my own body system. Talking to others is also talking to my own supersystem.

EDGINESS

Hot reactor	Gets on edge, ready to fight for his or her rights.
Reversal	I will realize that fighting for rights usually leads only to competition and territoriality. Is it worth dying for?
Warm self-talk	I will allow people to cut in front of me in line and to cut me out in traffic. I will allow hot reactors who are hurrying to kill themselves to get the advantage because I have transcended that level of competition in my life.
Daily living example	I will intentionally give an advantage to someone else and not take credit for it at a meeting or at home. If I am working at home, I will bake cookies and send them to the school fair with the name of one of my neighbors, anonymously giving her credit for the donation.

PERFECTIONISM

Hot reactor

Adheres strictly to all rules, or at least feels pressure to do so.

Reversal

Many rules have nothing to do with survival and wellness of persons. I will realize that although rules are not made to be broken, they must be considered with regard to their impact on the welfare of the world and myself.

Warm self-talk

I will not be bound by rules at the expense of the wellness of the world and myself. I will realize a morality that stresses that my rights end where someone else's nose begins.

Daily living example

I will strictly adhere to only those rules that seem to me upon contemplation to be relevant to the enhancement of the world. I will utilize rules to help me be more aware of others, not just more aware of rules.

PERFORMANCE ORIENTATION

Hot reactor

Tries to be "on," to be clever, quick, and funny, most of the time.

Reversal

I realize that it is not necessary to be on or to entertain everyone but myself. I am valuable in and of myself, and just by being present I am valuable to people.

Warm self-talk

I will not be aware of how I am coming across today. I will just try to be myself, to be open, to be sharing, and to be part of a system, not to direct the system.

Daily living example

I will start a project of collecting other people's jokes, and I will not repeat jokes of my own while I am collecting others' jokes.

ANGER AT LINES

Hot reactor

Becomes angry when waiting or standing in lines.

Reversal	I will enjoy standing in line, and while I wait I will learn to breathe deeply. I will realize that anger is one of the most dangerous things that can happen to me in terms of my health. I need anger only to attack a major disease; otherwise, my anger attacks me.
Warm self-talk	Lines are evidence that other people exist, and they are a way of training my immune system to realize my place in the universe. Lines are signals to my supersystem to slow down.
Daily living example	While driving, I will obey the speed limit strictly and try not to take advantage throughout the day. Driving is the perfect time to relax and be with me.

OVERTALK

Hot reactor	Interrupts others. Urgency of speech.
Reversal	I will not interrupt. I will focus on my listening skills. The rule of incomplete communication states that nothing is communicated until two people have shared their message.
Warm self-talk	I enhance myself by listening to others. When other persons are communicating, they are shouldering the work load in establishing a relationship, and relationships are important to my health. Listening is always healthier than talking, and talking always takes some toll on my health. I am much safer as a listener.
Daily living example	I will place a tape recorder in my office or at home, and I will listen to it at the end of the day to see how often my voice, compared to other voices, is on the tape.

ANGER AT TARDINESS

Hot reactor	Lacks toleration for lateness.

Reversal	I will view lateness as an opportunity to relax, to think, or just to do deep breathing. It provides a chance to be with myself for a while or perhaps to consult with my self-shaman.
Warm self-talk	Every delay I experience, including other people's lateness, will be an opportunity for me to have privacy and to be alone. It will remind me that time is relative.
Daily living example	I have learned that time does not really exist and that people are not really late— they are just not here yet. I will add up the time that people are late, in my view, and learn how much free "time" it provided me with rather than how much "time" it "robbed me of."

EXPIRATION OF TIME

Hot reactor	Believes time is running out; never has enough time.
Reversal	I will remember that time does not exist, so time can't run out. There is no logic to hurrying when time is not measurable anyway.
Warm self-talk	Today I will think only about people—not things, not time, not ticking, but being. I will think of beginnings.
Daily living example	I will make sure that there are three clocks in my office or in my home and that they are all set to different times. On various occasions during the day I will decide which clock is right on the basis of which one fits my needs at that time.

RUSHING OTHERS

Hot reactor	Accelerates others' life paces.
Reversal	I will not pay attention to other persons' paces of life, but I will attempt to find my own rhythm.

Warm self-talk	I will focus my alertness on my body rhythms, attempting to be aware of when I am hungry, sleepy, aroused, and peaceful. I may even eat only when I am hungry.
Daily living example	I will sit in a chair at least once today and snap my fingers to the rhythm of my life. If I repeat this opportunity, I will note that the rhythm changes during the day and that I, myself, can alter the rhythm at will, sometimes by just snapping my fingers more slowly.

INTERNAL VIOLENCE

Hot reactor	Thinks about violence. Has images of hitting, even of killing.
Reversal	I will realize that each time I think of violence I am doing damage to my health. Even the thought of aggression and violence is bad for me and my family.
Warm self-talk	I will not swear, curse, or threaten violence, even in jest.
Daily living example	I will not spank, hit, poke, swear, or in any way be aggressive or think aggressively during an 8-hour period. When aggression or violence occurs to me, I will immediately go on a hunt for someone to hug or to shake hands with. As phony as this may seem, the body will learn from this to control its violence and selfishness and to save them for the battle with a serious illness. There is no health advantage in "venting" anger.

SARCASM

Hot reactor	Puts people down. Communicates indirectly.
Reversal	I will not say negative things to people or about people. I will not plot clever manipulations or degrading statements.

Warm self-talk	I will realize today that every time I put someone else down, I put myself down further. I will not talk about people when they are not present.
Daily living example	I will not use sarcasm at all today. I will follow the old principle of not saying anything about someone if I can't say something nice about that person.

HARSHNESS OF SPEECH

Hot reactor	Engages in aggressive verbalizations and swearing.
Reversal	I will try to modulate my speaking and thinking by intentionally reducing my harshness and working on the quality of my voice.
Warm self-talk	I will make an effort to talk softly, even more quietly, censoring harshness and aggressive terminology. I will make sure words like "love," "caring," "joy," and "hope" are in my vocabulary.
Daily living example	I will sit privately and sing or hum to myself once today. Even though I feel I can't sing or hum, it is important that my body learns there is a magic to music. I might play a tape that I can sing along with as a way of decreasing my verbal aggression.

HYPERCLEVERNESS

Hot reactor	Makes statements containing double meanings. Hides true feelings through subtleness and manipulation.
Reversal	I will not be subtle or manipulative. I will be direct and open. Cleverness is usually manipulative.
Warm self-talk	I will not send covert messages. I will speak from my heart and soul. The principle of irreversibility states that no communication can ever be taken back, so I will be careful.

Daily living example	I will intentionally allow myself to be manipulated sometime during this week. I will not ruminate about this; I will learn that those persons who are manipulated may be healthier than those who do the manipulating. The puppeteer is fatigued sooner than the puppet. I will learn to cut my own strings, not to pull them.

NEGATIVE SELF-THOUGHTS

Hot reactor	Conducts internal dialogues of self-criticism and experiences dissatisfaction with self.
Reversal	I will value myself for I am the world. To devalue myself is to devalue everything in this world.
Warm self-talk	I am special. I am well, and I am valuable for who I am, for what I can do. I am always in-process.
Daily living example	I will surround myself with positive signs, notes, messages, songs, music, and people. I will realize that positives mean warm and negatives mean hot and that hot kills and warm can heal.

If all this seems impossible, unrealistic, ridiculous, absurd, Pollyannish, or silly, you are more of a hot reactor than you may be willing to acknowledge. Remember, as Neil Armstrong said as he took the first step on the moon, all change begins with one small step for mankind. Just reading through this list of reversals and strange-sounding assignments can help cool down the hot reactor.

BONUS COOLING-DOWN ASSIGNMENT: ZEN JUGGLING

I suggest to all my staff and students that they learn to juggle. It is a silly, useless, fun, challenging, distracting skill, and it teaches us to distract ourselves from the problem-focused hot world we live in. You cannot learn to juggle when you are running hot.

I suggest the book *Juggling for the Complete Klutz* by John Cassidy and B. C. Rimbeaux. The book comes complete with beanbags and funny suggestions for developing your first "jug." An office full of people learning to juggle is not an office that can run hot, at least not while juggling.

By the way, I hope you do not learn to juggle too quickly. If you are the first to learn to do it the best, you have managed to become a hot-running juggler. Slow down by juggling with someone who is much cooler, much more inept at the skill than you are. Perhaps you could look around for a few cold-running persons sitting and looking at the juggling bags, defeated before they begin. Maybe you could heat them up and they could cool you down. If they resist your invitation, tell them that this is Advanced Zen Juggling. That usually sounds more intelligent than asking them to toss some bags with you. On second thought, just toss them a bag.

You have now traced through 37 suggestions (and one bonus idea). Just reading through the list should have slowed you down. The idea, however, is not to accomplish a task but to learn a technique, to learn a cognitive change through which you take responsibility for your thoughts and no longer allow yourself to be stuck in a pattern of overheating. To help you with this, the last 3 of the 40 suggestions for going from hot to warm are presented below. These are the three *facilitating suggestions*.

First, if you are the partner, friend, or spouse of a hot reactor, as well as being a hot reactor yourself, it is important to know that role modeling is everything. There is nothing wrong with acting, and even though you feel hot, it is helpful to behave cooly. In my lectures I refer to this as the "phoniness-first" principle. The key principle of my clinic and my program for helping patients is "All motivation is preceded by change." Change before you really feel like changing, and feelings will follow.

This role modeling can be done through a quiet time together as a family before dinner, perhaps in the form of family prayer (saying grace) or of quiet contemplation with hands joined. Time to pause, even if it seems awkward at first, can be a constructive step for implementing the changes from hot to warm. Sometimes, if we allow our homes to be invaded by the heat of the overreactor or if we wait for motivation to change before altering our behaviors, we are supporting illness, not a person.

The second of the three facilitating suggestions is raised by the question "How do you feel?" Hot reactors must learn to stop talking about things and events and to focus more on feelings. Family settings and workplaces should encourage feelings as much as events. The most successful businesses in the United States are those that have emphasized caring, gentleness, and the quality of interacting with people rather than programs, memos, projects, and commodities.

In their business places and homes, hot reactors tend to recount work stories over and over again. These are sometimes referred to as "war stories," with the same characters causing the same problems and the same stress. Until American business learns that its survival, its profits, and the wellness of its employees depend upon caring, gentleness, and warmness, rather than projects and goals, it will continue to be trapped in the inefficient mode characterizing most American industry today.

When I pointed this out at a recent business meeting, one manager stood up and said: "I think you really are ridiculous. American industry is no worse off than anywhere else in the world." I suggested to this man that a slogan such as "no worse off" would not exactly be a successful advertising campaign for his company and that the negativism of this survival orientation, rather than a positive focus, was a risk to the success of his business and his own health. Imagine an advertisement stating, "We're no worse than anyone else."

It is important to reiterate feelings to hot reactors: Let them know you hear them, but do not get involved in a problematic solving of issues. This has been called the *reiteration principle* in my therapy programs. Hot reactors tend to try to solve things rather than just to listen, and this characteristic sometimes translates to those who work with them or live with them.

The final facilitating suggestion is always to maintain body contact with hot reactors when they are talking. They will resist this at first, but touching gently, holding a shirt lightly, or resting a hand on a hip can settle people down and slow their speech. If you are the hot reactor, reach out and touch someone while you are talking as well. It will feel awkward and uncomfortable, but behavior change will lead to feeling change.

When I lead discussion groups for heart patients, I attempt to use these three facilitating rules at each group meeting. We talk about problematic work or family issues only at scheduled and limited times. We talk about feelings at all other times, and we maintain touch within the group. We focus on the phoniness-first issue and the importance of using change to promote motivation rather than waiting for motivation to lead to change. Over time, these groups have been most successful in cooling hot reactors, perhaps because we can see in others that which we deny in ourselves.

One of the wives of a male patient suggested that it was "tough to maintain touch" with her husband because she had to "catch him first." I told her that the situation was serious and that she had better use the more severe technique of the "tightening" touch. This meant that if she attempted to touch her partner and sensed him pulling away, she was to grab on even harder with more firmness, grasping a button on his shirt or suit. She felt this would cost a great deal of money in terms of sewing on buttons, but she was willing to try the technique. She called to report that the tightening touch had not worked too successfully and that she had modified the assignment somewhat. She stated that she now carried a large old scarf with her most of the evening when her husband was at home. When she wanted to talk with him, she would walk up and place it around his hips and her hips and tie a knot quickly. Her husband had fought this at first, causing some stumbling and falling, but laughter had saved the day. The *change-first principle* is a key focus for changing the hot reactor to warm.

Warming up is the focus of the next chapter. Don't try to be a different person; just learn to have more control of your psychostat.

Chapter Nine

WARMING UP

WARMING COOL SUPERSYSTEMS

To ward off disease or recover health, man as a rule finds it
easier to depend on healers than to attempt the more difficult
task of living wisely.

RENÉ DUBOS

As I have just done with the hot reactor, I will reverse the characteristics
of the cold reactor to yield 37 suggestions for change. Following this,
I will provide 3 implementation suggestions, resulting in 40 specific
recommendations for warming the cold reactor. I have included a bonus
suggestion as well.

The reversal of the cold reactor to the cool-reactor syndrome is
accomplished by establishing the cool triad of optimism, confidence,
and energy. As with the hot reactor, the cold reactor must learn from
her or his syndrome and not feel defeated by it. Understanding the cold
syndrome provides a challenge, an opportunity for personal growth, not
an explanation for failure or disease. You must avoid the passivity of
the third arm of the cold triad, the defeatism that can only lead to further
disease.

Once again, read through the reversal process presented in the 37
categories. If possible, discuss this system of change with someone who
knows you.

READJUSTING THE PSYCHOSTAT—WARMING COOL SUPERSYSTEMS

SMEARING

Cold reactor

Disqualifies the positives and negates good things that happen.

Reversal

I will accept positives for what they are. I will not degrade others by assuming they are giving false positives and compliments.

Cool self-talk

I deserve positive comments. I will not seek additional ones by negating the ones I receive. This will only lead me to disappointment.

Daily living example

I will compliment someone in return as soon as I am complimented. I will not think about or compare the compliment paid to me, but I will immediately return the message. I will be a sender as well as a receiver.

THOUGHT STRAINING

Cold reactor

Engages in mental filtering, not receiving positives.

Reversal

I will be alert for positive feedback from my environment at all times. As Chesterton stated, "An inconvenience is only adventure wrongly considered."

Cool self-talk

There are a lot of happy things that have happened to me. I will start looking for more of them.

Daily living example

I will not compare and contrast positives today. I will accept them as is and at face value. I will not rethink or rerun them over and over again.

NEGATIVITY

Cold reactor

Personalizes. Sees everything as related negatively to self.

Reversal	I will realize that I am part of a whole cosmos and a supersystem, not a lonely person responsible for everything. Beard said, "The bee that robs the flower also fertilizes it."
Cool self-talk	The beauty of this world is that I am part of everything. It is not possible to be totally responsible or totally irresponsible. There is always the ultimate "us."
Daily living example	I will write a list of all the people I have related to, including coworkers, friends, and neighbors. I will see how much a part of their world I really am in spite of my feelings of loneliness. I will think about my contribution to others' lives. I will recognize just how many people I really affect.

MINIMIZING

Cold reactor	Minimizes and reduces life to oversimplified terms.
Reversal	I will not minimize myself, others, or this world. I will see them and myself as significant to the scheme of the world and the universe. I will wonder at the magnificence of the world.
Cool self-talk	I am significant, people around me are significant, and what I do and think will always be significant.
Daily living example	I will look at the pictures from my family life and write down significant events that I have been a part of. I will not compare them with events in other people's lives, or seek out sadness or loss, but will focus on the positives such as birth, jobs, picnics, and marriages.

THE ATLAS TRAP

Cold reactor	Lacks sense of closeness. Withdraws.

Reversal	I will find intimacy wherever I can find it: through friends, associates, involvements in social groups, churches, temples, volunteer work.
Cool self-talk	Hoping for closeness is not the same as looking for it. Finding it involves behavioral activity, not longing, thinking, and worrying about it. I have to act close to feel close. What I do determines how I feel.
Daily living example	I will join one group this month. I will not know anyone in that group in the beginning and will select a group that will require effort on my part to become involved actively with others already in the group. Even though I fear this and feel it may not help, I will learn, as the hot reactor must learn, that the phoniness-first principle applies. I can only feel close if I behave closely.

ECHOING

Cold reactor	Projects or blames others and things.
Reversal	I will realize self-responsibility in all that I do. It is not "it," "they," or "the world" that is responsible—it is I. I can be over-responsible if I do not share responsibility with all persons and things.
Cool self-talk	I have been and always will be responsible to myself in my day-to-day life. Others' failings cannot alter that fact.
Daily living example	I will avoid using words such as "they," "he," "she," and "it" in favor of "I" and "me." I will remember that I am no more a victim than anyone else is.

ARCTIC ISOLATION

Cold reactor	Thinks and fantasizes about withdrawing.

Reversal	I will realize the difference between loneliness and isolation, with "loneliness" meaning the choice to be alone and "isolation" meaning something imposed upon me through desertion by others. Isolation is rarer than loneliness.
Cool self-talk	I will realize that all of us have times of feeling totally alone and that this is not a sign of weakness or deficiency in me, but a realization that we all enter into different systems with different levels of intensity throughout our lives.
Daily living example	Today I will work on enjoying my loneliness and realize that all of us must be in touch with self. I can do a great deal to prevent isolation, but I must also learn to enjoy my loneliness. It has been said that when it is dark enough, one can see the stars.

THE DR. WELBY DILEMMA

Cold reactor	Engages in the overgeneralization technique, fantasizing about a perfection that can never be.
Reversal	I will realize that all generalizations about life are wrong. Life is made up of small events, positives and negatives. Eisenhower once said, "All extremists are wrong."
Cool self-talk	Today is today, now is now. The past and the future are made up only of nows. People are not all one way or another, and neither are time nor events.
Daily living example	I will write down the names of two persons who are outstanding, caring people. It does not matter if I know these persons or not. They can be movie stars or neighbors. Then I will write down some of the negatives that I think might apply to these persons.

I will note that as a cold reactor I may have tended to overgeneralize and idealize people and events. Everyone has deficiencies.

CRUMBLING

Cold reactor

Denies or avoids responsibility.

Reversal

I will realize that I am responsible for my life and not a victim of it. I will not negate everything that happens, and I will not avoid confrontation of my own flaws.

Cool self-talk

I will take my own life seriously and my own responsibilities seriously. When I know there are things I am responsible for, I will acknowledge my responsibility and not attempt to fool myself by denying reality.

Daily living example

As I consult with my own world's greatest expert, I will rethink some of the things that have happened to me and see how I may have avoided my own responsibility. I will spend time doing this today with my self-shaman, not in terms of more negatives but in seeing that I have more resources than I ever thought.

QUIET NOISE

Cold reactor

Exhibits what is referred to by clinicians as a passive-aggressive defense system, showing dissatisfaction through withdrawal or passivity.

Reversal

I will express my emotions and my needs directly and verbally to the appropriate persons in the appropriate ways, not by covert messages, withdrawal, or aggression by neglect.

Cool self-talk

When I am angry, I will state it. When I am happy, I will state it. I will not try to avoid a manifestation of my feelings.

Daily living example

If I feel like withdrawing, I will talk about the feeling rather than actually doing it. I will share my concerns instead of "demonstrating" them. I will be alert to my "cooling down" of others.

INSECURITY

Cold reactor

Checks and rechecks work.

Reversal

I will realize that if it's done, it's done. I probably did my best. It only pressures me more to keep rechecking and thinking about rechecking.

Cool self-talk

I will pay attention to what I am doing when I am doing it. Once it is done, it is done. I will not rethink each activity.

Daily living example

For a 7-day period I will complete a task and set it aside. I will not recheck and particularly will not rethink work activities. If I rethink something, that will remind me to do something new.

MORBIDITY

Cold reactor

Has a negative orientation to life. Thinks the worst.

Reversal

I will remember that speaking and thinking in morbid terms only negate life. Most of life is constructive and growing. Even loss is a part of our growth. There would be no life without death, no joy without sorrow.

Cool self-talk

I will talk in positives, in growth-oriented terms focusing on progress, movement, development, and change. I will not focus on loss and events I view as diminishing life.

Daily living example

At the end of each day I will focus on one growth factor that occurred, even if it may seem negative at first. I may learn that there are many positives that take place during the day if I focus upon them. I will not underestimate the problems of life or minimize my ability to cope with them. All crises are followed by some form of growth.

AMBIVALENCE

Cold reactor

Considers things as both positive and negative. Does not allow self a positive orientation. Is afraid to commit to an emotional position.

Reversal

I will take a stand, take a risk, even at the expense of being wrong. I will not continually vacillate and suffer by seeing things conditionally.

Cool self-talk

Today will be a day when I will reach out and take chances. Prior failures do not predict future failure. They are only the results of my life's behavioral experiments. Each day offers new opportunities for growth.

Daily living example

Today will be an experimental day. I will do something I have never done before, enjoy it, and finish it, all within one day. I will not look for problems with life events by overevaluation or overmonitoring.

CONTAINMENT OF EMOTIONS

Cold reactor

Constricts or holds back emotions.

Reversal

I will spontaneously express my emotions, not holding them in or waiting for others to elicit them from me. It is not childish to express emotions spontaneously.

Cool self-talk

I will be open in my emotional expression. I will begin sentences with "I" and share how I feel immediately and spontaneously with persons. I will not hold back or wait for invitation, hoping people will guess how I feel.

Daily living example

Particularly to myself, I will talk positively and share my emotions. I will verbalize out loud or in consultation with my self-shaman. When I overcontain myself, I overrestrict my supersystem.

CONVENTIONALITY

Cold reactor

Has a rigid and conventional orientation to life.

Reversal

I will be more spontaneous, less rigid. I will try to be unconventional and chance-taking once in a while.

Cool self-talk

Everything I do cannot be perfect and will not fit in with my perfect expectations. I will try things out and sometimes fail.

Daily living example

All persons fail. I will not allow other people's failures to bring me down or my own personal failures to devalue me as a person. I will do something today that is not at all like me, perhaps dance, sing, do a finger painting. I will not just avoid pain, but will also seek pleasure.

SELF-DEPRECATION

Cold reactor

Tends to be self-blaming and self-sacrificing.

Reversal

I will realize that I get nowhere if I sacrifice self, for then I have no self to give or to enjoy with others.

Cool self-talk

If I do for others, I am really doing for me. No one wants me if I sacrifice myself. *Altruism* means giving and sharing, not sacrificing.

Daily living example

I will receive help from others and not feel that I have accumulated emotional I.O.U.'s because of their sharing.

HELPLESSNESS

Cold reactor

Believes "There is nothing I can do about my situation." Lives in a state of stagnation.

Reversal	I will see that I am not helpless. There are always things I can do and things I can get others to do with me.
Cool self-talk	I am responsible. I have skills I have not begun to tap because of my cold style of thinking. I will try to use these skills and take chances.
Daily living example	People who act helpless very seldom get any help. As a matter of fact, people who appear helpless sometimes are viewed angrily by others because it makes other people uncomfortable. I will make a conscious effort to control my tendencies to act helpless or speak in a helpless fashion. I will be aware of my voice quality and posture, for these too send a message of strength or helplessness. I can feel as I act, walk, and stand. My body is a public advertisement of my personality.

HOPELESSNESS

Cold reactor	Believes "I am destined to a life of strife and struggle."
Reversal	I will realize that there is always hope. It is illogical and incongruent with the workings of the world to ever say there is no hope. Nothing is certain. Miracles happen.
Cool self-talk	I will hope for everything. I will not allow myself to succumb to the idea that there is no hope because, if that were true, it would only be true because I have said so and have convinced myself that it is so.
Daily living example	I will notice my vocabulary and monitor it for statements regarding hopelessness. I will realize that each statement of hopelessness only makes me more inadequate for solving problems. I can talk myself into being a certain way. How I talk is an advertisement of my inner self. My reputation with

myself is revealed by my expressed philosophy of hope or despair.

OVERCOMPLIANCE

Cold reactor

Believes "It is easier just to give in than to resist."

Reversal

I will not always comply. I will think, judge, and act.

Cool self-talk

People will not run me. I will not try to run people. I will work with people, not on them or for them. I have the right to question, to ask, to direct, and to cooperate by choice.

Daily living example

I will take responsibility for my life and all the activities that make up that life. I will behave as if I understand the fact that I should not be more compliant than anyone else. "Cooperation" and "compliance" are different terms, and I will be aware today of not mistaking my cooperative nature for a weak, compliant personality. I will remember that compliance can result in illness. I do not want my immune system simply to comply.

PROLONGED GRIEF

Cold reactor

Becomes overwhelmed by losses, even daily endings and changes.

Reversal

I will realize that there is always loss and that there is no gain without loss, no beginnings without endings.

Cool self-talk

All the losses I have experienced are a part of what I am now, and what I am now is a part of my future. In its most real sense, there is no loss, for everything is a part of me and I am a part of everything else.

Daily living example

I will talk to my self-shaman about the losses in my life, and I will ask what gains may come from even the deepest loss.

PROBLEMS WITH
INDIVIDUATION

Cold reactor	Experiences fear of separation.
Reversal	I will realize that there is no separation in this universe, that we are all a part of a large system. If we think separately, it is only a delusion.
Cool self-talk	The truth always begins with two, and I will always be part of everything. I can live on my own, and I will always be with myself, even if I am in a relationship.
Daily living example	I will go to a movie or a play alone. I will enjoy the show, a meal, and the travel without thinking how alone I am and without watching other people to see whether they all have someone else to enjoy.

ASSUMING THE WORST

Cold reactor	Assumes misfortune. Forecasts life hassles and disasters.
Reversal	I will assume that I will always have good fortune, for as I think, therefore I will be. I can create my own positive placebo effect.
Cool self-talk	Things are good and good things are going to happen. Good things happen to everybody. I have seen them happen to other people, and if they happen to other people, I am a part of other people and, therefore, they will happen to me.
Daily living example	I will talk to my self-shaman about some of the good fortune I have had. My self-shaman may see this more clearly than I do.

TRAGIC THOUGHT

Cold reactor	Thinks about ultimate tragedy. Believes life will end in crisis.

Reversal	I will remember that life is essentially beautiful, and good things and bad things happen through life. A positive direction to thought gives meaning to life.
Cool self-talk	I have and we all have misfortune. If life is a system, then misfortune will be balanced by good fortune.
Daily living example	I will behave as if I am moving in a positive direction. I will think of goals throughout the life process, including the later years of my life. The imagery I establish for my life can become reality, so I will create positive imagery.

PERSONALIZING FAILURES AND PROBLEMS

Cold reactor	Confuses influence with control. Overassumes responsibility.
Reversal	I will realize that everybody messes up part of the time. There can be no gain without pain.
Cool self-talk	If I mess up, at least it is a sign that I am doing something, that I am not just passive. Messing up will always beat boredom.
Daily living example	I will meet with my self-shaman regarding what I view as my mess-ups, and I will see what lessons I can learn from them rather than using them as points against me. "Failure" is a term that applies to tasks, not people.

FEELINGS OF INSIGNIFICANCE

Cold reactor	Experiences feelings of being ignored, unimportant, devalued.
Reversal	I will realize that whether I am ignored or not depends upon my own actions, ways of talking with other people, and ways of thinking about relationships.

Cool self-talk	If I pay attention to others, others will pay attention to me. I will not be on display if I become involved in the activities around me and try to create these activities.
Daily living example	I will invite people to my home. I will accept invitations. I will actively reach out to others, not passively sit back and think about how I am being ignored. Most people are too interested in themselves to ignore anyone intentionally.

LOOKING FOR WEAKNESS

Cold reactor	Looks for weak points. Sees a glass as half empty, not half full.
Reversal	I will look for strength in myself and others.
Cool self-talk	As a human being I have been given several blessings. I will look for these blessings as much as I can.
Daily living example	I will write down what I consider to be my weaknesses, and I will balance each one with a positive within me. The list should be equal on both sides. If it is not, I am distorting reality. I will look harder for positives.

"IT'S THE LAST STRAW"

Cold reactor	Feels overwhelmed. Lacks strategies for survival.
Reversal	I will remember that there is no such thing as a "last straw." The number of straws in life is infinite.
Cool self-talk	There is always now and tomorrow. The concept of giving up is useless for myself, for the world, and for those I love.
Daily living example	I will start as many new activities in my life as I can. I will not focus on endings, but on beginnings. When I come to my "last straw," I will just plant a new crop.

PREMATURE SURRENDER

Cold reactor

Gives up too soon. Escapes challenges by giving up.

Reversal

I will never give up. I will realize that stopping an activity is not the same as surrendering.

Cool self-talk

I will continue to try in any activity, including games and conversations. It is not the achievement that matters, but the activity itself. Life is a way of traveling, not a station I arrive at. I will learn to enjoy the trip.

Daily living example

When playing a game or discussing an issue with someone, I will not give up or give in, but give effort. "Giving up" means I have a goal that is not modifiable. "Giving effort" implies enjoying activity and interaction with ultimate assessment of goal attainment. Giving up will only distance me from others.

"NO ONE CAN HELP"

Cold reactor

Feels that no one can help and no one can understand.

Reversal

I will understand that everyone can help everyone. We are a system.

Cool self-talk

I have autonomy, responsibility, strengths, and a dependence upon others as well as my independence. I will not just look to others but will encourage them to look to me as well.

Daily living example

I will attempt to identify my resources, to reach out to neighbors, and not to be totally dependent on one family system. I will accept as friends those who are not perfect.

"THEY DID IT TO ME"

Cold reactor

Believes "It's never me that does anything; it's always them."

Reversal

I will remember that "they" is "me." I cannot externalize my world and continue to be healthy.

Cool self-talk

I will not just look outward. I will realize that I am a part of a whole system, and I will look within myself for a major part of that system.

Daily living example

I will write a list of things that I feel "they" do or have done better than I do. I will then write beside those items strategies I could engage in that would change "they" to "me." I will realize that involvement in government, local or national, is more important than the passive criticism and suffering from the ineffectiveness of "they."

OBSESSION WITH PERSONAL FLAWS

Cold reactor

Focuses redundantly on same personal flaws.

Reversal

I will realize that all of us have flaws and that few of them are major. Accepting these flaws as a part of the total person—with strengths as well as flaws—is more important than continually thinking about the flaws and their impact and surrendering to our inadequacies.

Cool self-talk

I am the total of my flaws and strengths. There will be no strengths without my flaws. I am as much my flaws as I am my strengths. I will be what I tell myself I am.

Daily living example

I will meet with my self-shaman to discuss how my flaws may be turned into strengths. Redundancy in thought patterns about flaws, and focusing on one major flaw, is a characteristic of cold reactors and can lead to the diseases from which they suffer. Focusing on major flaws is as destructive as looking for several small flaws.

"IT'S JUST NOT FAIR"

Cold reactor

Senses that there is no fairness in the world. Violates his or her own arbitrary sense of fair play.

Reversal

I will realize that's right—there is no fairness. There is no ultimate judge of fairness in the world; there is just the world itself. Things don't happen; they just are.

Cool self-talk

Fairness is not a concept that applies to our world. No one is in charge of fairness. Accepting life is maturity. We are not given fairness; we are given our inner strength, our basic humanness.

Daily living example

I will translate into challenges the injustices I feel I have experienced. Everyone asks about fairness as if someone were in charge of its distribution. This is an immature view of the world.

HESITANCY

Cold reactor

Holds in urgent messages while desiring to share them.

Reversal

I will not hold back. If I feel urgency, I will share it immediately and not continually think of how I can't share my intense feelings.

Cool self-talk

When I feel something urgently, it is a sign that it has been there too long and I must share it as quickly and openly as possible.

Daily living example

I will share first with my self-shaman, and I will practice sharing my urgent messages. I may find that they are not as urgent as I thought, that they are simply different forms of the same message I wished to share over and over again. They may be a symptom of my lack of action and tendency to think rather than to do.

AVOIDING ASSERTIVENESS

Cold reactor

Ends confrontations quickly. Fears self-representation.

Reversal

I will develop the ability to maintain confrontations and grow from them.

Cool self-talk

Confrontations are not a threat to me or anyone else unless I cause them to be so by my thinking patterns. Confrontations can be meetings between people, not threats to my integrity or safety.

Daily living example

I will practice assertiveness. Assertiveness is representing self. Aggressiveness is trying to control someone else. Self-representation is the most effective form of dealing with people who tend to be aggressive. Meeting aggressive people with more aggression is only a risk to my health and is always inefficient. I will listen to others and represent myself.

PESSIMISM

Cold reactor

Fails to anticipate the future with joy and the present with happiness because of thinking about the past.

Reversal

I will realize that enjoyment is behaviorally accomplished, not done for me or to me by some external system.

Cool self-talk

I will make every effort to enjoy my life. I will not wait for others to do so for me. I will realize the past has significance but the present and the future are important. My view of my history is probably distorted, so I will not allow it to dictate my life.

Daily living example

I will learn to anticipate small and daily events such as hobbies, projects, shows, music, time sitting alone. I will avoid the establishment of major life goals in favor of day-to-day enjoyment and a more general focus on the future.

PEACE AT ANY PRICE

Cold reactor

Keeps a low profile to avoid the need for personal sharing.

Reversal

I will understand that peace is received, not attained, and that it comes not at a price but from inside. It is up to me to be peaceful, not to find people who are peaceful.

Cool self-talk

If I think peacefully to myself, I am more likely to behave peacefully and find people relating to me who are peaceful themselves.

Daily living example

I will try smiling at as many people as I can during the day. Even though this is another example of the phoniness-first principle, it is more likely that I can feel better about myself by smiling than that I can smile because I feel better about myself. Doing nothing to maintain peace only guarantees the peace of nothingness.

DISGUST AT SELF FOR PERCEIVED FAILURES

Cold reactor

Believes in the law of unequal dispersal ("when something hits the fan, it tends to distribute itself all over me").

Reversal

I will realize that I am not the only one hit by material from the fan of life. All of us are affected by all negatives and positives in this world.

Cool self-talk

If I'm hit by material circulated by the fan, it's because I stand too close to the fan. I must be aware that I have control over my life. I am not victim to it.

Daily living example

Optimism is not attained, it is received by being open to one's inner feelings. The natural state of health is an optimistic state. Pessimism and feelings of being a victim are distortions, and result from lack of activity, behavioral change, and clear rational thinking.

Again, the act of reading through the above list of reversals helps in the process of reprogramming cold to cool.

BONUS WARMING-UP ASSIGNMENT: ZEN GARDENING

When my patients are running cold, they seem similar to plants that are failing to grow and barely surviving. They are psychologically withered, in need of sun, water, and nurturing. As happens with some plants, simple watering and placement in the sun seems to have little effect, for the nurturance that is needed must come from within, through a fertilization process stimulating the entire system of the plant.

I suggest to many of my cold-running patients that they purchase several plants. When I ask some patients to do this, they will respond in typical cold fashion, ''I haven't got a green thumb; everything I touch dies.'' I require that they purchase plants small enough to transport back and forth to their appointments with me. I point out that we will measure the plants' growth at each session and see what we have learned together. My patients report that the plants seem reactive to their own attitudes and feelings. Some of my patients begin to talk actively to the plants, and they notice that the plants seem to survive. This is not surprising, for plants are living systems with which we interact and upon which we depend. Sometimes, I am able to teach my patients to become gardeners instead of mechanics, to appreciate growth and even blossoming.

One of my patients recently brought his plant to his therapy visit, and before he could see me, he had called all the secretarial staff to him in the waiting room. He reported, ''Here it is the middle of February, and these flowers are blooming like crazy. I just can't believe it.'' One of the secretaries stated, ''It must be your personality; you just have the touch.'' The patient responded, ''I think you have a point.'' Even if the plants for the ''Zen gardening'' assignment do not flourish, even if they die, understanding the process through which the failure to flourish occurred can serve as a lesson to the cold reactor, a lesson about the limits of one's influence on life as well as the range of such influence. At the very least the Zen gardening assignment provides a focus away from the day-to-day ''awfulness'' of the cold reactor and toward the processes of life.

I avoid Zen gardening for hot-running people. They tend either to forget their plants, yell at them, or complain about the store that sold them or to start a contest for the largest, quickest-growing flower. They tend to measure their plants, rather than to love, smell, and talk to them.

One hot reactor said: "I tried the plant thing you had my uncle do. Mine died. I'm really surprised, because all the crap I have to put up with should have made some great fertilizer."

I asked how his juggling assignment was coming along. He reported: "I gave it up when I saw a guy on TV do it great. If I can't do it that way, forget it. Maybe I'll start juggling some plants. Nobody's done that. I could be the best."

As with the suggestions for the hot reactor, these ideas are so obvious and simple that we forget them in our daily lives. We then fall victim to our own intellectual neglect, a pattern of sick thinking.

I offer three suggestions for paying more attention to our thinking. They should help implement the reversals mentioned above.

First, avoid the blaming syndrome. Some popular books on cold-reactor diseases such as cancer suggest that one major life setback or personal failure may account for cell disease. This is absurd. You have heard about the complexities of the supersystem in this book. One event, one failure, does not ruin everything. Cell disease is a complex system occurring within another complex system. It is related to the whole system of the world, not to a periodic fault or one disaster in life. Cell disease does not develop over months or weeks but over years, and the right things and good things you have done are as significant as the negative things.

Second, it is important also to have a social support system. It doesn't matter where it comes from; it just matters that it is there. It is the surrender and boredom of passive longing for social support that is the danger, not just the actual absence of someone else in your life. You must seek some form of interaction with someone or a group of someones. If all else fails, go out and buy a pet. Just make sure it is a pet you can cuddle, hold, and interact with, not just take care of. A pet can be a break in the boredom sequence and can teach a form of contact and acceptance that is conducive to health.

The third facilitating idea and the fortieth suggestion for the cold reactor is that feedback is important. You need some form of information coming in all day long. Music, poetry, lectures, and books can help. The key is a feedback "loop," and you must be involved in activity, not just passively watching the glowing TV screen. You do come to feel as you behave, so dance, don't drag; hop, don't mope; sing, don't

TRIADS OF ILLNESS AND WELLNESS

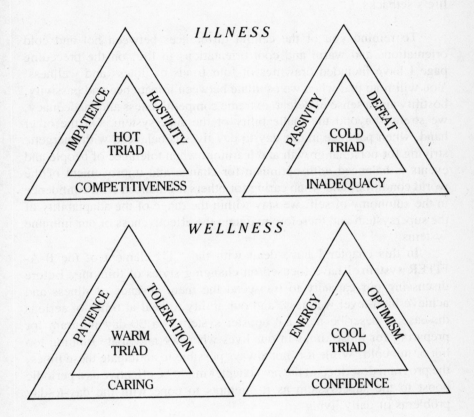

grumble. It's okay to be cool, just avoid being cold. Read poetry; look at art. The medical researcher Claude Bernard wrote a century ago, "I feel convinced that there will come a day when psychologists, poets, and philosophers will all speak the same language." When that day comes, it will be the language of the joy of living, not the misery of life's setbacks.

To remind you of the central differences between hot and cold orientations and warm and cool orientations to life, on the preceding page I have included drawings of four triads of illness and wellness. You will note that when we oscillate between impatience and passivity, hostility and a sense of defeat, extreme competitiveness and inadequacy, we stretch beyond the malleability of the supersystem. On the other hand, when patience in our day-to-day lives is balanced with energetic striving for personal growth and learning, when tolerance of people and events is balanced with optimism for change and improvement of the world condition, and when caring for others is balanced with confidence in the autonomy of self, we stay within the range of the adaptability of the supersystem and therefore maintain the effectiveness of our immune systems.

In this chapter I have dealt with the "T" element of the B-A-FITER system. I have focused on changing styles of thinking. Before discussing our capacity to transcend the mere absence of illness and achieve high-level wellness, and our ability to heal at times of serious dis-ease, I describe next a "booster system," a 30-day program for preparing for those times in our lives when we anticipate running too hot or too cold. While it is not always possible to anticipate these times, the program described in the next chapter might be effective as a periodic boost to the supersystem as it attempts to cope with the day-to-day problems of daily living.

Chapter Ten

A BOOSTER SYSTEM

Everything great in the world was created by neurotics . . .
MARCEL PROUST

A 1-MONTH IMMUNIZER PROGRAM: BOOSTING YOUR IMMUNITY

We all anticipate times in our lives when we will be going through particularly frequent and intense changes. We see hassles ahead, periods when we may temporarily run low on what we consider the uplifts that help us maintain our immunity. We know that we will be straining our defenses to the limit. Just as we might prepare for an intense physical exertion by a program of workouts, it is possible to enhance the supersystem, give it a boost, when we see challenges ahead. I suggest here a "psychological vaccination," a booster program of suggestions for strengthening the supersystem that integrates some of the points made in this book.

I have suggested 30 daily steps in this program. Many of my patients have used this system and found it helpful to them. Remember, the supersystem does not operate on its own. It is responsive to your thoughts, feelings, beliefs, and emotions, so strengthening the supersystem ahead of time is possible. Modify the following program to meet your own needs.

Day 1

Write down briefly and specifically the nature of the stress and strain that you anticipate in the future. Include when you expect the strain to start and when it may diminish. The entry in your "Immune-System Booster Log" should contain time of anticipated strain, source of the strain, and at least one major concern you have about the impact of the strain during this time. Take time and think carefully, because it is the thinking process itself, not the entry, that is the key. Here is one of my own entries in the immunity boosting program:

> From September 23 to October 29 I will be trying to finalize a manuscript. I will have to maintain my obligations at work and at home during this period. I expect time pressure to be intense.

Day 2

Write down a description of the most similar strain period that you can recall in your life. Again, include approximate time, source of the stress, and one major stress factor. Here is my entry:

> From May to June 1968 I had to complete my doctorate dissertation. I had to start a new teaching position and still find time to write and finalize my paper. I experienced conflict between trying to learn a new job and finishing a program that had taken years. Again, time pressure was the key factor.

Already you have helped your supersystem. You have compared your anticipated stressors with the past, much as a football team studies films from past events. As you continue to make entries in your log, it is important to allow yourself some brief time to sit and think about these entries, associate with them, and even discuss them with someone else in your life. Time for contemplation is vital.

Day 3

Write down the "uplifts," or the beneficial occurrences, that seemed to help you during the strain period that you identified on day 2. Include people or type of people who helped or things you did that seemed helpful in getting you through that stressed period. My entry:

> During the 1968 episode I played a lot of baseball and enjoyed the camaraderie of that team. In spite of intensive time pressure, I found the time spent playing ball to be well worthwhile in its relaxation and distracting effects.

No matter how stressed your supersystem was, you will be able to remember some things that were constructive to you. Even if the results of this past event were negative and may have included illness, some positive things probably occurred during that time, and it is important to have the supersystem recall those resources. The thinking process is the immune conditioning program.

Day 4

Write down your view of the present status of your supersystem as you prepare for the stressful period ahead. Are you running hot or cold? Use the tests in this book to help you with this. These tests are intentionally designed to be brief, with items drawn from research on the supersystem. Their simplicity and brevity will allow you to take these tests several times, even during a hectic schedule. My entry:

> I am running hot right now. I am highest on the hot scores even though I have elements of cold like everyone else. I realize that my running temperature changes, but I tend toward the hot side. I know I am overdoing it now with hospital work, teaching work, and worrying about covering as many research areas as possible so that my material will be thoroughly and currently documented.

Reading this entry after I wrote it, I could see that I felt frustrated. I was pressured by all kinds of obligations, lecture presentations, teaching responsibilities, and other professional and personal requirements. As I thought about this entry, I could see that my anger was aimed at myself for not taking full responsibility for my life and understanding that I cannot do everything and that some things would just have to go. I decided to cancel some of my lectures, substituting members of my professional staff to cover for me. I also decided to take vacation days to work on my manuscript a couple of days a week. I scheduled library time for journal review.

It is important as you make your entry for day 4 to look at Chapters Eight and Nine for suggestions on rational thinking and to check your cognitive errors. I also suggest reading the book *Feeling Good* by David Burns, which does an excellent job of identifying irrational approaches to stress in our lives.

Day 5

Now write down and study exactly what it is that you will be called on to do. Be as specific as possible. Include your emotions regarding what you will have to do. As a sample, here is my entry:

> I will probably have to rewrite, reorganize, restructure, and retype my entire book several times. At the same time I will have to see my patients, teach classes, prepare and present priorly committed lectures that I can't change, and still find time for my family. This means the number one thing I am going to have to do is structure my time instead of getting angry about there not being "enough time."

As I read over my entry, I noticed I was not specific enough. I still was not clear on exactly what I would have to do. The following correction resulted:

> I will need to spend several hours at a time sitting at my word processor typing, checking, and editing. I will also have to be driving back and forth to work, seeing patients, and every other week flying out of the city to lecture at other universities.

As I read over the second entry, I noticed that it would be necessary to sit down and write out a careful schedule and give copies to staff and family.

Day 6

By now you have been spending about 15 minutes a day writing and thinking and anticipating and trying to get the supersystem "in the mood'' for future stresses. For this sixth entry, it is time to replace emotions that are not helping to strengthen your supersystem with more effective emotions. My entry follows:

> It will help me to think of the enjoyment I get from writing. I enjoy sharing my ideas with others, particularly knowing that some of these ideas may help people who are sick to improve their condition significantly. I am not writing this book for a company or even for myself. Instead, I am doing it as a way of sharing some things with as many people as possible, and helping as many people as possible, giving them the chance to read an integration of some of the most interesting research I am aware of. I should be thinking of the opportunity to do this rather than the obligation to do this. After all, I chose to be an author, and if it is important to me to write and share with others, it is important to find time and structure my time so that I can do it without the negative emotions I am noticing in my log up to this point.

This entry should include hope and an attempt to ''positivize'' the upcoming stressful period. You have read that positive emotions are particularly constructive to the supersystem, and you may have to be a little phony to do this, a little bit of an actor. Pretend someone else is going to read your log for positives and signs of hope as you record this entry.

Day 7

At the end of this first week of preparation, it is important to identify your ''vulnerable system.'' Think back on when you have been sick, and write down how, where, and when. If you have had colds, flu, bowel problems, or headaches, ask where and why you think you became sick. My entry:

> I usually get a sore throat and a nagging cold when I am under stress. This means I might be running hot at times of several changes at once. It looks like my throat and respiratory system are particularly vulnerable.

By the way, it is a good idea to keep a supersystem record in your house for every family member. Write down not only what illnesses strike and what treatments are provided but also the emotions and pressures going on at the time. You will usually see a pattern over time. It is medically a wise idea to keep accurate medical records regarding treatments, medications, and health of all family members, but I am suggesting adding the emotional components as well for these are the markers of immunoefficiency.

Day 8

As you enter the second week of your 1-month preparation program, write down a one-paragraph imagery assignment that you feel will strengthen your supersystem, particularly in regard to your vulnerable system. Remember that all disease is metaphor. You may wish to check back in the book to review this idea. My entry:

> I have shown a remarkable capacity to bounce back from my sore throats and colds. My body's supersystem just rushes right in and protects me. Having a sore throat is a sign that my supersystem is at work and doing well. I congratulate my supersystem for its surveillance and effectiveness, particularly in my throat area.

Even if you have to memorize your entry, repeat this message in your mind for the last 3 weeks of this immune-system program. Find an imagery that is comfortable for you: white cells attacking viruses, your bowels being open and effective, your vessels circulating coolly and effectively. Think of an imagery aimed at the body part that had been vulnerable before, and make sure that you are commending yourself and your supersystem in that imagery.

Day 9

Realize that your body is a part of, not just a reaction to, your supersystem. It is important now to strengthen your body by paying attention to your physical health through nutritional and exercise approaches. This is really not as complex as it sounds. If you are being treated for a chronic medical condition, this would be the time to check with your doctor. Make sure your doctor is seen as a colleague and a helpmate in your healing, not as an expert. Describe to her or him what you are anticipating in several weeks, tell the doctor about your past vulnerabilities, and request a brief exam that rules out any present vulnerabilities. Unless you are being treated for a specific condition, such an exam will usually involve blood pressure, temperature, a blood analysis, and an electrocardiogram (EKG). If you have had a recent physical, you may be able to avoid this expense, but it might still be a good idea to call your doctor just to get his or her opinion as you anticipate the upcoming stress period. I suggest to my patients that they buy their own blood pressure gauges, for blood pressure can reflect a part of your health functioning.

Other things you can begin on day 9 are what I refer to as "the grandma rules." At one time or another your grandmother, grandfather, or parents certainly told you the following things, and research has supported their importance.

1. I will reduce my intake of toxic substances such as caffeine, chocolate, candy, sugar, salt, and artificial substances as much as I can.

2. I will increase my fiber and reduce the amount of fats that I eat as much as I can.

3. I will try now to establish a regular sleep pattern and develop a rhythm so that my supersystem itself can develop an effective rhythm.

4. I will walk a little more every day unless my doctors warn me otherwise. I will take stairs instead of elevators and park further away from my destination so that I get a little more exercise.

5. I will find time every day just to sit and rest, allowing my supersystem time to organize and center itself for future stress.

A word of warning here. As you write down some of your "body building" suggestions, you must be aware of the thin line between preparation and overpreparation. As I have pointed out, stress factors and change can have particular influence on the supersystem before the actual events occur. It may be that anticipation can be particularly problematic. For this reason, it is important that your preparation program be positive and hopeful and that you don't "play the whole ball game in practice," as one football coach stated. All successful trainers in athletics know that overtraining and overpreparation are as dangerous as underpreparation. This program is designed for fun and hope and relaxation, not overeager, wind-sprinting, huffing-and-puffing preparation.

By this time you have already done wonders for your supersystem. You are thinking more positively, you have learned from the past, and you have begun to prepare your body for a stressful period. Now it is important to make sure that your whole supersystem is integrated, not just focused on your vulnerable spots. A helpful assignment I have given my patients is as follows:

During your shower or bath every day, make sure you soap up and gently caress every part of your body. Talk to yourself while you do this. As strange as it may seem and in spite of the funny looks you may get from your family, speak out loud about your healthy foot, leg, body, head, eyes, back. In effect, you are integrating the supersystem and rewarding it. Our showers and baths should not be urgent preparation times, but chances for celebration of the miracle of the human body. We sometimes forget this, and day 9 is just a reminder to celebrate your humanness.

Day 10

This is the "nothing day." All day long, try to do as little as possible while still meeting your professional and personal obligations. Hang around, sit, walk, whistle, look, daydream, settle down, waste time, lower your consciousness, and try not to worry about anything. Skip all exercise programs, and even violate your diet just a little bit. This is a day to remember that you are not working for perfection, that moderation in all things is still an effective model.

You may find it difficult just to "diddle around," as one hot reactor described it, but this is essential for providing the supersystem with a chance to be itself, not to be hassled by some of the inappropriate ways we talk to ourselves.

It is important to enter the results of your nothing day in the log. You may not believe how nice it feels not to always be trying to improve, learn how to do something, progress, raise consciousness, eat right, jog, exercise, and essentially take a preventive mode of life. This 1-month program is an enhancing effort to mobilize internal healing strengths. My entry:

What a day! It seemed to last forever. No calls, no nothing. I didn't accomplish a thing, but I guess that really is a sign I did this day right. I also learned that this type of thing is tough for me—one of the reasons I must run hot so often. This is a good life lesson for me. I should take more time just to back off.

Day 11

This is the first of what I call "approximation days." For about 15 minutes, mentally rehearse the strain that you will be experiencing. Go through it in your mind and act it out if you can. My entry:

> I sat at my word processor and typed some tentative ideas for use in preparing my book. It's good to get back in the mood for writing and to establish some good practices. I also learned that I have a better place to put my paper and can arrange the computer screen better. I also learned that I need some new reading glasses, and I still have time to get them. Had I not rehearsed this, I wouldn't have had time.

I refer to this approach to preparing for stress as *successful approximations*. This is a way of identifying little conflicts and hassles before they occur during the stressful period. Had I not done my approximation, I would not be aware of the change in my glasses prescription that had taken place since I wrote the original draft of my book. You may find similar little hassles that can be avoided.

Day 12

This is "play day." Today's activity may be one of the strangest things I ask you to do in this 1-month immunizer program. The concept of *neoteny*, theorized by Ashley Montague, suggests that the survival of our species is dependent upon our ability to retain the characteristics of our young. We must maintain our ability to play, for play is energizing and healthy. I suggest you buy a puzzle and start it, and keep it going during the rest of the immunity preparation program. Perhaps you can buy juggling balls and learn to juggle. Buy a ball and jacks and go back to your childhood learning to play that game. What you need is a brief, silly, childlike activity that you relearn during this time, one that you can use during the stressful period ahead to distract you from the pressures you anticipate. My entry:

> I bought three beanbags and a book on how to juggle. I only learned
> one "jug," but it gave me something else to do other than worry
> about my upcoming pressures, and I decided to make sure I learn
> to juggle better by the time I complete my manuscript.

My patients have found that such activity has been particularly helpful to them. The key point is to choose an activity that is fun, a total waste of time, totally involving in its simplicity and repetitiousness, and one that you can laugh about. If you get upset and angry about it, it is the wrong activity. Pick something dumber.

Day 13

This is "intense imagery day." Today, practice for a longer period of time the positive imagery assignment you developed earlier. Think of the wonders of the supersystem, compliment it, salute it, and let it know that you are going to help it out. Even if you have been sick during the preparation program, commend your supersystem for staying on duty and helping you.

I suggest now that you select some special music for this opportunity, and perhaps repeat the self-shaman assignment I discussed earlier. Sometimes you need to consult with you about things and this is the time to do it. Set aside several 20-minute periods, if possible, to practice and repractice this assignment. Music to which you have a positive reaction is important here, for such music directly affects the biochemistry of the body and enhances your supersystem.

One of my patients enjoys the soundtrack from *Chariots of Fire* and plays this as part of his immune buildup program. Other patients have listened to Fleetwood Mac's "Don't Stop Thinking about Tomorrow" for they find its message and its sound to be uplifting. Now is the time to select your own "theme song."

I have assigned the theme song project to many of my patients, and they have found it something that stays with them for several years. Every time each of them hears his or her song in an elevator or on the radio, it seems to have an enhancing effect. Now is the time to match your song with positive imagery. This will take some time, but it is well worth it.

Day 14

By now you have a brief but interesting log with several entries, perhaps some new toys or childish activities, your own theme song, and some productive imagery to practice. Your supersystem is getting stronger every minute. Now you have to get a little bit more "intellectual." You need a backup plan. You need to have something ready should the stress become just "too much" during your anticipated period. My entry:

> If I cannot manage to meet all of my clinical, teaching, and writing obligations in the time I have scheduled, I will have to arrange for coverage of my classes to buy me more writing time. My patients are a given priority, but my students might even benefit from a temporary guest lecturer with a unique and specialized background different from my own.

Make sure you develop what I call a "cop-out system." You need something to fall back on that is preidentified before the stress period so that you won't view it as a total failure should you need it.

Day 15

Congratulations. You are at the midpoint in your immune enhancement program. You have done some miraculous things for your immunity and probably for the immunity of those around you. To celebrate, I call this the "mirth-burst day," a celebration of your "mirthday." This is a day when you plan a special party to be held at least once a year and hopefully more often. The drugs you take will be natural and from within instead of without—they are the natural opiates that flow when you laugh hard and well. Pick a day that will correspond every year to this day 15 of your immune program. From now on this will be your mirthday, requiring that you laugh as much as you can during the entire day.

If you have done several immune enhancing programs, you will have several "mirthdays," but since they are more important than birthdays, it's okay to have a lot more of them.

Buy a funny book. Watch some funny TV programs or videotapes. Be around friends whose laughter tends to "crack you up." If this is difficult, then go to a funny show at the theater. There is certain to be someone there whose laughter can set you off as well.

Some of my patients find it helpful to buy an album by one of their favorite comedians. Bill Cosby's albums, particularly his comments regarding parenting and family life, seem to be "mirthful" for my patients, and they are also free of the disruptive vulgarities that may affect some persons' supersystems negatively. So, "happy mirthday!"

You are now halfway into your booster program. You've played, laughed, done imagery, celebrated your body, and begun to learn or relearn some childhood skills. The last 15 days of the program are designed to make sure that your supersystem will remain within warm and cool bounds, not run hot or cold.

Day 16

This is what I call the "context day." In your supersystem log, make an entry which describes some things you are looking forward to which will occur several months or even years past the stress period you anticipate. This is to encourage the supersystem not just to get ready for one big "attack" but to place your life experiences in context. My entry:

> I hope to be an author who has done books that have helped as many people as possible. I look forward to receiving letters from people who state that they have gained considerable personal and spiritual strength from reading some of the material I have shared. I hope to speak with people throughout this and other countries regarding the material I have presented, and the stress period ahead will be just a small sacrifice in this overall program. I like to write anyway, and it will be even better if someone reads what I write.

As I read over my entry, I realized that I was viewing time in a very limited context. I reread some of my own ideas concerning space and time (discussed in Part Four) and reminded myself once again, in a more general context, of why I was writing this book.

Most of my patients report that this context day makes them feel much more hopeful and sometimes even diminishes their estimation of the difficulties of the period ahead.

Day 17

Today is "resuscitator day," a day when you make sure you have someone to "resuscitate" you during the stressful period should you need help. During our particularly stressful periods, we all need someone or several someones for social support. You will need what I call a *CPwR*. CPR is cardiopulmonary resuscitation and is used in life-threatening situations. My CPwR is a *caring person within reach*. Now is the time to make phone calls, talk with someone else about the stressful period you will be going through, and make sure the person will be available to you for talking, support, and listening.

Some of my patients report that they need someone outside the family. Sometimes a non-family member can be more objective. The person may even be a member of the clergy or a therapist if you feel this period is going to be particularly stressful. You may even wish to schedule an appointment with a professional person before the stressful period you anticipate, to talk about that period. Preventive psychotherapy is much more economical and probably much more effective than any other type.

It is important to be an effective consumer during this time. If you choose a psychotherapist, make sure you call ahead to describe exactly what you are doing. If the therapist thinks it is ridiculous, you know you've got the wrong person. If the therapist has a strict "pathological model" viewpoint and doesn't want to see you before you are "sick," this is not the person you want to be seeing anyway. I am reminded of the story told by one of my trainers in psychotherapy. A man called a psychologist's office and said, "I think I'm going crazy. How much do you charge?" The therapist responded, "One hundred dollars an hour." The man responded incredulously, "I'm not that crazy!" It is important to get your money's worth and to choose a therapist who follows a wellness model, not a sickness model.

Day 18

This is "ecology day." Research tells us that some persons are *meteorotrophic*, that is, hyperreactive to the environment, to rain, to storms, to cloudiness, to cold, to noise, to changes in the ecology. Now is the time to record in your log book, following your entry of the name of the support person you have consulted, the environmental changes that you think might help during this stressful period. My entry:

> I find relaxing music to be helpful when I am writing. I must make sure that I am able to play this music near my word processor. I'll have to spend some time setting it up now, because it is not as convenient as I'd like it to be in my study at this time. I will also have to talk to people at work and in my family about my time schedule and how they will be a part of my "working environment."

Do not underestimate the importance of ecology. Where we are is as important as who we are, and spending some time now on this can make your stressful period much less toxic. Even small changes such as having a small stereo with earphones, buying particularly comfortable clothes, or getting an air ionizer may help.

Day 19

This is "tender talk day," a day to analyze your vocabulary and to make sure that what you are saying out loud is something you want your supersystem to hear. Some of us become very careless in our speech, using many more negative words than we should. You might ask someone, perhaps that support person, for feedback on this or even tape yourself at work or at home to see whether you are a barometer within the house or at work, or actually the storm itself. My entry:

> From some of the tapes I have at work, I notice I use sarcasm as a form of humor. In the last several weeks I have not complimented other people very much, and I am going to have to make an effort to do it. I seem to take some of my colleagues' good work for granted.

This may not seem significant, and you may not notice that many negative words, but behaviors affect how we feel and we can change how we feel by talking the way we would like to feel. If it is true that people are what we tell them they are, then we ourselves are what we tell ourselves we are.

Day 20

Today is "touch day." This is a day to make sure that during your stressful period there is going to be someone around to hold and to touch. Research indicates that during particularly stressful times we pull away from others and suffer from a lack of body stimulation. Check your time schedule and be sure there is time for sexuality and sensuality. If you are making an entry in your log regarding this, make sure it is in code. People have a habit of looking over immunity logs, and you will probably consider this touch section to be not necessarily secret, but private.

Day 21

This is the day to seek invisible means of support. Now is the time to review your own belief system. If you are very religious, it is the time to assess the degree to which you are behaving in keeping with your religiosity. If you do not follow a formal religion, now is the time to examine what type of beliefs you do hold and, essentially, ask the question "Why am I doing this?"

This is the most complex of the assignments in the immune boosting program, but it may also be the most important. If there is no why, the stressful period you are anticipating will simply be stressful—without purpose, direction, and meaning within the context of the human community.

This assignment requires some quiet time and may require consultation again with a member of the clergy or someone else with whom you feel comfortable talking about beliefs. Most of my patients find this to be one of the most awkward steps, but they also tell me it is one of the most significant to them. If we know the why, the how is always much easier.

Days 22, 23, and 24

This is the 3-day warm-up: starting, doing, finishing. These three days are rehearsal days for the actual stress period. In addition to all the assignments initiated above, take time on day 22 to write in your log a role rehearsal of the stress period. My entry:

> I sit down and read my editor's suggestions, and I begin to work on them. I feel panicked that there is not much time, but I remember why I am doing it and this helps. When I get really panicked, I talk to my support system.

Day 23. My entry:

> I have been working now several days on my project. I am getting frustrated that I am not working fast enough. I must now remember that I could ask for an extension if I need one. Maybe I need some exercise, some touching, and some talking instead of just working harder and faster.

Day 24. My entry:

> At last. It's done. It's going in. Even in fantasy it feels good to think that literally years of work are finally over and the result will now be shared with others.

As you can see from my entries for days 22, 23, and 24, it is important to role-rehearse the entire event from start, through process, to end. This role rehearsal provides a practice period for the immune system. One of the most successful college basketball teams in the country was having considerable problems shooting foul shots. Every type of practice suggestion was made until someone finally suggested that the team spend some time just "imagining the ball going through the hoop" and rehearsing this before each game. Their efficacy increased threefold and resulted in a league championship. From that time forward, this team has spent time rehearsing the entire game from tipoff to half-time to end, imagining the course of the game to victory. Most successful athletes know the importance of this process, and most (particularly the Olympic athletes) will tell you that this is one of their "secret training techniques." Days 22, 23, and 24 are the warm-up exercises for the supersystem.

Day 25

Today is "life-system check day." Meet with those in your family and at work, and inform them that you are going into a particularly stressful period now. Let them know in detail what you will be doing and what might be happening to you during this time. Ask them what they will be needing from you during this period, and set the limits on what you will be able to do and not to do.

Many self-help books give suggestions implying that each person lives in a vacuum and that changes a person makes do not affect others. Every item of this immune booster program affects everyone in your household and at work. Day 25 should be a day when you sit with as many people as possible. Elicit their help and offer your help to them as well, for they too may be either entering, coming out of, or preparing for a stressful period in their lives. This is a day to remember your oneness with everyone else. If you lose sight of this fact during your stressful period, you will be much more vulnerable to illness. The supersystem needs to know that it has the help of its membership in the organization of all people and that it must also help other supersystems.

Days 26, 27, 28, 29, and 30

This is the 5-day immune-system deposit period, a period for rest, relaxation, exercise, and rerehearsal of all the items covered in the first 25 days. If there were elements that you could not get to in the first 25 days, use one of these days to do them. Perhaps you have not been able to meet with your family yet or find that support system person. This 5-day period is provided so that the immune booster program itself does not become a stressful period. On day 30 reread your log, congratulate yourself, and remind yourself that wellness is not something you get or do—it's the way you are.

So there you have it. A 30-day program for enhancing your immune system, your supersystem. If you take it seriously enough that some of the suggestions are helpful to you, but not obligatory and depressing, you are doing a good job. If you take it too seriously, and see these as impossible steps, then I suggest you reread parts of the book. Occurrences in life should not be viewed as final goals or destinations. To paraphrase Gertrude Stein, "Once we get there we may find that there is no there there.'' Life, after all, is always a way of traveling, not a station we arrive at.

As a review of some of the suggestions in this chapter, and as a quick guide for immune-system boosting in day-to-day living, review the following list as often as you find helpful.

Immune Booster Checklist

1. Am I attending to my sleep, getting at least 6 regularly scheduled hours of sleep a night?

   HINT: Sometimes a warm glass of milk (high in the natural substance tryptophane) before bed can help, as well as some soothing taped music. It does not matter whether you actually sleep, but that you are in bed resting regularly. Sleep will come.

2. Am I eating regular meals, including a good breakfast low in sugar? Am I avoiding processed foods and caffeine? Am I remembering that I am feeding my supersystem its fuel for health maintenance? If armies travel on their stomachs, the immune system certainly travels on a balanced diet.

   HINT: Vitamin C supplements at levels that do not disrupt the bowel habits may be helpful to the immune system. The same is true for the B complex vitamins, beta caradine, selenium, and a good broad-spectrum multivitamin supplement. As always, check with your physician regarding any significant changes in diet that you plan.

3. Am I making time just to sit and relax? Am I able to clear my mind for even a while? I do not need to meditate but simply to be able to sit down just for a while.

   HINT: Go ahead and watch some dumb TV programs. Just make sure these programs are absolutely of no intellectual value (this should be easy). Dr. Danilo Ponce, associate professor of psychiatry at the University of Hawaii, feels that we are overinformed about problems we can do little about. The national and local news abounds with such information, which may lead to the feelings of helplessness and hopelessness that depress the immune system.

4. Am I hugging and getting hugged at least once a day, if not more?

HINT: You may be surprised at how anxious people are to be hugged, and if you serve as the "hugger," you will no doubt end up a "huggee."

5. Am I getting some playtime every day?

HINT: The immune system seems to get some excellent rest and relaxation during happy, joyful play. Even if you have to carry along some juggling balls or other gimmicks, make sure to play just a little bit every day. All work and no play makes the immune system dull and unresponsive or overly excited.

6. Am I laughing a little every day?

HINT: The portable tape player can be very helpful here. Buy some tapes of your favorite comedian and have them at the ready. One of my patients taped himself laughing and also added some of the laughter of some of his friends. He finds this so strange to listen to that it almost always makes him laugh.

7. Am I stretching out all my muscles a little every day?

HINT: Work standing up as much as possible. If you have a desk job, walk while you talk on the phone. Take the stairs, not the elevator. Park far away instead of close. Take some time each day to stretch anything you can stretch from the forehead down to the toes.

8. Am I breathing instead of gasping?

HINT: If you answered "yes," think again. Are you really breathing deeply? Does your abdomen go out when you inhale? Can you feel the coolness of the air through your nostrils when you inhale, and the warmth when you exhale? Deep, relaxed breathing reduces SAM system activity.

9. Do I talk politely to myself?

HINT: At least once in a while, compliment yourself. Perhaps out loud, say something good about yourself. Your immune system is probably listening.

10. Have I made time for the spiritual part of my life?

   HINT: Say a little prayer during the day. No matter what you believe, say a prayer for your beliefs. Bow your head, whisper your prayer, pause, lift your head, and smile in celebration of the fact that you are alive and have within you a magnificent, wonderful super-system, working for your wellness and growth.

Remember, your supersystem is a miracle. It—you—can cope with anything.

Chapter Eleven

THE SUPERSYSTEM VERSUS THE DISEASE OF THE CENTURY

The major advances in civilization are processes that all but
wreck societies in which they occur.

A. N. WHITEHEAD

Acquired immune deficiency syndrome (AIDS) is a disease of civilization. It is dangerous enough to destroy the civilization that gave it birth. I believe the supersystem is capable of defeating this terrible invader, but only if several of the lessons that I have emphasized throughout this book are learned quickly and well.

Just over a year ago, a virus was isolated in France at the Pasteur Institute. It was named the *lymphadenopathy-associated virus* (LAV). At almost the same time in the United States, a similar virus was isolated in AIDS patients at the National Institute of Health (NIH) and named the *human T lymphotrophic virus III* (HTLV-III). It now appears that these two viruses are nearly identical. Much more work still needs to be done to understand more about the virus itself, but we suspect that it is a *retrovirus*, meaning that it can remain in a person's body indefinitely, to be activated by processes as yet unknown. This results in an as yet unknown but apparently quite long incubation period.

AIDS works its havoc through damage to the immune system rather than through a direct effect of the virus itself. In effect, it is an attack upon our defenses, as if our national defense system were attacked specifically and extensively, leaving us open for invasion. AIDS antibodies have been detected in a growing percentage of our population—more and more people are being discovered who have been exposed to the virus. The test for antibodies is itself not free of problems and not as reliable as some people believe. The Center for Disease Control in the United States now estimates that as many as 1 in 300 of us have been exposed to AIDS. Such information fuels the flame of panic, often without strong supporting data.

Far more individuals than those classified as having AIDS have *immunal suppression* and a syndrome that can include a reduction of our T helper cells, infection, fatigue, cough, diarrhea, and other symptoms. This has been called *lesser AIDS* or *AIDS-related complex* (ARC). Both AIDS and ARC affect the surveillance system and can destroy the supersystem itself. The virus, millions of which would fit in the period at the end of this sentence, appears to travel on our T cells, particularly the T helper cells that enhance our immune efficiency.

At the current time, it appears that the AIDS virus is transmitted through the exchange of bodily fluids. The virus has been found in blood, semen, and saliva and may also exist in feces and vaginal secretions. Theoretically, the virus is present in all body fluids, but many theorists believe that some opening in the body tissue is necessary for the virus itself to enter.

The general symptoms of weight loss, excessive fatigue, loss of appetite, loss of energy, night sweats, fever, and diarrhea not only are symptoms of AIDS but may be related to other diseases as well. This overlap causes even more anxiety.

During the initial stages of AIDS, the individual may only experience flulike symptoms, but this is a period when the immune system is being damaged. When this happens, the person is left open to secondary infections, most often *pneumocystis carinii*, or a parasitic infection of the lung. While the first attack of this disease may be successfully treated, the person is left exhausted and vulnerable, only to be infected again, perhaps fatally.

Kaposi's sarcoma, a rare form of cancer, is another infection that may result from AIDS-weakened immunity. This disease is characterized by small purple spots on the skin and internal organs that turn into a plaquelike substance that spreads through the body, eventually causing death. Although not a cancer in the truest sense of the word, it functions in much the same manner.

It appears that people must have a weakened immune system to contract AIDS, and for this reason the disease can teach us much about our supersystems. We know, for example, that malnutrition or the weakening of the immune cells by drug abuse makes a person more likely to contract AIDS. Malnutrition, for example, is frequent among Haitians and heterosexual men and women in Africa, who are a high-risk group for AIDS.

New evidence indicates that the use of petrochemical-based lubricants may relate to the transmission of AIDS. It has long been known that such substances weaken the immune system and are related to cancer. Research on mice has resulted in the death of all mice given rectal implants of petrochemical lubricants. In addition to this risk, recent work has indicated that nitrate inhalants, known as "poppers," weaken the immune system as well.

We know that anything that stresses the immune system increases our chances for AIDS. I believe that not only substances but also thinking styles which deplete our natural immunity make us potential victims of this dread disease. Research efforts are under way to wipe out AIDS by some miracle drug, yet the important issue of strengthening the immune system is being neglected. It is the message of this book, and a message that can be learned from the AIDS crisis, that enhancing rather than preventing, strengthening rather than only curing, should be our focus for wellness. If AIDS teaches us anything, it teaches us that a holistic approach will be the only answer for the ultimate survival of our civilization.

Dr. Robert Cathcart, an orthopedic surgeon in Los Altos, California, is attempting to strengthen the immune system by nutritional augmentation. He hypothesizes that the body is depleted of vitamin C when the immune system is under attack, either by substances in the environment, viruses, or any other forms of stress. Years ago, research indicated that persons with high levels of vitamin C intake produce more antibody molecules. It was also discovered that vitamin C enhances the action of prostaglandin, a hormonelike substance that can help the T lymphocytes and even increase the production of interferon, a substance in the body that can fight the spread of viruses. This concept of bolstering the immune system has not been popular in the modern medical approaches to the AIDS problem. Research in France has been aimed at administering immune-system-impairing drugs so that the AIDS virus cannot proliferate through the immune system. Dr. Cathcart and other researchers are suggesting that a bolstering, enhancing, strengthening approach is equal to or more important than the drug approach. If the immune system is where the battle occurs, that is where our strengths should be.

As an example, we know that some gay persons experience a high instance of internal parasites which can interfere with the healthy processing of foods, thereby inhibiting the immune system. Nutritional approaches are being devised to prevent this, including removing sugar from the diet; eliminating processed foods where possible; and, in the work of Drs. Orion Truss and William Crook, providing patients with zinc, vitamin A, selenium, and other components that can enhance the immune function. A balanced diet of protein, carbohydrates, ample water, and other nutrients is important for a healthy immune system. Beta carotene, vitamin B, vitamin B_6, folic acid, vitamin E, essential fatty acids, manganese, iron, zinc, garlic, and chlorophyll also seem to enhance the immune system. It is important to remember that in spite of the fact that I am stressing psychological approaches to protecting and enhancing the immune system, exercise, nutrition, and general healthy practices are equally important. AIDS may be teaching this lesson more clearly than any other disease in our history.

While researchers work fast and furiously for vaccinations, cures, and strategies for strengthening the immune system against the attack of AIDS, I suggest that the supersystem is already prepared to help us in this battle, if we will only pay attention to the lessons it teaches us. These are the lessons of the rules of the immune system, the ways in which the immune system is organized. I present here four lessons of the supersystem that may help us in this crucial battle: the rules of tolerance, specificity, holism, and balance that dictate the workings of the supersystem.

TOLERANCE

There is . . . an irreconcilable divergence of opinion as to
what is sense and what is nonsense.
ERIK TEMPLE BELL

The meaning of *tolerance* in the immune system is its selective capacity to identify and eliminate only antigens, the ''not self'' elements that enter the system. Essentially, the supersystem must be appropriately "intolerant," rejecting threatening others, but not attacking our "cells," or elements which are enhancing to us.

Unfortunately, our society's reaction to AIDS and particularly to AIDS patients has not been an appropriate intolerance of the disease itself or even an effective tolerance of patients suffering from this disease. The front-page editorial in the Manchester, New Hampshire, *Union Leader* warned that actor Rock Hudson "practiced a deviant sexual behavior" and that even though Mr. Hudson himself showed "courage and kindness," we should remember that homosexuality is an implied danger to all of us because of its relationship to AIDS.

The danger of AIDS is not homosexuality or deviance, but intolerance. Our society has failed to accept the sexual preferences of a large percentage of its population, thus driving some persons "underground" reactively to seek anonymous multiple sexual interactions. History teaches us clearly that repression always results in disease to our society. The fear of homosexuality, children with AIDS, giving or receiving blood transfusions, even being in the proximity of someone exposed to AIDS only develops an inappropriate intolerance, a further attack on our own systems and, therefore, a further weakening of our supersystems at a time when they are needed most.

The cure for AIDS, and the prevention of its further spread, depends upon our acceptance, not rejection, of others. The cure depends upon considering AIDS first and foremost a human condition, not a homosexual condition. The cure depends upon reminding and teaching our supersystems to accept, comfort, and help, not to fear, reject, and overreact. If we react too hotly or too coldly to AIDS, we will not be able to defeat it.

AIDS is transmitted during some forms of sexual interaction; it is not caused by that sexual interaction. Actually, it does not seem to be a very easily transmitted disease at all. Direct exposure to the body fluids of someone with AIDS seems necessary; the virus itself does not survive well outside the human body. Researchers are slowed in their efforts to solve the AIDS puzzle partly because the virus is difficult to keep alive for study in the laboratory.

So now is the time to increase our tolerance and focus our intolerance, for as Aristotle pointed out, "Anybody can become angry . . . that is easy. But to be angry with the right person, to the right degree, at the right time, for the right reason, and in a right way . . . that is not easy.'' Such appropriate anger on the part of our immune systems should be our focus in the battle against AIDS.

SPECIFICITY

A body of facts is needed to replace current supposition. All of us need more do's and fewer don'ts.

ARLIE V. BOCK, M.D.

The *specificity* rule of immunity teaches us that each alien substance elicits a response only from those immune cells uniquely prepared and designed to recognize and react to it. You may remember that every B cell has certain antibody molecules called immunoglobulins on its surface. These molecules have specific jobs to do, and the immune system continually learns, adapts, remembers, and grows in its identification and defensive skills.

The lesson of specificity for coping with AIDS is that, when a new challenge occurs, particularly one as complex as AIDS, we must teach our supersystem to focus, learn, and adapt, not to overreact, misidentify, and overgeneralize. For example, sexual contact does not transmit AIDS. Sexual contact which most likely involves some trauma to mucous membranes and/or exchange of body fluids transmits the infection. Even then, only some people actually become ill or experience the activation of the AIDS virus, for it may be that AIDS is *dose-specific*, or related to the amount of exposure, not just exposure itself, to the virus.

This specificity lesson implies not only that it is anonymous sex with large numbers of partners (homosexual or not) which increases the risk of AIDS but that only certain sexual behaviors seem involved. This may teach us a sexual warning list that contains more specificity.

1. Avoid exchange of body fluids when infection in the partner seems likely or remotely possible.

2. Cuddling, massaging, mutual masturbation, holding, and general touching may be emphasized in place of coitus and sexual intimacy in those interactions during which AIDS seems a risk.

3. The use of alcohol or other drugs may influence judgment. Therefore, avoid such substances, particularly when sexual intimacy is
   possible.

4. The use of condoms during intercourse can reduce the risk of other
   diseases, not only AIDS. Responsible interaction with others is a
   key to reducing all disease risk.

If our supersystems include our entire universe, all of us and each
of us, then the above lessons regarding sexuality have implications not
only for reducing the risk of AIDS, but for reducing unwanted preg-
nancies and other diseases as well. Syphilis, gonorrhea, herpes, ho-
mophilus vaginalus, and several other sexually transmissible diseases
are related to the above four lessons of specificity in our sexuality.
    "Dos" of intimate interaction emphasize the following suggestions:

1. Communicate *openly* with all potential sexual partners *before* intimate body contact.

2. Share your own health status first, as in "To my knowledge, I have
   never had or have never been exposed to any sexually transmissible
   disease. Have you?"

3. View sexuality as a totality of a relationship, not just body contact.
   Hugging, holding hands, cuddling, and other behaviors are possible
   even if one or both partners are ill.

4. Know the facts about all sexually transmissible diseases, their similarities and differences, and take responsibility for teaching these
   facts to others.

5. Discovery that a potential partner has or has had a disease should
   lead to more, not less, communication with that person. Teach,
   suggest, and give support, guidance, and referral for help if possible.

6. Remember, disease will either challenge and strengthen our immunity or diminish it. Learning, increased communication, and
   specific actions toward wellness are the enhancers of the supersystem.

HOLISM

Your theory is crazy, but is not crazy enough to be true.
                    NIELS BOHR, to a young physicist

The supersystem is a whole, integrating the mind, body, and immune system. Hope for defeating AIDS rests with our acceptance of and functioning within the principles of *holism*. Rest, sound nutrition, effective sanitation techniques, appropriate exercise, relaxation, meditation, and general overall integration of all body systems may be the significant factors that have restricted the spread of AIDS in western society. In most societies experiencing difficulties in the areas of nutrition and hygiene, AIDS has spread much more rapidly and much more directly to the heterosexual population. Rather than frightening us away from one another, AIDS should teach us the importance of drawing together to enhance our world condition, to reduce starvation and suffering wherever possible. When one of us is sick, all of us are sick, and this key lesson of AIDS cannot be denied. Physics teaches us that systems that adapt and evolve survive, and systems that isolate and separate deteriorate and eventually disappear.

AIDS will defeat the supersystem if we attempt to avoid it by isolation. The AIDS phenomenon should be a clear signal that disease and health are not only personal, but universal. When any of us starve, we all become just a little less healthy. If a child with AIDS is shunned by society, that society has taken the first step toward surrendering to the disease itself. AIDS may be seen as a symbol that our personal and social supersystem is not immunoefficient, not tolerant enough, not specific enough, and far from "whole."

BALANCE

We all need a balance within the supersystem, a balance between hot and cold that results in warm and cool functioning. This means that the SAM (sympathoadrenomedullary) system and the PAC (parasympatho-adrenocortical) system should work in coordination so that we do not run overly hot and overly cold for long periods of time, resulting in diseases unique to those psychological and neurophysiological periods of functioning.

I have related our psychological functioning, our "personality," to hot-and cold-running times in our lives. It is possible, since our immune systems are profoundly related to our thoughts and feelings, that vulnerability to AIDS is also related to our feeling states and general orientation of our supersystems.

A study of AIDS patients was conducted by Dr. Jeffrey S. Mandel at the University of California in 1982. Three findings emerged from that study that have relevance to the hot and cold theories I have suggested.

1. The AIDS patients tended to be overly dependent on "denial," that is, avoiding negative feelings such as anger and tending toward perseverance and emotional stoicism.

2. The AIDS patients reported a large number of stressful events in the year preceding diagnosis.

3. The AIDS patients in the California study indicated guilt about sexual identity and previous sexual activities.

Of course, these findings are preliminary and retrospective. That is, the findings have evolved from asking patients to look back on their lives, rather than identifying patients and then predicting the occurrence of AIDS. Nonetheless, such findings add credence to the importance of not only studying viruses, vaccinations, and biochemical approaches to AIDS but looking as well to psychosocial factors for the functioning and status of the supersystem.

Psychologist Dr. Gary Schwartz suggests that modern society has stressed the development of effective biomedical and behavioral procedures for repairing the body and ridding the system of distress. While important in the reduction of the immediacy of suffering, exclusive focus on this mechanical approach neglects the fact that "dis-ease" is a healthy response to "dys-order." Symptoms of disease enable us to detect that there are problems, disruption, and lack of regulation within a person's system and the system at large. AIDS should provide us not with the stimulus of fear and panic, but with the stimulus of more attention to intimacy, sexuality, and wellness of our entire society. In this context, AIDS and all diseases are not external events to be feared, but disruptions within the world system from which we must learn if we are to evolve and survive.

To emphasize the relationship between disease and wellness, I turn next to a discussion of wellness. As I have discussed in this chapter, disease is either a teacher or an executioner for the individual and for society. We must not turn away from the challenge of any disease, most particularly a disease as powerful as AIDS. As La Rochefoucauld points out, "There are two things we cannot contemplate with a steady eye: The sun and death." In the case of disease and wellness, we have to see only through our eyes, not with them. We can learn to think in ways that enhance the immune system, even help it to move beyond health maintenance to high-level wellness.

Part Four

THINKING FOR WELLNESS

It is probably true quite generally that in the history of human thinking, the most fruitful developments frequently take place at those points where two different lines of thought meet. . . One may hope that new and interesting developments may follow.

WERNER HEISENBERG

You have learned about the structure and function of the supersystem, two general coping styles of the supersystem, and how to take more control of this natural health maintenance system. Part Four describes a new view of the relationship between health, healing, disease, time, and living. Drawn from the ideas of some of the world's greatest thinkers and from ideas not traditionally related to the field of health, the material in this part will show that each of us is a part of a world supersystem, a system capable of God-given unity or hellish world destruction. The choice is ours.

Chapter Twelve

A DISTRESSING VIEW OF STRESS

If you haven't the strength to impose your own terms upon
life, you must accept the terms it offers you.

T. S. ELIOT

Have you heard these facts: Stress is bad for you. Agitated, hyperactive
people are more stressed than calm, quiet people. Busy executives are
more stressed than their less pressured employees. Major life events
such as death and birth stress us to the limit. Illness is caused by germs
and viruses. You have to change your feelings and attitudes before you
can truly change your behaviors. Some people are Type A and are
hurried, overwhelmed, ambitious, and worried, while others are Type
B and are more calm, easygoing, less ambitious, and more settled.
Some people are able to thrive and do their best when stressed. You
can be stressed for a little while without really affecting your health
negatively. Very young and very old people do not have as much stress
as middle-aged adults do. Depression and anxiety attacks are caused by
stress, as are mental illnesses that require professional help and medications. The only real way to deal with stress is to be more selfish, to
be more independent, eat right, and take charge of your own life.

Everything in the paragraph above has been written about in recent
books and articles on the popular topic of stress. The problem is, every-

thing in the above paragraph is untrue. The important topic of stress and its effects on personal wellness has led to workshops and programs designed to help executives, teachers, and laypersons meditate away their stress. We know now that for some people, meditation and relaxation are exactly the opposite of what they should be doing for their own health. Current interest in stress and its profound effect on all of us is high, yet there has been a lack of material available to the public that integrates research findings from medical and psychological literature. The public is left victim to the latest fads regarding stress. We are told that by hugging or loving or relaxing or eating the right vitamins, we will be able to reduce stress and lead lives of quiet, monklike existence. The fact is that the first step in dealing with stress is to identify your style of appraising events in your life, how you talk to yourself about what happens to you, and ways in which this causes your body to function compatibly or incompatibly with the possibility of longevity.

Eight myths dominate the writings about stress, each of which has resulted in recommendations for behavioral change that not only are incomplete and, in some cases, incorrect but also can be counterproductive and even detrimental to your health. I examine these now because understanding the hot- and cold-running immune systems depends upon not misunderstanding stress. Before you can mobilize the magnificent capacities of your supersystem, you must clarify the relationship between stress, change, and health.

MYTH 1: Stress Is Bad for You.

Come to the weekend workshop on reducing and preventing stress! For the last decade a carnival of stress-reduction workshops, self-fulfilling workshops, self-awareness workshops, holistic medicine workshops, and wellness workshops have flooded the consumer marketplace. Quick methods for going more slowly are offered to an eagerly awaiting public perusing the self-help book shelves for words from the latest guru on how to "pull your own strings" or "find sexual happiness."

Stress is simply change. Somehow that fact has been overlooked in a rush to offer solutions for stress. Stress is not something you do or your body does; it is something that happens or something that your brain tells you is happening which is different from what has been happening. Whenever you perceive change, your mind and body change too. Stress is change; *strain* is the reaction of the immune system and body. Stress is not bad or good—it just is. Strain can be bad, and the less strain over less time, the better.

To say that stress is bad is to suggest a life that one of my patient's called the *SSDD life*: "same stuff, different day." Think of the nature of your life if, every day in every way, your life became more and more the same. One of the surest ways to drive people insane is first to drive them "in same," that is, to allow no change in their lives at all. This is a primary theory behind brainwashing. Leave the prisoner alone, no calendar, no light, no noise, no change. Soon, no health, no strength, no will, no spirit. You don't get stress; you are not under stress or in stress; you don't do it or have it. A change simply occurs. The brain interprets this change and then tells the body what to do about it. The body reaction is *strain*.

To say that stress is bad, that change is bad, is like saying any natural life process is bad. For example, birth could be viewed as bad if one looked at the consequences of it. Child-rearing problems and child abuse would not occur without children. Without birth, no more people. Therefore, no more problems. Stress is the challenge of living, the fuel of life. Even plants and animals cease to exist without it.

Fact 1: Stress is defined as life change, and change is a measure of life in process. Strain is the body reaction. The supersystem is the guardian of equilibrium, the regulator within of those things happening without.

MYTH 2: Some People Thrive on Stress.

Patients who come to me reporting problems with relationships will sometimes state, "As for me, I am at my best when I'm under stress." It is difficult to understand what these people really mean by "at my best."

A salesperson called a recent radio talk show to respond to me by saying, "Doctor, I thrive under stress." When I asked what he meant by "thrive," he added, "I've won three straight sales contests, received two promotions, and, as a matter of fact, am making more money than ever." I asked how he was feeling, and he answered, "What do you mean? I just told you." He had mistaken changes in his environment for how he felt and described his thriving in terms of money or status, not general wellness. When I asked further about his health, whether he generally felt good or had headaches, colds, frequent illnesses, he added, "Everybody has those. I have an ulcer but it is under control, and my blood pressure is a little high." Yet this same man reported that he was thriving.

If what we mean by "thrive" is to make more money and get promotions, it is obvious that people will always think they thrive under stress. You can only get promoted and make more money through change. If what we mean by "thrive" is to be healthy, be happy, and live long in harmony with our families, then whether we thrive or not depends upon how and what we think about changes in our lives; whether or not our brains tell our bodies to prepare for fire alarms and tragedies when a boss presents the slightest change is a key question. What is our "self-talk"? Think of a fire department that mobilizes the entire squadron every time a match is lit, and you have some idea of poor coping.

Sometimes during my lectures, an audience member will stand up and announce, "Yes, I understand what you are saying, but I am feeling better than ever under all this pressure." Such people are "change addicts" who report getting high under rapid and recurrent stress. The problem with this strategy of life is that we have only so much body energy in the bank. It seems much easier to make withdrawals than deposits. One of my young students gleefully announced recently that she never slept, just studied, partied, and napped on occasion, and added, "I still feel high." Living on the energy of youth by withdrawing from a highly stocked account does not diminish the poverty of later years. As we do with financial planning, it is important to have some "stress sheltered annuities" for later life. Most addicts of any type die young.

An important caution! When the body adapts to change on signals from the brain and when the body is told, "You love it, you love it, do more," it seems to rally and take loans on its own energy account. This energy spurt can be addicting, feel energizing, much as racing a car engine can be exciting. The price for such wear and tear is likely to occur later, even several years later. Play now and pay later is the rule, and your health can suffer a decade later for asking too much too long from your body today. Your temper tantrum with your children today can predispose you to a serious illness years later.

Fact 2: Changes in life can be challenging, but no one can maintain lifelong wellness through constant adaptation to rapid and recurrent change. No one thrives on the unremitting spending of body energy.

MYTH 3: Agitated, Hurried, Pressured People Are Stressed People.

"Hyperactive" is one of the most overused, misused words from the field of child development and education. One teacher at a recent conference complained to me, "I've got this one boy who drives me nuts. He never sits down in class. Always out of his seat." I asked why she didn't consider having the whole class stand up while learning. After all, she stood up while she was teaching. She responded that learning is "a quiet, pensive, meditative, sedentary process" and that she hoped that the parents of this hyperactive child would consider medication to slow him down. I asked if she would consider medicating the remainder of the class to speed them up to the level of the hyperactive child, and she responded angrily, "Of course not, drugs are dangerous." That is exactly the point. Any teacher who assumes that "anyone who is more active than I am is hyperactive" is dangerous. Similar definitions have been used for the word "promiscuity" with as little fairness and accuracy. One cannot be overactive or underactive, for being hyperactive in one setting may not be hyperactive in another setting, and such descriptions are entirely relative.

Our bodies are capable of four major *whole-body reflexes*, reactions which take place rapidly under direction of the brain: the fight reflex, the flee reflex, the flow reflex, and "being" reflex. Hot thinkers fight and flee, cold thinkers flow, and fine-tuned, rational, clear-thinking persons can learn to "be." As mammals, it is in our genes to react physiologically to change. If the brain says that change means "look out, it's life or death right now," adrenaline increases, and the entire body mobilizes, the SAM (sympathoadrenomedullary system) syndrome goes into action. If the brain says, "No use fighting or fleeing; give it up; you are doomed," and tells the body to utilize the flow reflex, nausea and fatigue may set in, as we flow down the river and down the tube with the PAC (parasympathoadrenocortical system) syndrome.

Different hormonal patterns, different blood chemical levels, and different changes in our stomachs, our intestines, our bladders, and our bowels take place in response to what our brains tell us is happening. These responses were adaptive thousands of years ago. Fighting and fleeing helped deal with the lion at the door of our cave, and flowing could turn off preditors who may overlook the prey that appeared weak, ill, or even dead. To think that only the fight-and-flee response burdens the body is to neglect the burden felt when the flow-response occurs.

High level of activity is not stress.

Fact 3: The effect of life changes cannot be assessed by looking at activity levels. Fighting, fleeing, and flowing reflexes have been helpful in the past, but a being reflex is more adaptive in today's world.

MYTH 4: High-Level Executive Type of People Are under More Stress Than Those Lower on the Career Ladder.

The image of the overweight, cigar-puffing, hurried, clock-watching executive unknowingly toasting his inevitable premature death over a high-calorie lunch has been the model of the stress victim. Lower-level employees were seen as essentially protected by the principle of ignorance is bliss. Unburdened by the pressures of high responsibility, these people were seen as ulcer-free, enjoying a type of uninvolvement protection.

No doubt there are high-level executives who are in poor health due to the way they process changes in their lives. More frequently, however, level of occupation has little to do with general wellness. The pressures of trying to get to high-level jobs can be just as negative for the body as trying to maintain a high-level job. The pressure of trying to put food on the table can be just as excruciatingly painful as trying to protect large amounts of money in various stock accounts. Once again, the thinking style of the person is the key, and it has been found that thinking style is not dependent upon job classification. The negative aspects of strain are equal-opportunity employers.

We have learned that women are victims of stress and are not protected by some sexist view of female immunity to pain and disease. One of the tragedies of our times is the failure of women to bring to their newly found, if marginal, acceptance at higher levels of employment the uniqueness and equanimity of their gender.

I recently addressed the International Association of Professional Women. My first sentence in that address was, ''We do not need women in the business world.'' The audience fell silent in the anticipated attack from this sexist speaker. I quickly added, for my own survival, that experience is teaching us that we don't need women if they only bring a copy of the same egocentric male styles that have characterized the business world. Women enjoy a cultural permission to be more intuitive, creative, emotional, and group-oriented. Unfortunately, successful women, too, often abandon this strength to compete on a "male level." One woman recently pointed out that any woman who aspires to be equal to men has very low aspirations.

A "wonder woman syndrome" has developed. Work all day, cook all night, clean on the weekends, make every school conference, and parent not only your own children but perhaps even your own husband and parents—this is a partial job description of "the perfect liberated woman." Such an overburdening lifestyle affects not only the woman but her entire family. Negative reactions to stress or change are non-sexist, nonracist, nonageist, and not at all discriminating as to choice of victim.

Children can be victims too. Recent evidence shows that hyper-tension and cardiovascular disease are present in children as young as 5 years old. "Pedogenic illness," or illness caused by going to school, is well documented. One of the most significant threats to the wellness of our society is the lifestyle led by our children and an educational system that values being right over "being."

So men, women, and children, whatever the level of employment, unemployment, or school, all fall victim to stress-involved and strain-related illnesses. To assume that any group is immune to stress or more vulnerable to stress is to neglect the important finding that our bodies respond essentially in the same fashion. It is only how they are instructed to respond by our brains and our way of thinking that can be different.

Fact 4: All groups and all ages are victim to ineffective coping with change and the possibility of stress and strain-induced illness.

MYTH 5: You Behave According to How You Feel, so if You Calm Down You Can Behave Without Stress.

The first rule of effective therapy is to understand that you come to feel as you behave and that you behave as you think. Understanding why you feel a certain way and exploring the etiology of these feelings in long-term psychotherapy, while interesting, will not be immediately helpful in dealing with changes in daily life. In my clinic at Sinai Hospital of Detroit, we have found that transitional life events are best met by rational thinking, followed by concrete behavioral change, not by long-term exploration of feelings. Somehow, somewhere, the mythology in psychotherapy has been that "feelings are facts." Researchers now know that our feelings are dependent upon countless things and that the potential for clear, rational thinking is the one human gift unique to all of us and a possible source of strength in each of us.

Fact 5: You can come to feel as you behave, and your behavior is directed by how you think. Changing how you think about events is the greatest single hope for dealing with changes in our lives, for preventing illness, and for true healing.

MYTH 6: If Stress Really Gets Bad, You Can Go to A Professional for Help.

In the 15 years the Problems of Daily Living Clinic has been in operation, we have found that all we have to offer as psychotherapists is friendship and guidance in clearer thinking, followed by some behavioral recommendations on the basis of this improved thinking. In a minority of cases where a legitimate mental illness exists, medication can be helpful. In terms of holistic medicine, it has long been known, however, that all healing comes from the body itself and that the responsibility for wellness rests with the person, not the doctor. Psychotherapy is seldom helpful over the long term, and those who benefit most from psychotherapy are those who take most responsibility for themselves and work as colleagues with their therapists. A key principle of this book is that taking responsibility for your own life and your own thinking style is much more important than seeking out a professional to take responsibility for you and your life. No doctor ever healed anybody.

Fact 6: All persons are helped by themselves, not by anyone else. It has been said that we can no more control disease by external change than we can control the tides by an organized system of "mops." All healing comes from within, not without.

MYTH 7: Major Life Events Are The Ones That Really Put You under Stress.

It has been assumed that major events are the stressors of our lives. As pointed out earlier, the small day-to-day events, or what psychologist

Richard Lazarus calls "life's little hassles," are the most important changes to which we have to adapt. While a death itself can be a major crisis and cause the normal reflex of grieving and sadness (too often blocked by medications by insensitive physicians), it is the smaller events related to a loss that can cause most of the adaptation by the body. Funeral arrangements, readjusting the family, financial changes, parental changes, all the smaller components fatigue us and cause strain on our immune system. Learning to understand and cope with these small events is one of the key steps in thinking more clearly about changes in your life.

Fact 7: Transitional life crises on a day-to-day basis cause more profound changes for the body than do major life events such as births, deaths, and divorces.

MYTH 8: Illness Is Caused by Germs and Viruses of the Environment.

It has been estimated that medical expenses in the United States could be cut in half if people would understand that they have responsibility for their own wellness and that this responsibility centers upon how they think about their lives on a day-to-day basis, how they theorize and plan about life and living. All of us are familiar with people who suffered the insult of some environmental problem but who rallied to become even healthier than they were before they had become "sick." In my day-to-day practice, I see people with diabetes, arthritis, even cancer, who are happier and, in their own way, healthier than the 17-year-old with the God-given healthy body who abuses it daily with drugs, poor sleep, poor diet and who becomes depressed, agitated, and feels inadequate. "Dis-ease" is a process caused by how we interpret change in our lives, something that happens when we fall out of sync with the world. Getting back in sync is the key in taking charge of the supersystem.

As the stress of life is essential to the joy of living, so disease is but a dimension of our health experience. Without change, stress, loss, illness, and emotional and physical pain, the opposites of these elements of life could not exist, just as the concept of *full* has no meaning without its opposite of empty.

This book is not about prevention, avoidance, defensiveness, or fear. It is about hope, potential, strength, and the confidence we can experience when we learn that our supersystems can function in balance and return to balance following periods of crisis. If we can see stress and illness as a part of life to be understood and learned from, then we can enhance our immunity, our lives, our potential for superwellness. The next chapter will help you calculate your wellness quotient, to fit the concepts of disease, illness, and healing together toward a higher state of health.

Chapter Thirteen

CALCULATING YOUR WELLNESS QUOTIENT

I'm growing old! I'm falling apart! And it's *very interesting*!
WILLIAM SAROYAN

Disease is absolutely essential to being well. I have pointed out how even the terrible disease AIDS may teach us important lessons for the growth of society and of ourselves as individuals. All disease, all pain, and all discomfort represent a stimulus to our development. The prefix "dys" means broken, while the prefix "dis" means absence of. "Disease," then, means the absence of ease, the absence of balance between our hot- and cold-running times. "Dys-ease" means a faulty sense of ease, a lack of being in tune, of learning from challenges to our super-systems. In this context, it is true, as Dr. Gary Schwartz points out, that "disease is a special case of health," a lesson and challenge to lead to adaptation and growth.

My chronically ill patients and those patients who are struggling with the concept of wellness in their own lives have found my formula for wellness to be a helpful learning tool. I call this the *wellness quotient*, a simple formula comparable to the intelligence quotient formula, that illustrates the relationship between disease and wellness.

$$W = (D - I) + H$$

Just as the value 100 is typically seen as an average intelligence quotient, we can use 100 as a reference point for understanding wellness. It is important to remember, however, that there can truly be no measure of wellness and certainly no average wellness, for wellness is a concept of balance between mind, body, and spirit, all of which are concepts without limits, infinite as the universe, and forever intertwined. I use the value 100 for purposes of discussion and learning only. This is not a test on which you can get a perfect score!

D = DIS-EASE (LEARNING)

Are we to assume there are no hazards in inaction and pur-
poselessness? Does the body pay no price for emotional,
mental, and physical lethargy and stupification?

NORMAN COUSINS

Disease is our feedback system, the part of our humanness that functions as a thermostat does in response to heat or cold in a home. When it is too cold, the thermostat registers this fact and compensates for it by turning on the furnace. When it is too hot in the house, the thermostat turns on the cooling system.

So it is with disease. A sore stomach tells us that we are eating not only the wrong things but also the wrong way. A fever tells us that a battle is going on, and compensation for the heat is needed as well as more fuel and energy to support the battle. Without disease, we could never be well, for we would be without our thermostat of life, our monitor of our lifestyles, a sense of the meaning of our styles of inter-action with our world. I suggest that the experience of disease is an integral and indispensable part of wellness. This is not to say that we should not attempt to cure disease and reduce suffering, but we should be busy learning from our diseases, or what psychologist Dr. Gary Schwartz has called "the wisdom of disease."

Disease warns us against eating out of control, failing to attend to our sleeping habits, of losing the balance between rest and exercise. To experience and learn from disease is to evolve. If we fail to attend to and respond to the signals of disease, we fail to develop as a species. As a thermostat that cannot sense heat or cold, we burn down or freeze up when we ignore, run from, or attempt to overcome rather than experience disease.

I suggest that those of us who have experienced disease, rallied our forces for healing, and adapted and adjusted our lifestyles on the basis of signals from disease are capable of a higher degree of wellness than those of us who have never experienced disease or failed to learn from disease when it has been present.

Using a 100-point scale, arbitrarily assign yourself 0 to 100 points for the D factor. If you have experienced disease, learned more about yourself and your behaviors from this dis-ease and, in addition, learned about your relationships with others and your world from your disease, assign yourself several points. If you have not or do not remember having dis-ease, or were concerned only about the cure of disease rather than understanding the disease state, assign yourself fewer points for the D factor.

To illustrate this scoring system, I will use two patients I have worked with as examples. Mr. A had bypass surgery for clogged arteries surrounding and almost starving his heart muscles. He was hot-reacting on all counts and stated, ''I'm going in to get that old pump repaired.'' He never attempted to learn from his disease or modify the dangerous behaviors that contributed to his life-threatening situation. Instead, Mr. A was experiencing ''dys-ease'' and had disconnected himself from his supersystem, resulting in setback and interruption to a hectic, hot life-style.

Mr. B had exactly the same operation. In fact, he was in the bed next to Mr. A in the same cardiology unit. His reaction to his heart disease, however, was quite different. He reported, ''That does it. I can see that I really have not exercised, eaten correctly, and most of all, I have never taken any time for me and for those I love.'' Mr. B became pensive, talking with others in his life about the meaning and symbolism of his disease. Mr. B deserves several points for the D factor, for he was experiencing dis-ease.

Just for learning, we assign, say, 20 points to Mr. A, for after all he probably did learn more than even he knows from his disease. It is difficult to go through such a harrowing experience as heart surgery without learning something. We assign 80 points to Mr. B, for even though he is learning, he may be learning a little too hot and attempting quick solutions to his hot lifestyle. He is, however, making a conscious, cognitive, and emotional attempt to confront the metaphor of his disease. The exact points do not matter, but the direction of the scoring helps us understand more about the interaction between disease and wellness. The idea is to use the formula to learn, not to rank or rate.

The *D* factor is higher in someone who has had a serious disease than someone who has experienced a less debilitating problem. The challenge of attempting to rally in the face of major illness can be a strengthening event for the body and the soul, and those people who have grown through a major disease or have learned to cope and live with a chronic disease are capable of a level of wellness beyond those who have never known that experience. In this model of wellness, being sick or healthy is less relevant than learning and adjusting; therefore, the very sick can be very well. As radical as this may sound, disease is necessary to wellness.

I = ILLNESS (EMOTIONS)

For this is a journey that men make: To find themselves. If they fail in this, it doesn't matter much else what they find.
JAMES MICHENER

The *I*, or illness, factor represents the degree to which a person denies, panics, and blames during a disease experience. We are more ill when we deny disease, just as we can become overheated or underheated if we ignore our own body thermostat because of distraction or other involvements. We are ill when we blame others or ourselves, when we become disconnected from our society, when we blame government or "the medical establishment." We are ill when we simply comply or surrender to that medical establishment, instead of being an active partner, indeed a quarterback in the healing process. We are ill when we withdraw from others when we are hurt. And most of all, we are ill when we fail to see our disease as a part of the world system and proof of our own oneness with nature. It is likely that all disease is evidence of a break in our connection with our world, and illness is the inappropriate continuation of the separation in response to such disease when, in fact, disease should elicit an attempt to rejoin the system from which we have become separated.

Mr. A became angry at his doctors, his nurses, even himself. He suffered several setbacks during his recuperation and often complained about the "rotten food in today's society" as causing his heart condition. He added, "Pressures in today's workplace can kill anybody." He placed blame on others and situations for messing up, for causing his problems. For failure to learn about self, he is given a relatively high illness score, say 40.

Mr. B turned to social support systems before and after his surgery. He took time to meditate, to try to understand the metaphor of his heart problems, his "heart allergy." He receives fewer illness points, say 20. All of us have some illness when we have disease, for all of us become afraid. The trick is to learn from disease and see it as a part of a cycle and not simply as an invasion, to accept and learn and grow, not reject, withdraw, and blame.

So far, Mr. A has a disease score of 20 points from which we subtract 40 points for his elevated illness score. He gets some points toward wellness for having disease and experiencing an opportunity for challenge and stimulation to his wellness system. By subtracting 40 points, Mr. A is now actually "in the hole," with a minus 20. His negative score is the result of his negative emotional state, his poor coping strategies, which increase the deductions for illness. We will, then, be subtracting points from his H, or healing, factor once it is calculated, to determine his full wellness score. We already see that his wellness quotient (WQ) will be below average on the arbitrary scale of 100 points as a theoretical average.

On the other hand, his hospital roommate with the same disease had a D score of 80 points for his self-reflection and responsive, connecting adjustment to his disease. We subtract only 20 points, for even though he did some self-blaming, he has sought social support and maintained some optimism instead of defeatism. Both techniques result in subtracting only a few illness points from the positive aspects of his disease experience, for a partial score so far of 60. We can see that Mr. B will most likely be above average in his wellness quotient due to his self-reflection and self-responsibility.

Remember that the actual numbers do not matter, but the degree and direction of the scores give some indication of the wellness in your life, your capacity to *heal*.

H = HEALING (IMAGERY)

There is a part of the mind that we don't really know about, and that is the part that is most important in whether we become sick or remain well.

NAVAHO MEDICINE MAN,
quoted by Dr. Jeanne Achterberg

Unfortunately, the concept of the *H*, or healing, factor has fallen on hard times. Some health care professionals regard the term "healing" with suspicion, as if it represented some prescientific form of shamanism. Dr. Jean Achterberg points out in her recent book *Imagery in Healing: Shamanism and Modern Medicine* that "the shaman's work is conducted in the realm of the imagination." The shaman, the healer, has a long history. The witch hunts were aimed primarily at "healers," usually women, and the aftermath of the witch hunts has been an antifeminine, antihealing bias that continues in modern medicine. In reality, all medicine is shamanism, for all medicine is about or should be about healing.

The *H* factor refers to the ability to be a "self-shaman," the ability to mobilize your thoughts and imagination to rally the supersystem to return balance and achieve growth within the human system. You have learned in this book about the power of the supersystem to direct the most complex of healing processes. Your healing factor is high if you are able to use your imagination, to dream, to fantasize, to believe, to feel, to think rationally, and to embrace the concept that body, mind, and spirit are one. You receive more points for hope than self-blame, for acceptance than self-doubt. The B-A-FITER factors (*b*eliefs, *a*ttitudes, *f*eelings, *i*mages, *t*houghts, constructive *e*motions, *r*emembrances) are all subcomponents of the *H* factor.

Research has shown that neutrophils, the powerful little killers of abnormal or overgrowing cells and other invaders, are under the control of our own imagination. Even one little cell can be controlled by our thoughts. The healing factor refers to the attempt and ability to mobilize this control system, to be able to feel, sense, and experience disease, and to relate that disease to our total life experiences and, in turn, to attempt to mobilize the self-shaman actively within ourselves.

Mr. A receives only a few points for the healing factor. He states, "Cut me open, patch me up, and sew me up, Doc." He denies any possible value in imagining a clearing of his vessels or imagining the coming together of the skin at the site of his surgery. He is not a dreamer, a self-shaman, but rather an object within the medical system, a recipient or someone to be treated and done to. We assign Mr. A only a few points for healing, say 40. He receives some points, after all, for he probably has healing powers he is not yet aware of that are at work, perhaps his humor or his feigned self-confidence offers some self-shamanism in spite of himself.

Mr. B spends several minutes each day imagining his heart clear from obstruction and becoming stronger and healthier. He laughs instead of mocks, shares instead of criticizes, and touches his wound, forming a connection with the supersystem that can reestablish ease. He is high in self-shamanism and receives high points, say 90.

Mr. A must have 20 points subtracted from his 40 healing points, as he failed to score many points for his D factor, and was penalized heavily on the I factor. His WQ is only 20. With an IQ score, this would be in a severely impaired or vulnerable range, and so it is with Mr. A. In fact, the course of his disease was an unhappy one. He had several complications and had to be returned to the operating room to have several areas of leakage repaired. Angina, or pain in the chest, continued. And though he continues to survive, he is not high in wellness, not only in this wellness scoring system but also in his own view. He now comments, "They really cut the heart right out of me. I am weaker than I ever was." His need for counseling, for support, and for sharing is high, and hopefully he will seek this out. Unfortunately, his heart dis-ease has not helped him recognize his human potential for growth.

Mr. B adds to his strong H factor of 90 points his 60 points for his learning orientation to his disease and his low penalty points for illness or negative emotions. His WQ is 150. In IQ comparison, this would be a wellness genius. Mr. B's response to his surgery reveals his genius for wellness. He has altered his entire work schedule, now spends several evenings a week with his family and friends, regularly meditates about his wellness state, and sees his physician regularly for follow-up, working as a colleague with his doctor.

The WQ concept is a dynamic, changeable, adaptable one, open to the improvement by anyone willing to view health, disease, mind, and body as one. As it should be with the concept of intelligence, wellness is not something you are but something you do. Take the time to calculate your own wellness quotient now by arbitrarily assigning scores based on your recollection of your disease experience, your illness penalty points, and your capacity for healing. You receive more illness points to the degree that you are high on the hot and cold scales I described earlier. Think of diseases you may have had and your ways of dealing with those diseases. Think about the message of this book: the oneness of all of us and the importance of gaining control of the immune system and your brain, which may otherwise become a potentially fatal self-maintenance system at the expense of this oneness. Have someone else calculate your wellness score with you, for the person may have a more accurate view of some of your strengths and liabilities.

My prayer for you is that this book will have nudged your imagination just enough to free your spirit from the fear of disease and the harness of illness, thus giving free rein for the supersystem to do its miraculous work.

SUCCESSFUL SICKNESS: THE NECESSITY OF DISCOMFORT FOR DEVELOPMENT

I'm not OK . . . you're not OK, and that's OK.
        WILLIAM SLOAN COFFIN

There is a big difference between self-blame and self-responsibility. The greatest danger of this book is that you will look for fault in yourself or your loved ones, some way in which you have caused your own or their own diseases. I hope instead to focus on an understanding of our potential for the control of our supersystems as the greatest hope for humankind. Converting this understanding to a set of accusations or a type of psychological autopsy of self-recrimination only results in dysease and interferes with our natural healing powers.

To help remember this point, think of your own experience of disease. If you look closely, you can see that experience as a key part of who you are now. In fact, if that experience was removed from your life, you would be an entirely different and in some ways less of a person than you are now. This is not to say that you would not wish away much of the pain you had experienced, but it is true that there is no gain without significant strain.

It is likely that discomfort and personal disruption have been key factors in the development of our civilization. Perhaps a look at some of our most creative and productive people will support the hypothesis that the D, or disease, factor in the wellness formula is necessary for personal, social, and even world development.

Albert Einstein. Often seen as the greatest genius of our time, he suffered throughout his most productive years with continued stomach pain, which was most likely due to gallbladder trouble. Einstein refused to follow his doctor's recommendations for cure. He wrote to one of his close friends, ''At least the gods seem well intentioned toward me when they squeeze the gall bladder.'' By this he meant that he worked "more successfully when I suffer an attack." Disease for him was a learning, energizing factor.

Beethoven. His deafness motivated his compositions, including the *Pastoral Symphony*. He stated, "To be forced to be a philosopher at the age of 28 is not easy, least of all for an artist." Again, suffering contributed to growth.

Sigmund Freud. Seen as the founder of our present approach to psychology and psychiatry, he felt that one of his classical works, *The Interpretation of Dreams*, was subpar because "I was feeling too well physically; I have to be somewhat miserable in order to write well." Freud was bothered with several illnesses throughout his life, and his biographer Ernest Jones feels that "happiness and well-being" were not helpful to Freud in completing his most successful works.

Franklin Roosevelt. The ravages of polio and other related complications left President Roosevelt severely crippled and in pain much of the time. In spite of this, he guided the United States through some of its most difficult days.

John Kennedy. Effective as a president in many ways in spite of his serious back problems, John Kennedy was known to be in severe pain daily. It seems clear that his pain and disease in no way limited and in some ways motivated his high energy level as he attempted to compensate for this pain with exercise and social involvement.

Paul Klee. He stated, "I create . . . in order not to cry."

Abraham Lincoln. President Lincoln suffered throughout his life with a serious heart and circulatory disorder compounded by recurrent bouts of depression. All these conditions did not prevent him from carrying the United States through perhaps its major developmental crisis.

Molière. His creativity through illness was revealed in his statement, "I'm not strong enough to stand the remedies, it's all I can do to stand the disease."

Charles Darwin. This genius who developed the often questioned but important theory of evolution was bothered throughout his life by several diseases. In fact, he became a classic hypochondriac.

Florence Nightingale. This pioneer in the health care system was bedridden herself throughout most of her life. She suffered from several chronic illnesses but continued to be creative.

Thomas Edison. He worked around the clock, ignoring his health in spite of the fact that he suffered from continually nagging health problems.

Mary Baker Eddy. This creative woman founded Christian Science, but she was sick most of her life with bouts of colic and chronic pain.

Phillip Sandblom's *Creativity and Disease: How Illness Affects Literature, Art and Music* describes the role of disease in the creativity of people across the spectrum of the arts. Most meaningful to me was Sandblom's quote of Graham Greene: "Writing is a form of therapy; sometimes I wonder how all those who do not write . . . can manage to escape the madness, the melancholia, the panic and fear inherent in the human situation."

This is only a partial list of names of people who experienced disease but contributed creativity to our world. I am sure you could make your own list. Study the life of one of your favorite artists, and you will see the relationship clearly.

Health is not the absence of disease; it is the capacity to experience and learn with disease. We must learn to function relatively well no matter what happens to us, to learn to accept and receive, not just fight and overcome. Sociologist Renee Fox reports that if we include objective and subjective symptoms of disease, then almost everyone in society could be regarded as "sick." Studies indicate that up to 90 percent of apparently healthy people have some physical problem. The more intensive the physical evaluation, the more likely it is that we will turn up some problem. Disease is actually normal, even statistically.

So, once again, take heart. Do not blame yourself or others, do not despair at what you have done or failed to do to enhance your supersystem. Instead, rejoice! You are and will be sick like the rest of us. The supersystem knows that, and your mind is made even more ready for your humanness when you remind yourself daily that you, your mind, your body, and your immune system are one within itself and with the universe, with disease and with health. The universe is as much disease as it is wellness or, as the Chinese say, as much yin as yang, an unending circle of universal experience.

I received a phone call from a patient who stated hurriedly, "I can't make it today for my appointment. I have to go to a stress-reduction program sponsored by my company. I hate these things, but I'll get canned if I don't show up."

I asked if there was not some way of avoiding the program since this man clearly did not want to go. "Oh, no!" he responded. "The mood ring I got at the last company stress program is turning black. That means I'm really stressed. I can't get it to turn blue or even green. I've got to go and get *de-stressed*." The phone disconnected before I could respond, and this man was probably out the door before the dial tone started, running as fast as he could to chase health. He may never be home when health arrives at his doorstep.

Our immunity is enhanced when we learn that our mechanistic, dualistic, simplistic thinking is not in keeping with the laws of the universe. Time, space, speed, life, death, beginnings, and endings are viewed in the context of our hurried lives. Forever is how long we wait for a tax refund. Time is measured by electronic pulses strapped over our own pulse.

The geniuses of our time tried to tell us that there is a new way of thinking, a way in keeping with the rules of the stars, not the rhythm of traffic lights. Such ideas as Einstein's relativity theory have been dismissed as relatively impossible to understand, yet his thinking and that of other new physicists holds a promise for a better understanding of our supersystem, for that supersystem functions by the rules written in the stars. The next chapter looks at some new thinking that transcends the limits of our mechanistic world, for the supersystem is impaired when one attempts to understand it or make it function by rules it will never be able to embrace.

Chapter Fourteen

NEW THINKING
FOR A NEW TIME

All I really ever have is time.
PATIENT IN INTENSIVE CARE UNIT

WHO'S GOT THE TIME?

The waiting room was full of nervous mothers and confused children. This was testing day for a large metropolitan school system, and each child had been brought to the public school offices for a day of psychological examination. It was hot and humid, and the room smelled of peppermint and chocolate from the candy bribes offered by mothers willing to sell their souls for some sense of control.

I stood in the door of the waiting room and looked for the child I was to harass for several hours with a series of problems and puzzles designed to determine why he was harassing children at his school. As I called the name, the secretary looked up and talked through her large desk fan, giving her voice the sound of a person riding on a roller coaster over extremely bumpy track. "Your appointment is late, Dr. Carter's is early, Dr. Smith's will come later, Mrs. Green thought she was supposed to be here yesterday, your appointment may not come until tomorrow, and Dr. Carter started his testing ahead of time. By the way, if you have a minute, I need to talk to you now." In one secretarial report, the complexity of our view of time was illustrated by this over-worked, overheated, time-ridden secretary.

Each style of supersystem I have discussed has included problems with the perception of time. Our entire existence is dominated by time, as if it actually existed as a real thing, as if it could be measured by the tiny death monitors ticking over the pulse of our wrists. We can only understand the supersystem and assume control over that system if we understand that time is really only a matter of theory, a hypothesis, a conjecture, an individual viewpoint, and that this conception is dependent upon long-established scientific views of what constitutes reality and our world, the theory of life, a way of thinking of our world.

The hot waiting room grew hotter as more mothers and more children arrived. Some were late, some early, some on time. Mothers looked at their wrists as soon as they entered the room. The secretary looked at the large pendulum clock on the wall. By size, if nothing else, this wall clock became the *real time*. Arguments ensued over who had the right time, with admissions of being a little off, a little ahead, a little behind, or truly out of time issued by various parents. In all disagreements, the biggest clock was the final arbiter.

This tiny waiting room provided a perfect example of how perception of the meaning of time is taught in our society. Researchers more than 40 of what we call "years" ago established that perceptions of time are different between different social classes and that such perceptions are taught through daily life activities. In this small waiting room it was clear that various parents had different concepts of time and were busy teaching their individual time lessons.

Some of the parents were teaching that there is only *now*. No future, no past, just the immediate here and now was the lesson taught by "cut it out" punctuated by a slap on the child's rear end. That the future is all important and should determine your present behavior at all costs was being taught by the parent yelling across the room to her child removing a fish from the lukewarm water of the fish tank: "Don't do things like that, or you will never do well on your test later." Another mother based her interventions on the past and tradition as she firmly sat her daughter beside her and scolded, "Your grandfather would never have said something like that." Present, past, and future were modeled within the same room, all at the same time. Our own view of time and its impact on our wellness was largely learned through these same child-parent interactions.

HOT TIME AND COLD TIME

You are ushered in according to your dress;
Shown out according to your brain.
                    YIDDISH PROVERB

You may remember that hot-supersystem people live in the future. Their philosophy is always be aware of the impact of now, so that later on you can get more from tomorrow. Cold-supersystem people live in a distorted now, which moves slowly or, seemingly, not at all: Right now seems so long that no future seems possible. The hot reactor resembles the orientation of the mother warning about having later trouble on a test due to present behaviors. The cold reactor resembles the traditional orientation of the mother invoking the sanctity of an ancestor or grandfather, the family tradition, looking back for an understanding of now. It is not that the cold reactor's perception of time is immediate but that the cold reactor is living in a past that is mistaken for the now. Both the hot reactor and cold reactor fail to develop an adequate sense of personal time in tune with their own supersystems. They both suffer from a type of temporal arrhythmia, and unless they find and reset their own unique internal clocks, they parade in and out of life activities as the wooden characters on an old Swiss clock enter and leave their house on the assigned hour.

The concept of time itself is a new concept related to the physics of Sir Isaac Newton and the invention of the pendulum clock which gave one consistent market for counting. Against the count we called "seconds" (and interestingly not "firsts"), both the hot and cold reactors gauge their lives. The hot person looks forward, ticking faster and faster. The cold person looks backward, listening to what seems to be a slower and slower unwinding of the clock. The hot person eats quickly while doing several things while eating. The cold person eats strictly by a traditional time plan at long-established dinner and lunch "periods." Neither of these types eats when he is hungry, and is not able to realize the true state of hunger due to his future- or past-oriented time. Both lack a sense of personal time and are likely to develop their own characteristic versions of time illness.

Hot people tend to be what Dr. Richard Restak calls "owls." They maintain their body temperature late into the evening, signifying an alertness of mind and body. Cold reactors tend to be "larks," rising early but losing alertness as the day progresses. They experience a decrease of body temperature and feel sluggish. Research has shown that owls tend to be more extroverted and active, while larks tend to be more introverted and passive, characteristics related to hot and cold styles, respectively. It is possible that the immune systems of hot and cold people correspond to the owl and lark patterns, perhaps resulting in deficiencies and vulnerabilities to disease correlated to time of day and exposure to different viruses.

It may be that one determining factor of hot or cold time orientation is a tiny part of the hypothalamus called the *suprachiasmatic nucleus* (SCN). This tiny part of the brain possesses a natural rhythm of its own separate from all tissue around it. It is particularly sensitive to signals from the eyes regarding light and darkness.

Researcher Dr. Norman Rosenthal has identified a condition called *seasonal affective disorder*, a depression in some people that sets in during the long winter months. Rosenthal suggests that lack of sunlight results in this disorder, and he has successfully treated people by exposing them to high-intensity, full-spectrum lighting similar to that used for indoor plants. As if in hibernation, the person with seasonal affective disorder tends to withdraw, overeat, and underexercise. A brain chemical called *melatonin* is secreted by the pineal gland in the brain in response to signals from the hypothalamus, and this hibernation chemical is reduced by exposure to light. It is clear then that our brains control not only our immune systems but the rhythmicity of our lives and our emotional swings to and fro in search of the nurturing sun.

Personal Sense of Time Test (The PSTT)

Time out!
ATHLETE IN TROUBLE

To help you understand your view of time, rate yourself from 0, meaning not at all, to 12, meaning almost always. By the way, it is important not to time yourself on this test.

1. Do you check the clock by your bed as soon as you awaken in the morning?

   0   1   2   3   4   5   6   7   8   9   10   11   12

2. Do you put on your watch as soon as you get up in the morning?

   0   1   2   3   4   5   6   7   8   9   10   11   12

3. Do you find yourself sneaking a look at your watch, even when talking to people?
   0 1 2 3 4 5 6 7 8 9 10 11 12

4. Do you find yourself drawn to clocks as you walk or drive?
   0 1 2 3 4 5 6 7 8 9 10 11 12

5. Can you preset yourself to wake at a specific time?
   0 1 2 3 4 5 6 7 8 9 10 11 12

6. Do you find yourself awakening in the middle of the night but almost always at the same exact time and, as you do so, looking quickly at the clock?
   0 1 2 3 4 5 6 7 8 9 10 11 12

7. If someone asks if you are hungry, do you find yourself looking at your watch for the answer?
   0 1 2 3 4 5 6 7 8 9 10 11 12

8. If asked if you have the time, do you give the exact time? Instead of a more general answer such as "a quarter past," do you respond "1:14 P.M."?
   0 1 2 3 4 5 6 7 8 9 10 11 12

9. Do you consider someone late if he arrives more than 5 minutes after the agreed-upon time?
   0 1 2 3 4 5 6 7 8 9 10 11 12

10. Do you talk about time racing, fleeing, flowing, sailing, going by?
    0 1 2 3 4 5 6 7 8 9 10 11 12

11. Does the clock in your car keep accurate time, and if it hasn't, have you insisted on its repair?
    0 1 2 3 4 5 6 7 8 9 10 11 12

12. If someone's watch disagrees with yours, are you sure that he (not even necessarily his watch) is fast or slow and not you and yours?
    0 1 2 3 4 5 6 7 8 9 10 11 12

Now, ignore all your answers marked "5." Count the number of items to the right of 5, and subtract the number of items to the left of 5 from that number. Now place yourself on the following scale:

Cold time   0 1 2 3 4 5 6 7 8 9 10 11 12   Hot time

Related to our earlier discussions of hot and cold supersystems, you are more likely to be in balance, to experience the Goldilocks phenomenon of just right, if your score is 0 or near 0. A zero score would mean that you have developed a personal sense of time, free from the limits of the old physics and in keeping with a set of universal rules proposed by the pioneers in the new field of science—a science that suggests an entirely new world view. Cold reactors lean toward the left on this time scale, toward a cold time that drags slowly, bound by a stagnant historical orientation. Hot reactors cluster toward the hot time score and are in a race against the clock that may end up counting them out. Both types need to understand that our world functions by laws that exceed the complexity of our sixth-grade science classes.

In the remainder of this chapter, I will speculate about the relevance of a new world view, the science called *new physics*, which has gone beyond the Cartesian-Newtonian science that has dominated our thinking for decades. The new physics suggests a system that alters every preconception of our day-to-day lives.

I will be speculating about a new paradigm, a new model of understanding that is in keeping with the new theory of physics, a physics that talks of oneness, of simultaneity, of transcending our "clock-hour" view of time, of particles and waves in a world system that is changed when the smallest particle within that system changes, of a world of relationships, integration, and energy flow. We run too hot or too cold when we are not "just right" with the world, and the functioning of that world may be very different from what you and I were taught in our high school physics classes. We may have been taught, and therefore lead our lives by, rules that "ain't necessarily so."

I suggest that the development of a superimmunity depends upon developing our capacity to help our supersystems function by a new set of rules. I suggest that by attempting to regulate our supersystems by the mechanical, mind-body dualism of Cartesian-Newtonian science, we have restricted them from their as yet unmeasured capacities, for our supersystems do not operate by such a limited set of explanations.

THINGS WE KNOW THAT AIN'T NECESSARILY SO

"The Ancients have stolen our best ideas."
MARK TWAIN

To learn more about hot and cold supersystems, it is important to understand that the world we think dictates our lives is an illusion. We sometimes function as if we were separate from the things we see. In the early 1900s, Einstein and others stressed that the observer is part of the world and that perception is indeed everything. We, in fact, do not believe something if we see it, but we are more likely to see it if we believe it.

A grandfather walked through the woods with his young grandson. The sun screened through the tall trees creating a dreamlike haze. The grandfather looked up and saw a squirrel flying from tree to tree. He grabbed the shoulder of his grandson: "Look, a flying squirrel." "Grandpa," frowned the boy, "squirrels don't fly." "Look, there he goes again," said the grandfather, gesturing firmly. "Grandpa," said the boy, "squirrels are a different class from birds. We just studied that in science. They don't fly. They climb."

"I know," said the grandfather, "but this is a kind of squirrel with extra skin between his legs and body. He can open his legs and glide like a plane, like this." The grandfather illustrated the gliding of the squirrel with his arms, holding his jacket out at the side to become the skin of the squirrel, moving to and fro as a human glider plane.

"Grandpa," responded the boy, "squirrels climb, birds fly, humans walk and run, unless, of course, they use an airplane." The grandfather surrendered, placed his arm around the boy, and the pair walked on.

The grandson stopped suddenly, gasped, and pointed up toward the trees. "I see him, a flying squirrel, look, I see him!" The boy had changed his perceptions because of his grandfather's demonstration. Squirrels could now fly. The boy's linear experience of if-then had changed, not the squirrel. The observer became part of the event and had actually helped create the event. You, too, will bring your personal experience to our discussion as you bring your personal experience to your illness and wellness. In Lewis Carroll's *Alice in Wonderland*, Alice stated that she found some things very hard to believe. "Really," the queen said pityingly to Alice, "Close your eyes, take a deep breath, and try again." Take a look at five things we think we know that are not necessarily so. If they are hard to accept, perhaps it will help if you close your eyes, take a breath, and try again.

1. If It Exists, It's Measurable. If It Is Not Measurable, It Does Not Exist.

We were taught in school that space is infinite, parallel lines never meet, and a straight line is the shortest distance between two points. These and other ideas come from Euclidean geometry. This is a geometry named after the man who developed a set of ideas that explain the see-touch world of the concrete. It is the same geometry we took home and asked our parents or some engineering friend to help us understand. It all seemed so concrete, so real. The rulers, protractors, compasses, pencils, and the right or wrong check marks from our teachers made these measures seem the ultimate reality. In fact, good teachers know there is no right or wrong in a world of individuals, even if an individual flunks a course teaching one form of measurement in that world.

In 1916, Einstein published his theory of relativity. The world had not changed, but we now had a more complete and unique understanding of our world available to us. Einstein showed that space is not infinite, but had a finite radius. That is, if we could shoot a powerful light ray off into space and if we had time enough to wait and could shoot it fast enough, it would eventually return to shine in the middle of our back. It would not just go out "forever." What goes around comes around, although round is not really the shape of most things in this world of new physics.

The shortest distance between two points near a star is not a straight line at all, but something akin to the dancing path of a firefly on a warm summer evening. We are, after all, living on a perpetually moving plane, not on a dot circulating within a black sphere as may be seen in some "old" science demonstration.

A boy was asked to learn the configuration of the stars and to name some of the constellations. To do this, he was given several sheets of black paper through which he punctured several holes in the patterns of major constellations. He then put these patterns in a shoe box and shined a flashlight from the other side so he could see the light shining through the holes. He asked the teacher, "Is this how it is? Is this how the stars shine?" The teacher said, "No, stars exist, they have their own light, and they are real things out in space. This is a demonstration. It is not real." The teacher was wrong. By the time we see a star, it is quite likely it does not exist at all, for the speed of light sometimes exceeds our capacity to understand and to know. It certainly exceeds the capacity of flashlights and shoe boxes. Perhaps the teacher should have asked the boy about his perceptions of the stars, how he experienced them, what his reality was, and what he felt, believed, and perceived.

The apparently impossible has now become possible. Observing from outside, from an abstract set of rules, would never again be intellectually or personally honest after Einstein's contributions. Models of wellness and illness based on Euclidean or yardstick measures are only partially correct, yet cosmopolitan medicine clings to numbers and linear measures. We still count cells, read temperatures, and measure almost every body function by computer. In spite of this, there is a whole other set of rules governing the cosmos and our wellness. While we need our blood cell counts, our blood pressure indications, and our thermometers, we must realize that these are not indications of wellness, and are no more real than a thought, an idea, a hope, or a prayer. They are simply inaccurate means of communication, a form of medical charades with physician and patient guessing together the meaning of all these numbers.

It is the message of the new physics that we are the cosmos, and there are many sets of rules that govern us. We are not a demonstration, a blood pressure, or a blood count; we are the stars. Measurement is not the final criterion of existence.

2. All of Us Are Separate from Everything Else.

If the new rules of functioning of the world were to be considered in our understanding of our lives, it would become necessary to understand that we do not see the cosmos, but that we are the cosmos. Think back to the cancer patient with her hand held firmly against the window near the icicle. She asked if she or the sun melted the icicle. I had responded, "Yes," not only to get her attention and to engage her in dialogue but to illustrate that we are not separate from anything. It is the brain's illusion that it is separate, and if it persists in this illusion, it will kill the person.

Medicine has come to value the individual, to look at illness as the perturbation of an individual system. Medical school teaches only the importance of the individual patient. The more liberal medical schools pride themselves on "paying attention to the individual." In fact, we should be busy teaching that we are all a system and not individuals. Even though the brain seems to enjoy this separateness and individuality, it is just not accurate. It is "us" who get sick or well. Patients with doctors, staff within hospitals, hospitals within communities, communities within the world—all interact. Certainly when one person in a family is ill, the whole functioning of that family changes. We assume that this is because of small germs being transmitted within the family, but this is really due to the universal rule of oneness.

I have lectured throughout the country and talked with hundreds of patient groups about these issues. It is a consistent finding that patients talk less of the technical, mechanical skills of hospitals and hospital staff than they do about the caring or lack of caring of the people in the hospital itself. Ask patients who was most important to them during their stay in the hospital, and they will typically identify not their doctors, but a nurse or someone on the hospital staff. It is not just a single nurse, but the interaction among the nurses who have day-to-day and night-to-night contact with the patients that determines the nature of the hospital experience. We are sick in direct proportion to our failure to function with awareness of our fit with all others.

3. If I Do This, Then I Know That Will Happen.

We are also taught a view of wellness that suggests an accomplishment mode of health. Jog enough, eat enough, swallow enough vitamins, meditate enough, and you will be healthy. If you do this, then you will be that. Self-help books promise techniques for finding, achieving, getting, maximizing, and discovering health. I am not aware of one of these books that is titled "receiving" wellness. This is because history and the philosophers taught us that everything unlimited or boundless and not "earned" is evil.

Aristotle wrote that evil is anything unlimited or boundless. Good is always limited, achieved and controlled. Good is accomplished and achieved by limiting and controlling one's self and one's desires. Socrates taught us that we should work to exclude the unconditional, for it is corruptive. Plato saw the unconditional, the free and spontaneous, as evil and related to the sensory, the sensual, what he called *esthes*, or the female orientation of life. He saw the logical or *logus* or limited as a male characteristic, a principled good life. All of us have been taught to "get ourselves under control," not to lose control, to become aware of control, and to work toward and for health.

A little boy I tested in that same public school building mentioned earlier was sent to me because of emotional problems. These problems were indicated in the teacher's view by his continual masturbatory behavior in the classroom. He would rub his genitals so that other students became aware of this, giggled, and began teasing. In spite of disciplinary attempts, the boy stated that it was impossible for him to stop. He had been sent to two psychotherapists and spent hours sitting in the principal's office and alone in the hallway as punishment. He had even been sent to talk to the school nurse about this "unnatural behavior." Because of the school personnel's discomfort and the threatening nature of this behavior, emotional problems were assumed. No one had thought to give him a complete physical examination. Such examination revealed that he had a mild *urethritis*, or an infection of the genital area. His masturbation was a symptom of an irritation within his body, not an emotional problem. All this is not surprising until one considers this young man's statement as he left my office: "I don't know why people get so upset about this kind of thing anyway. My teachers are always saying, 'keep your hands to yourself,' and that is all I was doing."

This student had been a victim of circumstance and perceptions of "where" he did, "what" he did, and "why" he did it. He had not shown appropriate control or conditionalism—a limited approach to life. In fact, one of the most significant criticisms we can level about someone has become, "You have lost emotional control. You are now too emotional." We speak of emotional distance as if even our emotions are measurable. One wonders how far an emotional distance is, how it is maintained, and how and if it should be maintained.

We are not well if we can demonstrate an absence of fever. We are not sick if a glass tube shows mercury moving beyond an arbitrary number. Our illness and wellness is a result of a dialogue with ourselves and our interactions with others, including the person who places the thermometer in our mouths. We know that blood pressure rises simply by a doctor entering the room. Medication given by one doctor has one outcome, while the same medication given by another has a different outcome. This is determined by our perceptions, expectations, and communication with that doctor. As psychologist Lawrence LeShan states, "There is a healthy way to be sick." That healthy way depends upon understanding that health is not achieved but that it is received. If we can learn to stop fighting, fleeing, and flowing, and to just "be," health may find us. It is received through a self-awareness of our inner dialogue, not through discovery of some outside manipulation or new vitamin. Outside manipulations of the body will never achieve what inner and spiritual growth can do much more powerfully. It is no coincidence that some physicians and nurses see their patients get well very quickly, while other physicians and nurses see their patients fail to respond, assuming that all external ministrations have been tried and all that is left is the appropriate reflex action by the human system. After all, if a stitch in time saves nine, then nine stitches in the abdomen should save anybody if they only learn to ''respond'' appropriately.

One of my physician colleagues raced into the lunch room and tore open his paper bag to get at his sandwich. ''Mrs. Smith thinks she is some kind of a spring chicken. She is acting like she doesn't have a damn thing wrong with her. She has congestive heart failure, and after lunch I am going to let her have it. She will never improve until she knows how sick she is and takes this whole thing seriously.''

How wrong he was. This patient would only improve if she knew how well she is and can be, and how she could learn from her condition at this present time. She would become well only if she was not affected negatively by her hot-reacting doctor who felt he had to first convince her how sick she was so that he could mechanically manipulate her system to health. Hospitals and schools are places where ''labelers'' work to convince ''labelees'' of the validity of the labelers' view, rather than places where self-learning regarding human potential takes place. The enhancement of self-esteem has to be smuggled into hospitals and schools.

4. Opposites Are as Different as Night and Day.

The health business is our largest and most rapidly growing industry. Billions of dollars are invested in this largest of all conglomerates. Billions of prescriptions are written annually. Drug companies are multimillion-dollar conglomerates. It seems to be our financial and political goal to end all disease. Even if this were accomplished, it would be the worst thing that could happen to humankind, for without disease there would be no wellness, as there is no sunlight without shadow, no happiness without sadness, no life without death.

Think of times when you have had severe flu. Nausea, fever, weakness, and fatigue took over, and you realized how wonderful it was when you were able to eat a meal, take a long walk, and smell the fresh air. Philosophers have often stated that the greatest truths are those for which the opposite is also true. If happiness makes us smile, then smiling might make us happy. If illness and wellness are seen as life processes, part of the whole, then illness can be a way of enjoying wellness, as wellness can teach us how to cope with illness.

Illness and wellness are both natural parts of life, as night follows day and day follows night. In this view, health is our view of the world, including our theories about, and interactions with, that world. It has been said that there are no atheists in foxholes, and since most doctors, nurses, and patients find themselves in a type of medical foxhole, they typically report the need for some transcendent belief. In spite of this, such beliefs are typically given only token acknowledgment in most hospitals.

If we learn to view ourselves as a whole, as a part of our cosmos, and realize that our universe does not value suns over moons, then we understand along with the new physicists that opposites are not opposite but that they are part of our total experience. Opposites apply a linear structure, a continuum of the universe, a left and right. Einstein and the new physicists taught us, as did Columbus, that we do not sail off the end of our world into sickness but instead move around from distress to strength back to distress in a continuing ballet of life.

"I never knew that the air smelled so good or felt so good. I could feel it going in through my nose and really enjoy it," said the patient who had experienced an allergic reaction to a seafood dinner and had been rushed to an emergency room. He could barely breathe and had to be placed on a respirator. He watched in horror each day as the alarm that signals malfunction of this life-support system was turned off while the machine was cleaned and reset. He dreaded the possibility that the technician would forget to turn the alarm back on, leaving him vulnerable to any machine malfunction. The patient had become dependent upon the annoying alarm as his ultimate life saver. His worst fear came true one day as the technician forgot to turn the warning device back on after a cleaning. The machine malfunctioned this same day, and no alarm was sounded for the nursing staff.

Following a several-hour shift, one nurse was walking to her car but decided to check the patient's room just one more time. As the nurse entered, she found the patient dying. The respirator sat useless as the patient suffocated, and there was no warning tone. The nurse took appropriate measures and saved the patient's life. She received an award from the hospital for her rapid behavior and her technical skills at reviving the patient. But these were not the elements that saved this man. It was her caring and concern that revived him. It was that immeasurable moment when she decided to check just one more time, that magical "oneness."

The patient told me that there was never a day now that he does not give thanks for his ability to breathe. As there is no exhaling without inhaling, there is no health without the experience of illness, no sense of safety without the knowledge of our ultimate vulnerability. The patient asked me, "I wonder why she decided to stop by on that night. She had never stopped by before. It's kind of eerie, isn't it?" It is unfortunate that we label as eerie or strange the reality of the world that contains feelings, instincts, beliefs, hopes, fears, joys, and miracles.

5. What Is, Is.

The world is not made up of objects. In his book *Quantum Reality: Beyond the New Physics*, physicist Nick Herbert discusses the new physics research supporting the contention that the world is not hard objects, but is instead a quantum world of rules that transcend our limited view of reality. For example, electrons and particles in this quantum world cannot be seen. There is no single image which corresponds to an electron. An electron is not a thing but a field, an occurrence. The quantum world of which we are a part is constituted by events, waves, fields, and perceptions, not hearts, lungs, and tumors.

Sigmund Freud, always the analytic, rational scientist, considered that mental telepathy or the sending of feelings and thoughts was not only possible but in fact did occur. In spite of Freud's ultimate rationality, his respect for the human system left him no alternative but to conclude that communication beyond our units of measurement was possible. All of us report experience with occurrences that are not measurable by the Euclidean yardstick mentioned earlier. Sir Isaac Newton's apple fell, and a whole set of rules relating to a concept of gravity evolved. These rules of gravity are accurate for our see-touch world, but they do not apply to our personal world and to the world of quantum mechanics or Einstein's cosmos. Modern physics teaches that gravity and concepts such as falling, up and down, in and out, are relative to the eye of the beholder. A passenger on a train sees the world as passing. Those watching the train see the train as passing. Who is right? For the people on the train, they are as right as the people watching that train roar by.

A very famous finding called *Bell's theorem* is seen by some scientists as the most significant discovery in the history of science. As significant as this finding was, it has failed to find its way into our modern medicine. In very complex ways, it demonstrates that particles once in contact with one another are forever affected by one another. This finding, supported by detailed research, indicates that the speed of light could be exceeded, that the concept of "simultaneity" was indeed possible. If this is true for particles, it is equally true for thoughts. Einstein himself had trouble believing this, stating that "nothing could go faster than the speed of light, therefore things could not happen at exactly the same time." But Bell's theorem showed that they do. We do sense "vibrations." We do get "in touch" with one another, feel one another, sense people, groups, and hospitals, and feel that we are going to get sick and going to get well above and beyond concrete measurements. If two particles once in contact can change simultaneously even though they are millions of miles apart, then feelings and thoughts can change and be sent and received. We are all one anyway, and a change in one of us is a change in all of us. What is left is to develop our senses and our sense, to take control of our supersystems, to be more aware of ourselves as participants in the quantum universe. A modern medicine that struggled to accept the fact that invisible germs could cause illness has so far refused even to wrestle with the idea that invisible things such as thoughts and feelings can cause illness and wellness.

Every nurse knows that the particular mix of a patient's personalities, nurse morale, physician attitude, and countless other factors influence not only the general morale of the hospital but the frequency of complications following surgery and the rapidity of healing. Nurses know that they can sense when a patient is going to go bad or rally. Some nurses sense this through their eyes, through their noses, through just "a feeling." This talk, however, is seen as unscientific "soft talk." Courses dealing with these issues are seen as soft curriculum courses. When I am asked to speak throughout the country, I am often asked to do either a soft presentation on feelings and attitudes and the new physics or a hard presentation on the so-called real world of the endorphins and the biochemistry of the brain. We continue to cling to the concept that what we can touch is real and what we can feel is mystical.

If the only trace of an electron's existence is a smear across a special instrument measuring what the electron did, where it was, and where it went, but never the electron itself, then we had best understand that wellness is not a thing but a sense, not a state but a theory, not accomplished but lived, not an event of the mechanical but a process rising from the garden of the soul.

PHYSICS LESSONS FOR THE SUPERSYSTEM: THE COSMIC SEVEN

It takes at least fifteen years before a major scientific discovery
penetrates the public consciousness.

SCHRODINGER

Seven men have provided profound conceptualizations about our world,
concepts that have direct relevance to understanding our supersystems.

Albert Einstein. While everyone knows his name and recognizes him
as one of the greatest geniuses of all time, few people realize that his
work has direct implications for our health. His special theory of relativity and his new way of looking at electromagnetic radiation became
the underpinnings of atomic theory. Both these contributions suggested
that all events in our world are interconnected, not in the linear causal
sense of the old physics, but connected relatively or with direct influence
upon one another, including the observer as well as the observed. Einstein's theories tell us that mass is but a form of energy, that a rock is
really resting energy potential.

EINSTEIN'S SUPERSYSTEM LESSON
Einstein's theory taught us that all perturbations to the human system
and to the world in general are problems on the energy level. Even
though modern medicine looks for tumors by x-ray and diagnoses disease
when a lump is present, early formation of disease actually takes place
as a problem with energy flow, much as traditional Chinese medicine
suggests. If doctors were trained as physicists and not biologists, they
would likely be trained to read energy flow more often than to read
slides under a microscope. We must learn to view our supersystems as
a form of energy interacting with everything within and about us, not
a "something," a collection of organs and secretions.

Max Planck. The founder of the theory of quantum mechanics, he
taught us that a whole new world of relationship exists on the level of
the very, very small going very, very fast. In this world, the laws of

our day-to-day, see-touch world do not apply, for they are much too limited to explain the miracles that take place at the quantum level. The *quantum effect* is the theory that the more a particle is confined, the faster it tends to move around, and quantum theory suggests that our concepts of inside and outside, beside and next to, are insufficient to explain the functioning of the human system.

PLANCK'S SUPERSYSTEM LESSON
Quantum mechanics suggests that openness and growth are healthier than confinement, limitation, restriction, and imprisonment. Every component of our systems is in constant motion, running hot, cold, warm, or cool. The hot reactor experiences the quantum effect of an accelerated particle, the cold reactor the isolation of planets scattered in a wide universe. Somewhere in between rests the balance of health.

Neils Bohr. Dr. Bohr introduced the theory of complementarity. As with the well-known yin-yang polarities, this complementarity theory suggests that one explanation of anything is inadequate. In Dr. Bohr's study of particles and waves, he discovered that the possibility of understanding one element of particles left much more not understood in the area of waves. The more we learn on one level, the less we know on another.

BOHR'S SUPERSYSTEM LESSON
We have learned more and more about cell biology and the functioning of organ systems. In emphasizing this approach, we have neglected the importance of thought, spirit, and feeling. Cells and thoughts experience complementarity. They interact directly. To study one in detail without the other violates the theory of complementarity.

J. C. Bell. As stated earlier in this chapter, Bell's theorem is viewed by many scientists as the greatest scientific breakthrough in history. His theorem, or set of explanations regarding the world, shows that instantaneous events can occur. Electrons planets apart change the direction of their spin simultaneously with the change in another electron, as if they were together. In effect, the whole determines the functioning of the parts; things within the system are affected by any change anywhere in the system. The universe is not some mechanical system, but a concept, a perception. As James Jeans states, "The universe begins to look more like a great thought than like a great machine."

BELL'S SUPERSYSTEM LESSON
This view means that feelings, beliefs, and the entire B-A-FITER system influences our health immediately and totally. It is impossible to change just one part of ourselves without changing our entire selves and effecting others. Modern physics has taught us that all change is universal and simultaneous.

Ilya Prigogine. This Nobel laureate details ideas regarding what he called *dissipative structures*, which suggest that all development is due to breakdown and that self-renewal, not gradual disintegration, is the rule following any breakdown. We are not gradually working toward destruction but working toward integration. In effect, falling apart is only a phase of falling together.

PRIGOGINE'S SUPERSYSTEM LESSON

Our view of wellness is affected by the theory of dissipative structures, for this theory implies that a medical model which emphasizes illness, deterioration, aging, and a problematic focus is not in keeping with the rules of the universe. The supersystem is designed to follow the laws of enhancement, of gain, of growth, of development, of building. For the supersystem, all change leads to challenge and growth.

Ludwig Von Bertalanffy. This German biologist formed a new science he called *perspectivism*, later referred to as the *general systems theory*. This theory sees all elements of our world as influencing one another in a chain reaction. A change in governmental policy affects a given state, which, in turn, affects a workplace, which affects an employee who takes such an effect home to his family, which, in turn, affects a child, which affects the parent, who, in turn, changes his or her work performance, in turn affecting the workplace, in turn affecting the state economy, which affects the government. Reverberating circuits of interactions between all elements of the system continue. Concepts of feedback, integration, rhythm, and equilibrium originate from the general systems theory.

VON BERTALANFFY'S SUPERSYSTEM LESSON

If there is a unifying concept to the supersystem, it belongs under the heading of general systems theory. As the waves of the ocean strike against the beach, so do changes within the supersystem cycle infinitely from the cellular level, to the family, to the nation, to the world. The slightest governmental policy change eventually has its effect upon the lymphocyte. This is Larry Dossey's concept *biodance*. He states that there are actual elements of the stars within our bones, for we are not just a part of the universe, we are the universe.

Werner Heisenberg. This researcher expressed the limitations of many of our most basic ideas about our world in precise mathematical formulations, now called the *uncertainty principle*. He essentially showed that the more we emphasize one aspect of our description of something, the more uncertain we become about the total of all else. This is the central rule for all physics and is directly related to the theory of dissipative structures. New research into the connections between any elements of our world show that the more we focus our study on one part of our world, the less we realize that much more needs to be known about other parts and their interactions.

HEISENBERG'S SUPERSYSTEM LESSON

The uncertainty principle tells us that by our very focus on any element of our system, we are pointing out a need for more knowledge in another. An integration between the mechanical wonders of modern medicine, the remarkable cellular biology discoveries capable of saving countless lives, and the power of the mind over immunity requires our time for understanding and our recognition that by focusing on any one of these, we are neglecting the other; the more we know, the more we are uncertain.

So there you have it: a quick lesson in the new physics, with seven lessons that apply to our supersystems. We really do have to begin thinking in new ways about ourselves and our wellness, our concepts of time, matter, and relationships. If we are able to change our thinking, maybe someday we will move toward a definition of wellness that transcends the absence of symptoms and realize our own relativity and the fact that everyone in the world is as much a part of our supersystems as any white blood cell.

The table on the following pages summarizes the impact of the cosmic seven's thinking for a superimmunity. As you study this chart, remember that the new physics is not the last physics and that each of the seven men and other pioneers in the new physics will suggest that their work is only a part of a continuing and broadening spiral of understanding on levels as yet to be explored.

The final section of this book examines some practical ways in which we can implement the ideas presented in this chapter. I will attempt to translate theory to day-to-day suggestions for applying the unity, intimacy, and growth emphasis of the thinkers described in this chapter.

As a reminder of the importance of a practical perspective, one of my patients related the following story. He was a college professor and had taught philosophy for several years at a major midwestern university. He had gone on his own pilgrimage in search of the truth. Following several years of travel and study, he found what he felt to be one of the leading gurus in the world. He saw this man as all wise, all knowing, and "one of the most profound thinkers I have ever met." The guru stated, "I am willing to answer one well-thought-out question for you.

The professor paused, anxious to use this golden opportunity wisely. He then questioned, "Yes, guru, tell me the meaning of death."

The guru paused, looked down, looked up, hesitated for what seemed like hours, and then responded, "I don't know."

The professor was stunned. Forgetting the status of this great teacher, the professor responded, "You don't know? I can't believe that. You are one of the wisest gurus in the entire world."

"Yes," responded the guru, "but I am not a dead wise guru. You would have better asked how to catch the next plane home. I have been to the airport."

THE COSMIC SEVEN'S RULES FOR SUPERIMMUNITY

New Physicist	Old Physics	New Physics	Rules for a New Superimmunity	Super-immune Thinking
Einstein **Relativity Theory**	Cartesian dualism; separateness.	Oneness: all things and events connect, are relative.	Mind-body are one; all events in our lives are interconnected; our immunity interacts with everything and everyone.	"Holism"; connections; relationships
Plank **Quantum mechanics**	One world—operating with one set of rules.	Many worlds and levels of functioning with many rules and concepts.	Our immunity cannot be understood by any one set of rules. Mechanical-Newtonian laws do not adequately explain the quantum and universal nature of immunity.	Multilevel; several ways of knowing

Bohr **Complementarity**	Either-or concept — an explanation is either right or wrong.	Our world is unified—all parts of that world always compliment one another.	Our health is an indivisible, dynamic whole. All parts of our body work together—health and sickness are both natural and necessary—immunity allows for both.	Dynamic; adaptive
Bell **Bell's theorem**	All things happen in a cause-effect, before-after, now, later sequence.	The whole determines the actions of the parts—things happen faster than our concept of time.	There are no limits on our wellness and healing. Miracles happen every day. It does not take time to heal; it takes hope and belief beyond time.	Belief as important as thought
Prigogine **Dissipative structures**	The world is gradually breaking down, deteriorating, burning up.	The world evolves through all change—stability is not balance but change.	Symptoms are always signals of stability, not breakdown. They are teaching signs of the inherent organization and adaptability of life.	Hope; positive view

New Physicist	Old Physics	New Physics	Rules for a New Superimmunity	Super-immune Thinking
Jon Bertalanffy Systems theory	The world is hierarchical—organized on separate levels.	The world and persons are an interconnected dynamic system.	Our entire body system is interrelated with the world system. Any change on any level causes changes on all levels—in the whole system.	Relatedness to all things and people
Heisenberg Uncertainty principle	With enough study, we can become sure, certain of events.	Every explanation is limited; the more we learn, the less we know.	There can be no final diagnosis; no certainty in the area of health. The more we learn of one disease, the more we need to know of other diseases and wellnesses.	Constant relearning

Part Five

TOWARD SUPERIMMUNITY

And could you keep your heart in wonder at the daily miracles of your life, your pain would not seem less wondrous than your joy.

KAHLIL GIBRAN

This final part presents suggestions on living for a superimmunity, a way of living on the basis of intimacy, unity, and growth even at the time of apparently unrelenting grief and pain. I will discuss the importance of touching, healing emotional states, and enhancing of immunity and the supersystem at times of challenge. Most importantly, I will discuss the discovery of a magic healing place, a place where immunity means tolerance, acceptance, balance, growth, and oneness.

Chapter Fifteen

THE INTIMACY FACTOR: SENSUALITY AND WELLNESS

Sex isn't the best thing in the world, or the worst thing in the world, but there is nothing quite like it.

W. C. FIELDS

"Multiorgasmic?" she gasped incredulously when her husband asked her about her sexual responsivity. "I'm not even uniorgasmic."

The couple had dreaded coming for therapy for their long-standing lack of sexual fulfillment. They sat tense, embarrassed, and angry at each other and themselves. The husband, a successful 45-year-old accountant, had suffered two heart attacks in 3 years. He now bragged that he jogged every day while listening to stock market reports on his portable tape player and had watched "TV shows on sex for some ideas."

"I work on you for what seems like hours," he responded to his wife's statements regarding her orgasms. "Now you tell me that it's all for nothing."

The 40-year-old wife was now accused of being a failed sexual project. She described her own career as a teacher as "six hours of boredom punctuated by five minutes of panic." She appeared fatigued.

Her shoes were stained with dark blue paint, and her black blouse showed the reverse chalk image of the day's assignments on the upper back and right arm. Her reading glasses hung lopsided around her neck, and one of the stems was bent. She often described a day's teaching as the experience of driving a stagecoach with a thousand "deaf, hungry, and untrained horses."

"Work on me? Maybe if you would stop trying to erase my genitals and really touch me and hold me, we could make love instead of doing it." Her voice was shakier now, as if she was on the verge of crying.

This combative, accusatory, and painful attempt to find sexual intimacy characterizes the sexual problems of many couples coming for marital help. The hot-reacting husband and the cold-reacting wife in this example both had unmet needs for intimacy, and both were made vulnerable to physical disease because of their frustrations, helplessness, and lack of effective strategies for accomplishing their goals.

The wife had initially come to my office with a self-diagnosis of arthritis. On some days it was an effort for her to walk the halls at school. She was often jostled by the hurried hot-reacting children and found herself so sore in the evening that she was unable to sleep. Following several visits to specialists, it occurred to her that her arthritis may be related not only to physiological factors but also to her own cold-reacting supersystem that she had heard me describe at a recent teachers meeting. Further interviewing revealed that sexual problems existed, and these were the reasons for the couple coming to the clinic at this time. All disease emanates from systems, not things or people. This couple was producing illness in themselves and in each other. The husband's accelerating and isolated heart had combined with the wife's restricted body movement, and both persons were as affected by their hot and cold supersystems as they were by their failure to communicate effectively.

After more than 15 years of working with couples, I believe it is clear that our immunity to disease is related not only to our ability to reject other but also to accept other. It is interesting that we almost always go to the doctor alone when, in fact, the most important systems are not our body systems but our belief systems, our healing systems, and our interactional systems. This chapter is about the importance of these systems and, particularly, the significance of physical touch of and by someone we love.

To love and be loved is perhaps the single most important result of being healthy. When we fail to love, our supersystem is jeopardized.

As physician-philosopher Paracelsus stated, "The main reason for healing is love."

The results of loving, of touching, holding, and relating are tangible. Researcher David McClelland of Harvard showed that students
watching a film showing love experienced immediate increases in their
levels of immunoglobulin A (IgA), one of the immune defenses against
colds. Just the act of watching selfless love was immunoenhancing. I
will show you in this chapter that sexual love is important to all loving
and that touching and sensuality directly enhance the supersystem.

THE BUFFERING HYPOTHESIS

To love is to be lonely. Every love eventually is broken by
illness, separateness, or death.

CLARK MOUSTAKAS

Researchers at Boston University School of Medicine have studied what
they call *conjugal bereavement*. They have suggested that social support,
the presence of caring persons, reduces the impact of the loss of a loved
one on our immunity. The equivalent of 12 football stadiums full of
people will lose a spouse each year in the United States. One-half of 1
of these 12 stadiums equals the number of bereaved spouses who will
die in the same year following the loss of the loved one. Thousands of
suicidal attempts per day are directly attributable to a death of a spouse.
Certainly there is something basically human, basically essential to our
survival, that is related to interacting intimately with others and to the
experience of losing someone close. In spite of our brains' selfishness,
there is something within us that is keenly aware of our unity with all
others, our belonging to a system.

Separate a mother monkey from her baby monkey, and she will
angrily attack the wall placed between them. Following several minutes
of fruitless attack on this wall, she will surrender, withdraw, and become
physically sick. This *rage-withdrawal* sequence is noticed in our own
lives when we lose someone. The heat of rage and the cold of withdrawal
relate to the illnesses we have described earlier in this book, and whether
we are hot or cold is intimately associated with our abilities to maintain
our present relationships and develop new relationships. The *buffering*
hypothesis suggests that the most important buffer we have against

illness is our social-support system, the presence of and contact with others.

There is new physiological evidence supporting the significance of loss to our general health. If our reaction to loss is extreme—with rage, anger, or hostility being the primary way in which we demonstrate our reaction to loss—the hypothalamus will stimulate the pituitary gland to release a substance called *ACTH* (adrenocorticotropic hormone) in the blood. This results in stimulation of the cortex, or outside of the adrenal gland. Two hormones that may be released by the cortex are called *mineralocorticoids* and *glucocorticoids*.

If mainly mineralocorticoids are released by the cortex of the adrenal gland, this is indirect evidence that the brain has made a decision to fight the loss, to rage, and resist its reality. The body is left vulnerable to the diseases of the hot reactor typified by this hormonal pattern.

If mainly glucocorticoids are produced, this is indirect evidence that the brain has decided to coexist with the loss, perhaps surrender in a form of despair, despondency, and helplessness. This may make the person vulnerable to diseases of the cold reactor. Several researchers have documented this phenomenon. Dr. D. M. Kisen has researched a characteristic of lung cancer patients. As a group, he has found, they tend to suppress their emotions. In a book entitled *Psychosomatic Aspects of Neoplastic Disease*, edited by Dr. D. M. Kisen and Dr. L. LeShan, cancer patients were seen as ignoring their negative feelings such as depression and guilt. When we withdraw from the system, our own supersystems may withdraw as well.

The physiological evidence of the presence of specific hormones related to hot and cold reactions to loss illustrates the disruption of the Goldilocks phenomenon. If things are not in just the right balance in terms of our reaction to loss and we are not able to maintain a social-support system at times of loss, there is little to buffer us against grief disease.

The whole story of our supersystem is about its ability to protect self, to recognize and dispose of other, but it is also about the brain's ability to realize that it is not alone, that it should allow "chosen others" to create an "us" of daily living. We are invaded by our own defense systems if we fail to teach our brains their place in the universe and their dependence upon other. The overheating of our supersystems in reaction to loss results in circulatory diseases or diseases of "overkill" and overmobilization, while cold supersystems result in the boredom diseases of rapidly growing cells, the stagnancy or lack of physical and emotional movement. I suggest that our supersystems must learn to cope much more constructively with the concept of us, not just other, and to maintain a sense of us even in the face of insult and challenge to our supersystems imposed by the disruption of a paired bond.

Dr. Christopher Coe of Stanford University reports that separating infant squirrel monkeys from their mothers suppresses the immune system. A 1 percent increase in unemployment, another form of bereavement and grieving, shows an immediate increase in disease rate on a national level. Dr. Saul Shonberg at Duke University has shown that human touch is essential to the growing child, and in the absence of such nurturance, growth hormone levels may be insufficient and the child will fail to thrive. We are all one another's buffer against illness and avenue toward personal development.

Touching others is a signal to our immune systems to relax, accept, and stay in balance. Throughout this chapter I will focus on the touching and sensual dimension of relating, for this dimension has been neglected in work in the area of wellness. Certainly, love is much more than touch and sexuality, but without physical closeness and fulfillment, the full range of love is restricted.

The number one question I hear from my seriously ill patients is almost always about the future of their sexual lives, their future potential for touching and being touched. Questions before and after surgery are almost always related to the maintenance of intimacy, if only the professional person is open and comfortable enough to hear the question. Every physician knows that it is impossible to separate the emotional from the physical. Every patient knows that the emotional cannot be separated from the need to touch and be touched.

THE HEALING TOUCH

There is no greater or keener pleasure than that of bodily love—and none which is more irrational.

PLATO

The first barrier of the supersystem is the skin. This largest of all body systems in terms of inches is activated immediately when it is touched, stroked, disrupted, or gently stimulated. The brain is activated as well. It reacts to the signal of touch with an interpretation that the touch represents the presence of other. It has to be taught that touch can also mean us, can also mean that it is okay to allow this other to join the system, that it is okay not to reject or attack this other.

Sex is actually the experience of touching, and the instinct of touch is evident in our day-to-day lives. It provides the first and lasting link between mother and infant and is the only tangible way we have to confirm our existence in our world. Hot reactors seem challenged too much by touch and tend to disregard, rush past, or overreact to touch. Cold reactors long so for touch that they never seem to get enough and, paradoxically, find themselves alone and untouched, much as the over-demanding child becomes alienated from the mother.

Our first reaction to pain is to touch the area of the pain as if the brain was pointing out the location of disruption or the site of the pertur-bation. The mother or father who offers to kiss the "ouch" of the child seems to know that to touch an injured area can help it heal. Faith healers are well named, for their effectiveness rests with the faith of the healed and not the healers themselves. It is interesting that the word "healing" has been banned from most medical discussions, other than its specific use as healing a given wound. Most people in medicine see the term as related to shaman, witch doctors, and others outside the scope of what they call traditional medicine. In reality, healing always comes from the people themselves and is related to the verification that someone other than ourselves cares about us and can enhance our wellness.

way of making another egg." He meant by this that Darwin's theory of survival of the fittest, or what he called natural selection, was in-complete. The idea that our world is made up of countless individuals struggling for their own survival as separate entities seems inadequate when we think of the supersystem and its innate intelligence. Such a view has trouble explaining the concept of *altruism*, or giving others priority over self. If the supersystem is dedicated to its own survival, why are some of us able to put others' needs before our own? Certainly within families, parents are capable of putting their children's lives and survival before their own. Some researchers suggest that this is due to the fact that the selfishness of the supersystem and the selfishness of genes that precode that supersystem direct us to promote the survival of those who have genes in common with us, such as our families. According to this view, our brains and our genes are always attempting to guarantee their own survival through their temporary hosts—us. This was why Spencer felt that the hen is only the egg's way of guaranteeing the existence of another egg. This new field is called *social biology*, and whether or not it is correct in its assumptions, I suggest that our innate selfishness can be controlled and directed in favor of our own wellness through the lesson of love and loving. The love guru Leo Buscaglia suggests that we are all angels with only one wing. We fly only when we join together.

One of the earliest researchers on the concept of stress, Hans Selye, suggested that a necessary factor to the maintenance of our health was to achieve the paradoxical sounding state of altruistic egoism. This was his concept of the beneficial integration of *other concern* and *self-concern*. He pointed out that the only distinguishing factor between a cancer cell and a healthy cell is that a cancer cell cares only for itself. The other body cells, at some point in the past, gave up their independence to form a stronger and more complex being. The golden rule which suggests that we do unto others as we would have them do unto us is not just a nice way to be; it is an essential way of enhancing and preserving our well-being. Just think of any time in which you went the extra mile and helped someone push a car from a snowbank, and remember the good feeling you experienced. This is an example of enhancing self through enhancing others. Even if our "genes are wearing us," we still are capable of caring for others.

In a society where "putting the touch on somebody" has negative connotations, it is important to learn the relationship between sensuous, tender touching and our health. I pointed out earlier that researchers have documented a risk to our physical balance, our health, from two "selfishness factors": first, seeing oneself in narrow, egotistical terms, as if separate from others, results in alienation and associated stress; second, when we identify strongly with our narrow, self-centered view, we behave more hostilely, aggressively, possessively, and impatiently. Both these factors are risks to our supersystems.

Bereavement is a term for loss. Grief is our natural psychological and physiological response to bereavement. Grief always challenges our supersystem. We have all heard the words "heartsick" and "crying our hearts out." If we do not take rational control of our brains, they will select their own way of dealing with loss, and their own way may be creation of a replacement other in the form of disease. If our brains continue to build walls between us instead of bridges toward each other, we will ultimately end up alone and more vulnerable because of this aloneness.

SEX TALK

Lovers never get tired of each other, because they are forever
talking about themselves.

FRANCOIS LA ROCHEFOUCAULD

Pioneer sex researchers William Masters and Virginia Johnson have
established that over one-half the couples in the United States experience
sexual problems. Most if not all of these problems are related to failures
of talk, failures to communicate with comfort, openness, and vulnerability.

One of the first couples I treated for sexual difficulties was the
quietest, most staid, reserved pair of people I had ever met. Yes or no
were long drawn-out answers for each of these people, particularly in
the area of sexuality. Discomfort was high and even yes or no was
replaced with singular head movements from side to side or up and
down. Indeed, if as much circulation of blood had occurred in their
genitals as occurred in the cheeks of their faces each time they were
asked about sex, they probably would not have needed to come to my
office at all.

Each therapy session was a struggle to collect the basic information
with which to begin making suggestions for improvement. The wife
grew frustrated with the slow pace of therapy and sent me a confidential
note. This quiet, reserved woman revealed a sharp wit, with her brief
statement of her problem:

Dear Dr. Pearsall:
My husband feels that the magic has gone out of our marriage.
He is totally wrong. Sex did a complete disappearing act years ago.
It has disappeared with a thoroughness that any magician would be
proud of.

(Signed)
The magician's assistant

We do often laugh for fear we might cry, and the humor of this
note masked a despair at the trap that this couple had fallen into, the
years of isolation and loneliness that resulted from their lack of sexual
fulfillment. It was not instruction for some type of sexual intimacy
presented by some "sexpert" that was needed by this couple, but a
course in what was for them a foreign language, the language of sex.

Sexuality is the totality of our maleness and femaleness. It is everything about us as men and women, including the masculinity and femininity within each of us. It is the reputation we have with ourselves. It includes the way in which we think, feel, and behave. It is inextricably entwined with the supersystem, for it is truly the us part of the supersystem, the part of self that goes public.

A second phrase in our sex talk system is the word "sex." One of the most important lessons of our childhood is the learning of the importance of sensuous, tender touching to our general health. Sex is one of the ways in which we express our sexuality, typically involving the erogenous zones, or areas of the body that feel good when they are touched or do the touching. We convey our sexuality through intercourse, talking, walking, writing, sitting, or just being. Sex is not something we have; it is the way we share about ourselves, the way we get in touch with others. Even though we seem forever trying to get more of it or have some of it, the it is a process of sharing and signaling about our sexuality including but not limited to our genital interactions. Having sex with someone would be like having tennis with someone. It is not consumed or accomplished. It is a process of sharing, and as I said earlier, disruption of this sharing process always results in an impact on our wellness.

Sensuality is the third part of our sex talk vocabulary. It is the part of sex that has to do with sending and receiving messages. It is our ability to mobilize the supersystem. To touch, to receive touch, to listen and be heard, to react to odors, to sense and be in tune with vibrations are all part of sensuality.

Sensuality is the movement part of the sex vocabulary. Francis Gaulton in 1884 wrote, "When two persons have an 'inclination' to one another, they visibly incline or slope together when sitting side by side." We use phrases such as falling in love, being inclined toward someone, close to someone, getting next to someone, moving together or apart. Sensuality is the ultimate communication system, for it has to do with the establishment of paired bonds, of relationships that last over time.

Sensuality Survey

To assess your sensuality, rate yourself from 0 to 10 on each of the following factors: 0 represents never, 10 always.

1. Are you aware of the texture of things in your environment, such as the steering wheel of your car, articles of clothing, the wind in your face?

    Score_____

2. Are you aware of pleasing odors and a range of odors from trees, flowers, and the aroma of air after a thunderstorm?

    Score_____

3. Are you sensitive to music, your body swaying almost involuntarily with the beat of songs, even in shopping malls, in your own car, in a waiting room?

    Score_____

4. When you share a sexual response, do you leave a soft light on or a door from an adjacent room ajar, so that light will allow you to see your partner?

    Score_____

5. Do you enjoy watching your own body in sexual experiences, perhaps watching in a mirror or glancing at shadows?

    Score_____

6. In a sexual encounter, is touching as important as sexual intercourse? Is play of value in itself and not a foreplay or a type of getting ready for the main event?

    Score_____

7. Do you hold, touch, caress, kiss, interact, and talk sexually with your partner without proceeding to actual physical sex?

    Score_____

8. Do you continue to caress and be caressed after sexual intercourse, enjoying the warmth and intimacy of the presence of another person (do you avoid the PON reflex, or the *post-o*rgasmic *n*ap, in favor of the POS, or *post-o*rgasmic *s*haring)?

    Score_____

9. Do you bathe with your partner and use lotions or oils as a part of your sexual encounters? (One of my male patients resisted this, responding to his partner's suggestion of using oils, by asking, "Are you trying to cook me or to have sex with me?)

    Score_____

10. Do you undress and redress your partner in a sexual encounter? (One of my patients described sex with her husband as "one big reverse fire drill. Clothes off, get off, get your sleep, and get to work.") Do you spend as much time dressing your partner as you do undressing him or her?

Score_____

Any less than 70 points on this test, and it is likely that much more sex talk is necessary with your partner for you have become victim to a genitalized, mechanical approach to interacting with others sexually.

In understanding more about sensuality, it may be helpful to make sure that you are treating the outside-observable parts of the supersystem with the respect it deserves. When couples talk about sex, sooner or later body shape enters the discussion. Issues regarding obesity can cause pain and block open communication. Our standards of beauty are extremely limited. They are determined, not by our own sense of self and self-worth, but by our brains constantly comparing us to commercially created images. Try now to free yourself of such images, and not think of what others expect, but answer for yourself in your own appreciation of your body. If people tend to be what we tell them they are, then our bodies, the socially advertised part of our supersystems, may be affected by how we think about them.

Take some time alone, and after a relaxing shower, stand nude in front of a full-length mirror. Lock the door, give yourself some privacy, and take a body journey. Remember, do not compare yourself to someone else's standards. How do you feel about your body?

Body Quiz

On a 0 to 10 scale, 0 stands for personally displeasing and 10 stands for personally pleased. There are two scores for each item. The second score also uses 0 to 10, with 0 standing for seems unhealthy and 10 standing for looks hardy and healthy. You will be checking your looks and your health appearance.

Appearance   *Health*

1. How do you feel about your hair, its texture, its shape, its color, its style?   Score _____   Score _____

	Appearance	Health
2. How do you feel about your eyes, their color, shape, general mood they seem to convey? (Do you see the low energy of *sanpaku* eyes mentioned earlier?)	Score _____	Score _____
3. How do you feel about your nose, mouth, ears?	Score _____	Score _____
4. How do you feel about your neck, its structure, its relationship to your body, the presence of wrinkles?	Score _____	Score _____
5. How do you feel about your shoulders, the message they convey about self-reputation?	Score _____	Score _____
6. How do you feel about your breasts? Remember, men, you have nipples too! Also remember that breasts come in more than the two sizes of too big and too small.	Score _____	Score _____
7. How do you feel about your stomach and its proportion to the rest of you, including the texture of the skin of your stomach?	Score _____	Score _____
8. How do you feel about your hips and rear end? (One of my patients complained that her rear end was in the rear because God protected her self-esteem by hiding it from her forever.)*	Score _____	Score _____

*Self-deprecating humor can mask real embarrassment about our bodies. Humor stemming from our collective mockery of our hypercritical approach to our self-images can help us remember that none of us is perfect.

	Appearance	*Health*

9. How do you feel about your legs, thighs, calves, and feet? (One patient said that she did not have thunder thighs—she had standing-ovation thighs because they clapped so loudly and consistently.)*

             Score _____   Score _____

10. How do you feel about the appearance of your genitals? If you have never done so, take a mirror and look. When you do, remember that genitals are as different as fingerprints, and the range of normal is much wider than you may imagine.

             Score _____   Score _____

Less than 70 total points in either of the two categories and you should think of providing some positive feedback and attention to the part of your body that diminishes your score the most in either category. Even if you have physical impairments or scars from major or minor surgery, it is important that you think and feel about your body constructively, appreciating its beauty. Whether or not you appear beautiful depends upon whether or not you think you are beautiful. If you disagree with this, think of times when you have met someone and noticed that they seem to become much more attractive as you learn more and more about them. Of course, people can become much more unattractive in this same way.

You will also note that healthy looks and good looks are most likely scored very close together for each subscore. Health, sexuality, positive body image, and touch are inseparable parts of an intact supersystem.

HOT AND COLD SEX

The meeting of two personalities is like the contact of two chemical substances; if there is any reaction, both are transformed.

CARL JUNG

The term "philia" is Latin for love. Without love or aside from love is the word "paraphilia." "Hypophilia" means less than love or underloved. Hot-supersystem people are characterized by paraphilia, or a sexuality of the neglect of closeness, intimacy, and caring. Too rushed to pause for caring, the hot reactor regards sex as a release, even an obligation, an expectation of self and others. Fulfilling sexuality is the capability of generating the secretion of healthy chemicals within the supersystem, a type of internal symphony of wellness. For the hot reactor, however, the symphony is a 3-minute popular song, a 45-minute record played at 78 rpm. The player wears out and the music loses its beauty.

The cold reactor experiences hypophilia, or a deficiency of love. Although the cold reactor longs for closeness, sexuality becomes a missed opportunity, a privilege for others to enjoy. The cold reactor reacts to sexuality as something from the past, with slim hopes for more of it for the future. They may find themselves sexually abused, used, or taken for granted. They may seek sexual interaction as a negotiation for closeness or remediation of the boredom that seems to dominate their lives.

The hot reactor has problems with intimacy, and seems to fear closeness as a slow encroachment on the speeding rhythm of life. The cold reactor has problems with autonomy and individuality, and fears isolation as the ultimate state of life; the end result is a protective withdrawal from sexuality because of the fears of the isolation that may follow. Both hot- and cold-supersystem people have problems with the natural role of sexuality in their lives, the roles of growth and sharing, and the affirmation of self, other, and us that can be accomplished through sex, sexuality, and sensuality.

The Hot Sex–Cold Sex Test

Man is the only animal that blushes, or needs to.
MARK TWAIN

In order to determine whether or not you are oriented toward the hot or cold style of reaction with regard to touch and sexuality, take the following test. It is important to take this test three times (this includes the hot-reacting reader who may have just panicked at the thought of all the time this may take). First, respond to each item as you yourself feel. Second, respond as you think a partner would score you. Finally, respond as how you would score a partner. Use the following scale:

1—Almost never

2—Seldom

3—Sometimes

4—Almost always

1. Do you think about touching and intimacy only after all other responsibilities and activities have been completed, settled, or put out of your mind?
   Self___ Partner's perception___ Perception of partner___

2. As a man, do you have trouble with achieving erection or controlling your ejaculation or with being unable to ejaculate?
   As a woman, do you have pain in intercourse or trouble with lubrication?
   Self___ Partner's perception___ Perception of partner___

3. Does sex seem to be the furthest thing from your mind, so that even question 2 seems inappropriate, embarrassing, shocking, or out of place?
   Self___ Partner's perception___ Perception of partner___

4. Do you masturbate or stimulate yourself sexually to relieve tension or frustration or to help you fall asleep?
   Self___ Partner's perception___ Perception of partner___

5. Did you react to questions such as item 4 with surprise, even shock, and consider masturbation childish or a sign of unhappiness and loneliness?
   Self___ Partner's perception___ Perception of partner___

6. Do you fantasize about romantic places, sunsets, palm trees, walking hand in hand on a moonlit beach with a caring, tender person?
   Self___ Partner's perception___ Perception of partner___

7. Do you prefer to cuddle after sex, to talk quietly, and to hold and be held?
Self___ Partner's perception___ Perception of partner___

8. Does pornography disgust you and seem to be a deprived expression of lust without love?
Self___ Partner's perception___ Perception of partner___

9. Do you feel more sexually aroused after you have exercised or accomplished some major project?
Self___ Partner's perception___ Perception of partner___

10. Do you feel more sexy during vacations or with a change of scenery or environment?
Self___ Partner's perception___ Perception of partner___

11. Does pornography turn you on, allowing you to identify with one of the characters?
Self___ Partner's perception___ Perception of partner___

12. Do all the sexy fashions and sexy toys on the market today seem foolish, even disgusting?
Self___ Partner's perception___ Perception of partner___

13. Do you feel sleepy after sex, experiencing what I refer to as the "beached whale phenomenon"?
Self___ Partner's perception___ Perception of partner___

14. When you see two people kissing and embracing in public, do you feel envious, stopping to take a quick and even conspicuous look?
Self___ Partner's perception___ Perception of partner___

15. Do you look at parts of people, such as their legs, breasts, and rear ends?
Self___ Partner's perception___ Perception of partner___

16. Do you cry, even a little, while watching a love scene, a play, or a movie about caring interaction between people?
Self___ Partner's perception___ Perception of partner___

17. Does your language include "sex words" several times a day, so much so that you are not even aware of it until someone points it out?
    Self___ Partner's perception___ Perception of partner___

18. Do you watch one or more soap operas regularly?
    Self___ Partner's perception___ Perception of partner___

19. Do you find a need for variety in sex by place, posture, and partner?
    Self___ Partner's perception___ Perception of partner___

20. Are you willing to exchange sex to get love, seeing an affair as a source of comfort and intimacy rather than just a sexual liaison?
    Self___ Partner's perception___ Perception of partner___

Now add up your scores. As you will see when I discuss the concept of sexual wellness, right or wrong in sexual matters is exclusively a matter of one's own morality. If no one is emotionally, physically, or spiritually hurt by your actions, the only unnatural sex act is one you cannot do. If you can do it, it is human or natural. Whether it is right or wrong is a moral decision, not just a psychological one. This test is intended only to promote discussion and attitude examination; it is not diagnostic.

There is actually a potential of six scores yielded by this test. Draw six columns on a piece of paper. At the top of each column, write the titles for "Self—Hot," "Self—Cold," "Other's Perception—Hot," "Other's Perception—Cold," "Perception of Partner—Hot," "Perception of Partner—Cold." Under each heading there will be 10 numbers, each representing a number related to the hot or cold style of sexuality. The *hot* numbers on this test are 1, 2, 4, 9, 10, 11, 13, 15, 17, and 19. Total your scores on those items, and you will have a *hot* score for self, from someone else, and how you perceive someone else. More than a total of 20 on any of these sets of numbers would indicate that you view yourself, you think your partner views you, or you view your partner as a hot reactor in terms of sex.

The *cold* numbers are 3, 5, 6, 7, 8, 12, 14, 16, 18, and 20. Over 20 points as a total of these numbers would mean that you consider you, you think your partner considers you, or you think of your partner as a cold reactor in the sexual area.

Sit down with someone and discuss the six scores, item by item. If you can do that, you have already made great progress in improving your health, for you have opened up communication channels in this vulnerable and sensitive area of human interaction. You may, however, find it very difficult to talk openly about sex. To help with this, I will look in detail at the issue of sex talk.

Hot and cold styles of thinking and feeling result in impairments in intimacy, the failure to experience fulfillment in sexual relationships. I have spent more than 15 years counseling people with sexual problems and have noted in almost every case supersystem status is related to the nature of the diagnosis of the sexual problem.

The hot-reacting male has problems with ejaculatory control, tending to ejaculate too soon for himself or his partner to be fulfilled. The cold-reacting male tends to have trouble ejaculating at all, or may not maintain his erections.

The cold-reacting woman has trouble with orgasms, unable to reach fulfillment or trust enough in self or partner to surrender fully to the orgasmic experience. The hot-reacting woman has trouble with lubrication, sometimes experiencing dryness, or even has a spontaneous tightening of the vagina called *vaginismus*, which restricts the possibility of intercourse.

Both hot and cold reactors have problems with total fulfillment in a sexual experience. During hot-reaction times when the SAM syndrome dominates, the fight or flight response is dominant. This premature and overwhelming discharge of hormones is related to the anxiety, fear, and guilt associated with the hot-reaction syndrome. Anxiety relates to the impatience and rush past intimacy that is characteristic of this type of thinking. The fear rests with the loss of self, of getting too close, of losing the baton used to accelerate the rhythm of the symphony. The guilt comes from the inner sense that even at the most intimate of human moments the hot reactor is somehow not really involved, not really there.

The cold reactor is characterized by the PAC system domination and a pattern of withdrawal and depression of secretion of hormones. This is related to the emotional states of anger, disgust, and ambivalence. The anger is an ubiquitous and strong sense that true sharing seems beyond the cold reactor's grasp. The disgust is at self and other for failure to really merge through an emotional and physical exchange, for the negotiation of love seems to result in a loss of that love, a sense of emptiness. The ambivalence comes from the awareness that this most special of human moments is somehow removed from the possibility of continued generation of intimacy, a feeling of being used instead of the comfort of sharing.

Healthy sexuality involves the opposite emotions from those accompanying hot and cold reactions. Anxiety should be replaced by comfort. Fear should be replaced by an ultimate sense of safety and security. Guilt should be replaced by a sense of giving and taking balanced with personal needs and awareness of the needs of others. Anger should be replaced by joy and the intimacy of life. Disgust should be replaced by rejuvenation and enhancement of self-esteem growing from deep and meaningful interaction with another person. Ambivalence should be replaced by a confidence and assuredness that sexuality is a form of confirmation of humanness, of a merging of self with other and the establishment of an us that transcends the immediacy of the genital interaction.

Sexuality is the most intimate of tests of style of the supersystem. It is ironic that hot reactors end up having cold, meaningless sex and that cold reactors end up experiencing hot sex that displeases, alienates, and separates them from their need for closeness. What is needed is a sexuality that generates a temperature from the interaction of two people themselves, a mixture of cooling and heating that is more than the individual temperatures brought to the act by the players. As when boiling water is combined with cold water, the result can be a pleasant new temperature of water yielded by the new combination of supersystems.

QUANTUM SEXUALITY

Personal relations are the important things forever and ever.
                                        E. M. FORSTER

Timeless Sexuality

Both hot and cold reactors view sex as being bound by time. The hot reactor is done quickly, having had it "better before" or getting it "better later." The cold reactor longs for a past sex, fantasizing for "the way it was before" or "the way it seems it could be" if based on some soap opera or romantic novel. These are both linear concepts of time. The more unity-oriented, nonlinear view of time I discussed earlier suggests sexuality free from hours, second hands, and timed orgasms. There is no *fore*play in a time frame for love in which there is no before or after, only the now. How many times a day, week, or month becomes a meaningless question in a view of time that has no such reference points. Planned sex, arranged affairs, and quickies are replaced by a sense of each other instead of the clock. The point is not only making sure that there is no time measurement instrument nearby during a sexual encounter that serves as a ticking parking meter of parceled-out intimacy, but also freeing ourselves from our internal timing devices by joining with someone else.

Some people are industrial lovers. They are on the night shift, making love only at bedtime; indeed, they *make* love instead of experiencing each other. They tend to count orgasms and sexual experiences as if paid on some type of sexual merit plan. They may find themselves "laid off" with long periods of sexual deprivation, alienation, and loneliness. They may even lose their jobs to someone else better able to meet the requirements of the activity. Endocrinologists and others who study our hormones know that late morning and the afternoon are the times when our sex hormones are at their highest levels. Although sex is far more than our hormones, the only reason people relate sexually at night seems to be because that is when they *make time* for it. This is when we take time to make time to make it. Even such terms as premature ejaculation suggest that there is such a thing as a mature ejaculation. Failure to experience orgasm means only that time and maybe even your partner "ran out."

Every diagnosis of sexual dysfunction is bound by time, including failure to have orgasm within a given time frame, failure to maintain an erection long enough, failure to respond in the expected time limit, and the inability to have sexual desire often enough, frequently enough, or long enough. Concepts of beginning and ending of the sexual encounter, phases of the sexual response from excitement, through plateau to orgasm, to resolution or resting phase, tend to divide the sexual relationship into a four-quartered athletic event. The end of the event may even resemble the hurry-up offense of professional sports.

Researchers use the term *sexual cycle* as a framework for sexual interaction. One assignment I give my patients is to have intercourse "backwards." That is, rest, sleep, rest again, touch, cuddle, have intercourse, then have what is called foreplay, dress one another, go out the door, go on a date, and become more familiar with one another as if meeting for the first time. I call this the *sutioc* technique ("coitus" spelled backwards), and I use it to point out the time limitations and other artificialities of our sexual intimacy.

Books on sexuality have been so popular that most of my patients are keenly aware of the Masters and Johnson sex cycle of arousal, plateau, orgasm, and resolution. To help them rethink their time limitations to their sexuality, I suggest they score themselves on this 10-phase model. How do you ''score''?

	Not Very Much	*A Lot*

1. DESIRE   0 -1 -2 -3 -4 -5 -6 -7 -8 -9 -10

This relates simply to the number of times one has a sexual encounter. It has nothing to do with wishes, wants, or motivation. It is simply a frequency count.

2. INTEREST   0 -1 -2 -3 -4 -5 -6 -7 -8 -9 -10

This is our cognition, our thinking about sex. It is possible to think a great deal about sex yet have a low desire (frequency) or to have high desire and not think about sexuality a great deal.

3. AROUSAL   0 -1 -2 -3 -4 -5 -6 -7 -8 -9 -10

This is our emotional reaction to the interest phase. Some people become aroused as they think about sex. Other people experience a problem at this phase, and this can become a focus for discussion in enhancing sexuality. This may be seen as your HQ, or your happiness quotient.

4. READINESS   0 -1 -2 -3 -4 -5 -6 -7 -8 -9 -10

This is the actual response of the body system, the erection of the penis, the lubrication of the vagina, the hardening of the nipples, the tensing of muscles, the engorgement of vessels in the pelvis, the development of a sex flush in the cheeks and upper chest. Some people have a difficulty with the connection between readiness and arousal, and by viewing the phases I am presenting here, partners can have an open discussion between themselves within a framework that does not follow a biological clock but allows for variations in desire, interest, arousal, and readiness.

5. EXCITEMENT   0 -1 -2 -3 -4 -5 -6 -7 -8 -9 -10

Excitement is the emotional reaction to readiness. This is being in touch with the body, experiencing a sense of joy and celebration at the changes taking place. Some people also experience a difficulty at this phase of the sexual cycle, and various opportunities can be shared by the couple to learn to tune in more fully to the body's readiness.

6. PHYSIOLOGICAL ORGASM   0 -1 -2 -3 -4 -5 -6 -7 -8 -9 -10

Although essentially orgasm is a release of tension accompanied by muscular contractions, some people are unaware of the nature of this response and the various types of orgasm possible. Education along these lines can be most helpful.

7. PSYCHOLOGICAL ORGASM   0 -1 -2 -3 -4 -5 -6 -7 -8 -9 -10

Psychological orgasm is one of the most controversial concepts for my patients. It is likely that more men than women have difficulty with orgasm, for they mistake their physiological orgasm for a psychological experience. Essentially, orgasm is the ultimate freedom from time, a sense of merging with another. It is an ultimate manifestation of wellness, for it involves the body, the mind, the spirit, and truly merging with "other," a transcendence of space and time.

8. REFRACTORY PERIOD   0 -1 -2 -3 -4 -5 -6 -7 -8 -9 -10

This is a physiological period during which both men and women may feel the need just to lie still and not experience any additional physical input from partner. This can also be a period of timelessness. Although it is important to share this phase of the cycle, most couples seem to skip or see it as unnecessary, an imposed time out, instead of a timeless *in*.

9. AFTERGLOW   0 -1 -2 -3 -4 -5 -6 -7 -8 -9 -10

Afterglow is a period during which the entire experience can be relived verbally and mentally by the partners. Many partners are so rushed by the time concept that they skip the afterglow period, either returning to more sex, dressing, or falling asleep.

10. SATISFACTION   0 -1 -2 -3 -4 -5 -6 -7 -8 -9 -10

It is a sad comment on sexuality research that the word "satisfaction" has been absent from most sexuality textbooks. Most researchers seem to assume that if people engage in a sexual encounter, they must be satisfied. This again is a time concept; something happening within a time frame between two people is supposed to mean that its success and significance is obvious, a foregone conclusion. Feeling enhanced by a sexual experience is what is meant by satisfaction.

A score over 70 generally indicates effective, sensuous, sexual communication, a balance between hot and cold orientations. A score of less means that you need more balance, that you need to spend more time communicating intimately.

Think of sexuality without a beginning or an end, without foreplay, without turn taking, without accomplishment, goal, fulfillment, or completion. Think of the sexuality of interaction in the now without an end, but governed only by the interaction between two persons, their needs and respect for one another, their own communication. Think of sexuality that is a part of our lives instead of an afterthought, allowable only after meeting our other daily obligations. Think of sexuality acknowledged by society as natural and beautiful, something people do in privacy to protect their own dignity, not in secrecy to hide their basic humanness. Think of sexuality as an option, including within it the option of celibacy, that is, not a time-constrained sacrifice but a choice by some people within their lifestyles.

Non-Euclidean Sex

The sex of hot and cold people is a measured sex, a sex compared against the standard of an ideal partner, the perfect fantasy, or a living up to expert advice in some reference book or popular talk show. The advice of sex therapists has taught us to count the brush strokes of a fine oil painting instead of appreciating the painting itself.

Euclidean geometry is a geometry of lines, proofs, and limits. To impose such measurements on our intimate lives is to do injustice to our humanness. Size of genitals, size of breasts, height, weight, attractiveness, and ugliness are all discussed as if they were absolutes and actually existed, just as Euclidean geometry made the mistake of equating number with reality. Perceptions of the sexual encounter which are free of imposed standards and expectations are those encounters most likely to lead to joy, growth, and a sense of well-being, not some goal of "good sex."

Discussion of postures are often represented as a geometry of love in some textbooks which may lead us to a form of sexual break dancing, with postures assumed much as theorems in some geometry equation leading to proofs of fulfillment. Imagine the first reports from the space shuttle of the new "astronaut's gravity-free posture." Who will be on top in an outer space in which concepts of time and position have no meaning?

SELFISH SEX

Giving the gift of self, sharing one's own fears and hopes, is the most constructive avenue to sexual fulfillment. Rather than guessing at the needs of another, it is better to share your own needs and hope that such sharing sets the model for others to follow.

"If he really loved me, he would know what to do and know how to please me. If I have to tell him, he probably doesn't love me at all." This is a common statement heard from many of my patients. In fact, if you truly do love, you would not allow for guessing or testing of love by waiting for behavioral evidence. You would guide, ask, show, and teach. If you have ever had your back scratched, only you know exactly the magical spot that rewards you with the response, "Ahh, right there." So it is with sexuality. A test of your willingness or ability to give the gift of self and to enjoy the wellness that comes through such giving can lead to a discussion between yourself and your partner.

The 10 T's Test

Using our 0 to 10 scale again, 0 meaning never and 10 meaning always, respond to the following items.

1. TALK
   Do you talk during a sexual relationship, sharing your needs and conveying your satisfaction? Would a tape recording of your bedroom behavior be full of discussions and talks, moans and groans, or a blank tape punctuated by an occasional murmur or sigh?

   Score_____

2. TOUCH

   Do you touch and promote touching? Do you touch all over the body, not just places you consider erogenous zones?

   Score_____

3. TENDER

   Are you gentle, caring, careful, and alert to yourself and your partner during a sexual interaction? It may be possible to be too soft or too gentle but not too tender or alert to feedback from your partner.

   Score_____

4. TEASE

   Do you allow for an ebb and flow, a buildup and return, a stop-start technique, or do you proceed on a step-by-step cyclical process toward an end point? Are you able to stop, start, stop, and start again?

   Score_____

5. TOTAL

   Do you interact with your partner as a person, not a gender? Do you focus on every aspect of him or her as a person, not just as a body part?

   Score_____

6. THOROUGHNESS

   Are you aware of feedback from your partner? Are you aware of your partner's needs, not just as a sexual being but as a person in his or her own world? Thoroughness implies a full awareness of the person, an awareness of his or her sexuality, his or her experiences in life. In this orientation we do not do sex to or for someone, but always with them.

   Score_____

7. TIMING

   Are you free from trying to match responses, attempting mutuality, always following a turn-taking scheme? Does there seem to be a natural give and take, rather than a planned system for trying to last, holding back, getting ready, preparing someone else?

   Score_____

8. TRUSTING

Are you confident with your partner, and do you work toward enhancing the trust in your partner? I talked with two of my medical students, and one student said disappointingly to the other, "You told me you loved me once." His woman friend responded, "I did, and that was the once." The absence of mutual trust between these two "lovers" was apparent.

Score_____

9. TENSENESS

Although it may sound paradoxical, a mutually fulfilling sexuality depends upon enhancing the circulation and muscle tension within the body, the readiness phase we talked about earlier. As Victor Frankel once pointed out, "What is to give light must experience burning." Are you aware of a buildup of tension, of a constructive tension enjoyable through the trust that mutual communication will relieve the tension?

Score_____

10. TEACH

Do you continue to teach your partner during your sexual interactions? Do you avoid patterning and setting of achievement-oriented tasks so that each new sexual encounter is a new learning experience, not a turn-taking reenactment?

Score_____

Once again, under 70 points and considerable effort toward improvement is needed in the areas discussed above.

Quantum sexuality has to do with sharing self. I have emphasized the dangers of an immune system overly prepared to shut out all "others." Sexuality provides the single most profound opportunity to thrive beyond self, to teach the supersystem to accept as well as reject, to join as well as repel.

If a partner is not available, the importance of touch dictates that touching yourself and being comfortable with your own body are still necessary for your wellness. Unless your morality system excludes it, autoerotism can be a significant contribution to a healthy sexuality. Too often, physicians fail to discuss the importance of self-touch, somehow viewing such behavior as degrading or immature. Evidence is clear that pleasuring self is one of the most significant gifts you can give yourself. Those people who can love and admire themselves are more able to touch and be touched, to admire and be admired by others. It would seem that our society tolerates "musturbation" much more than it tolerates masturbation. Sexual wellness and total wellness depend on acceptance and pleasure with self and others.

TOWARD SEXUAL WELLNESS

I believe the greatest gift I can conceive of having from anyone is to be seen by them, heard by them, to be understood and touched by them.

VIRGINIA SATIR

Sexual wellness is an ability. It is the ability to take responsibility for self and to share that responsibility with a partner of choice, in a manner congruent with one's chosen lifestyle. This same definition applies to the attainment of general wellness. Rather than being a victim of your supersystem, you must assume control over that system lest its effort to prevent invasion will lead it to attack that which it is designed to defend. The best sex education is an education for a personally responsible life, one of sharing, of giving, of a sense of us, a sense of altruism, not just an exchange of skin contact that our modern-day society considers sex.

I use a cartoon in my lectures that shows a pencil sketch of a little boy standing on the shoulders of a little girl. Both are naked and both look perplexed. The confused face of the little girl looks out at the audience. The boy looks out at the audience in equal confusion and wonders out loud, "Well, I took my clothes off. You took your clothes off. I got on top of you. How soon till it starts to feel good?" The answer is that it starts to feel good when we take charge of our supersystems, when we realize and behave as if sexuality was not a series of acrobatic postures and maneuvers, but the ultimate means of combining supersystems.

A second slide shows the same posture of the little boy standing on the head of the little girl. The girl's response to the boy's wondering as to when it starts to feel good is, "I don't know, but now I know why mommy gets a headache." I use this slide to illustrate that actual physical symptoms result from sexual frustrations, from the pressures not only of this cartoon figure standing on the head of another but the pressures of lack of intimacy, lack of a sense of being with another. In almost 20 years of working in hospitals, I have never seen a patient who did not also share problems in the sexual dimension of his life. In this same period, I have never seen patients who have not been helped by attending to the sexual dimensions of their lives as a strengthening factor in the rallying of their immune systems. The healing touch is not speculation, but fact.

Returning to the couple I described at the beginning of this chapter, their 1-year follow-up visit to the clinic revealed that significant gains had been made. The wife responded when I inquired about her orgasmic status, "I'm not uniorgasmic or even multiorgasmic; I guess I'm sort of omniorgasmic." Her husband laughed with her and stated, "What we mean is that we have both stopped trying to 'come' and are trying instead just to be. The magic in our marriage now is that we seem to actually have become part of each other."

If unity and intimacy are key components of wellness and super-immunity, there are concepts thousands of years old that can also be resurrected in favor of our immunity. The next chapter describes some ancient principles of healthy living stated in modern-day terms. They are principles common to all major religions and only now being re-discovered by modern psychology that form a psychology that goes beyond behaviorism, psychoanalysis, even humanism, to a transpersonal and transcendent psychology of daily living.

Chapter Sixteen

BEYOND HEALTH: THE SUPER SUPERSYSTEM

The known is finite, the unknown infinite; intellectually we
stand on an islet in the midst of a illimitable ocean of ex-
plicability. Our business in every generation is to reclaim a
little more land.

ALDOUS HUXLEY

The world partly . . . comes to be how it is imagined.

GREGORY BATESON

Psychologist Abraham Maslow once stated, "If you deliberately plan
to be less than you are capable of being, then I warn you that you'll be
deeply unhappy for the rest of your life." Dr. Maslow called our failure,
even fear, to be all that we can be the *Jonah complex*. As Jonah fearfully
fled the presence of the Lord, we sometimes fail to realize that life is
much more than just coping, just avoiding illness, more than preventive
medicine. We are capable of a level of health that somehow seems to
frighten us as Jonah was afraid of his potential. We can practice enhancing medicine and extend the capacities of our supersystems beyond
survival and protection to growth and transcendence.

This chapter is about some ways we can learn to be *super well*, to
bolster our immune system to new levels of efficiency and, by so doing,
enjoy being very, very well. The description "hale and hearty" is

seldom used now by doctors. More often we are "without symptoms," free of positive results on tests to detect illness, or, heaven forbid, as "sound as a dollar." How many tests for the presence of super wellness are on the shelves of drugstores, as compared to the tests for covert signs of disease?

In this chapter, I share a few examples of some unusual ways in which you can enhance your immune system by promoting more positive emotional states, by developing more positive imagery, and by looking back thousands of years for some ideas that have a new meaning and context for today's lifestyle. The focus throughout will not be on avoiding sickness but allowing ourselves to be free of the Jonah complex, for wellness depends on how we are, not just what we do. The speed of healing of surgical wounds in the immediate postoperative period is much more rapid for those patients who showed faith, trust, and confidence in their doctors, nurses, and themselves. A careful study by Dr. Jerome Frank, at the Johns Hopkins Medical School, showed this relationship between how a person is and how fast he or she heals. This chapter is about some ways of being that may promote a super supersystem.

A WARM HEART AND COOL HEAD

A merry heart doeth good like a medicine; but a broken spirit
drieth the bones.
                          KING SOLOMON, PROVERBS 17:22

You have read about 80 ways to be a liver. Your reaction to life is volitional before it is emotional, and the style of cognition illustrated in the 80 suggestions is achieved by a gradual reprogramming, an alteration of the information supplied to the brain, a continual reviewing process.

I have pointed out throughout this book that there is no such thing as Type A vulnerability to disease, infection-prone people, or cancer-prone people, but rather styles of thinking and feeling that relate to immunosuppression or immunoaggravation, hot and cold styles of immunity resulting in our failure to "be," to live in a state of just right, a life of balance. The research listed in the reference section of this book documents the fact that links between the emotions and illness are never simple. We are just beginning to learn about the subtle, complex processes influencing our wellness.

The *New England Journal of Medicine* recently contained a detailed project by Dr. Robert Case of St. Luke's Roosevelt Hospital in New York. He has discovered that the demoralized or joylessly striving person who is cynical about life is actually more vulnerable to heart disease than the so-called Type A personality. He found that it may not be Type A behavior but a cluster of thoughts and emotions that can alter the immune system and cause it to overmobilize or demobilize.

George Solomon, at the University of California in San Francisco, has reviewed 93 research projects in a recent issue of the new journal *Advances*. He hypothesizes that autoimmune disease (or the attacking of the body by its own immune system), rheumatoid arthritis, cancer, and other cold-reactor diseases are related to such personality factors as self-sacrifice, compliance, subservience, depression, withdrawal from assertiveness, and even left-handedness (which relates to the right-hemisphere dominance of the cold reaction). His review suggests that it is not personality style but immunity style affected by thinking and emotions that relates to disease vulnerability.

But what about the positive emotions? First of all, it is important to remember that positive emotions are not just the pleasant emotions. We have already learned that appropriate anger and assertiveness can help mobilize and direct the immune system. Positive emotions are those that maximize the supersystem's capacity to function in the day-to-day world. Thinking clearly and rationally and taking control of the head can result in positive "just right" emotions.

Dr. Naomi Remen at the Soybrook Institute and Dr. Paul Eckman of the University of California at San Francisco have shown that our emotions actually last less than 10 seconds and usually not more than 4 seconds. While our moods can last for hours and even days and our traits can last months or a lifetime, it is our emotions, these little spurts of affect, which can help or hinder our immune system most dramatically and immediately.

Remember that I have suggested that the immune system can be an angry, edgy, protective system in close allegiance with the selfish brain attempting to maintain its own information flow at all costs. Dr. Nicholas Hall of George Washington Medical Center in Washington, D.C., has demonstrated that cancer patients who practice positive imagery, similar to the self-shaman technique illustrated earlier, actually increase the level of lymphocytes, or fighter cells, to combat disease. These people also experience an increase in the level of hormone produced by the thymus gland (the gland so crucial to our immune system in its production of T cells and other immunity factors). This hormone, called *thymosin-alpha-1*, not only facilitates the functioning of our supersystems in the production of T cells and T helper cells but causes a sense of well-being when it is secreted. Since we know that this thymosin is important in our immunity and that practitioners of transcendental meditation show a rise in this hormone, we are beginning to learn how imagery and a positive emotional state can make us and keep us well.

I suggest that positive imagery—whether the self-shaman exercise, the return to a womblike healing darkness technique utilized by Dr. Remen, a technique suggesting images such as "powerful sharks destroying weak germs," or good white cells eating up bad cancer cells —actually provides an instruction manual for the immune system. Perhaps a combative, aggressive, assertive imagery will help with diseases such as rheumatoid arthritis, autoimmune disease, and cancer, while the more peaceful imagery of a quiet stream, healing womb, or warm campfire will help with the immunoaggravated supersystem of the hot reactor. In either case, the self-shaman imagery suggested will provide clues as to forming an imagery program suited to your own immune-system style.

People who are out of touch with or unaware of their emotions and have trouble accepting particularly negative emotions are more prone to the cold diseases. They tend to suffer from something called *alexithymia*, or the inability to find words to express feelings. Hot reactors may suffer more from a form of *hyperthymia*, or the expression of an overbombardment of emotions, too much aggressiveness and assertiveness. As we have learned, the task is to bring things into balance, to provide a map for the immune system by freeing ourselves from the innate anger and selfishness of the brain and immunity system itself.

We know that the left hemisphere of the brain deals with the so-called positive emotions such as joy and love. The right hemisphere deals with the negative emotions of depression and sadness. Dr. Pierre Flor-Henry of the University of Alberta in Edmonton, Canada, has presented evidence supporting this lateralization of emotions. By administering barbiturates, he sedated and thus blocked one of the brain's hemispheres, and was able to determine that the left hemisphere has to do with the positive emotions of joy and love and the right hemisphere has more to do with the depression and despair emotions. This left-love, right-rotten relationship may relate to the hot reactor's deceptive euphoria and typically left-hemisphere-Apollonian cognitive style. The cold reactor's depression and despair may relate to the Dionysian right-hemisphere style.

This book is about the fact that we are not victims but masters of our supersystem. If we understand the preliminary findings about the supersystem as discussed in this book, we can begin to do something to protect and enhance our health, even though all the evidence is far from in. This book is an attempt to share in summary form a preliminary report so that all of us can benefit from findings that may alter the way we view wellness, illness, and healing. As an example of one way we can control our supersystem, I offer the following test.

Double-Dozen Emotion Test

Complete this test without stopping to think about each item. Beside each emotion on the list, put a check if you have felt that emotion in the last week. Remember, we need *all* emotions for a full life.

Dis-ease	*Ease*
1. _____ Fear	1. _____ Love
2. _____ Dread	2. _____ Joy
3. _____ Disappointment	3. _____ Acceptance
4. _____ Sadness	4. _____ Eagerness
5. _____ Disgust	5. _____ Titillation
6. _____ Contempt	6. _____ Pride
7. _____ Anger	7. _____ Anticipation
8. _____ Vulnerability	8. _____ Celebration
9. _____ Remorse	9. _____ Surprise
10. _____ Repulsion	10. _____ Awe
11. _____ Grief	11. _____ Optimism
12. _____ Despair	12. _____ Caring
_____ Total	_____ Total

Scoring Directions for Double-Dozen Emotion Test

Count the number of checks you have in the "Dis-ease" column and the number of checks you have in the "Ease" column. If you have more checks in the "Dis-ease" column, it is likely that you are vulnerable to illness, for these are the general emotions related to the invasion from inner space I have been talking about. If you have more checks in the "Ease" column, then your immune system is likely to be stronger. If the checks are about equal, then you are probably similar to most people in our society in that you are not well but not ill either. Instead, you may be in the long, lingering, and vague process of not feeling too good.

If, under the "Dis-ease" column, you had checks next to numbers 1, 2, 3, 5, 6, and 7, you are more vulnerable to the diseases of the hot supersystem. If your checks were by 4, 8, 9, 10, 11, and 12, you are more vulnerable to diseases of the cold supersystem. Checks anywhere on the "Ease" column are good for you and for all of us. It is a comment on our cosmopolitan medicine to know that the feelings in the "Dis-ease" column are typical of patients in hospitals, for very few of the emotions from the "Ease" column are elicited by a stay in our modern health care system. As Norman Cousins has said, "Much grief results from the physicians dealing with patients as if they were things."

Our emotions are constantly changing from the emotions of ease to dis-ease. Remember, also, that illness and injury can lead to the emotions of dis-ease as well as dis-ease emotions can lead to illness. The issue of being well is not a linear direct cause-and-effect relationship, but an exceedingly complex system of interactions, of checks and balances, of ease and dis-ease.

The 80 suggestions presented earlier are attempts to elicit the ease emotions. Dr. James Henry of Loma Linda University has researched the specific hormonal changes that accompany positive and negative emotions. He has shown that shifts from feelings of security to feelings of helplessness are accompanied by rises in the adrenal corticoids in one's blood, or activation of the PAC system. The shift from social success to social failure can cause a drop in levels of the *gonadotropins* in the blood, which are hormones related to reproduction and parenting drives. His work, and the work of many others, has suggested that the last decade's focus on stress and negative emotions and their impact on health has neglected the significance of positive emotions which can prevent illness by offsetting negative consequences of behavioral change and strain on the body system.

In our efforts to be scientific and objective, we have neglected some of the more subtle, difficult areas of study, such as altered states of consciousness and high-level well-being. Psychologist Joseph Royce has said, "The most important issues go begging. I have a rough rule of thumb which says the more important the problem, the less we know about it." We have failed to study exceptional health. Our cosmopolitan medicine is based on an illness model and the study of the sick. Dr. Roger Walsh and Dr. Deane H. Shapiro ask, "Are we all that we can be? Or are there greater heights and depths of psychological capacity within us, undreamed of by most, glimpsed by some, and nurtured and brought to fruition by but a few?" As Louis Mumford has said, "Every transformation of man has rested on a new picture of the cosmos and the nature of man." Recognizing the relevance of emotion to our health requires such a new picture of our own nature.

THE SNIFF, SPURT, SIP, AND SWITCH TECHNIQUES: CREATIVE IMMUNITY

Each dream contains images which we literally did not conceive that we could conceive.

DAVID FOULKES

As an example of the application of some preliminary findings regarding the supersystem, here are four techniques you can practice today. I cannot prove they work, but I can promise they will give you an emotional boost, and that's nothing to sniff at.

Technique 1: The Sniff Technique

Dr. David Shlannahoff-Khkalsa of the Salk Institute has shown that a 90-minute cycle exists in a type of cerebral swaying from right to left. The hypothalamus, the brain of the brain, allows one hemisphere to dominate for about 90 minutes and then the other hemisphere takes over. Hot and cold reactors tend to allow this swaying to get out of sequence and the oscillation of mind rhythm becomes disrupted.

Dr. Shlannahoff-Khkalsa's research has shown that constriction or dilation of vessels within the nostrils gives evidence of this swaying: The SAM system, or activating arm of the nervous system, causes the right nostril to allow more air to enter for a period of time, and then the PAC system, or relaxing arm of the nervous system, causes the left nostril to allow more air to pass. Right-nostril breathing relates to more rational, logical thinking and more positive emotional states, while left-nostril breathing relates to imagery, spontaneity, and more negative emotional states. By blocking one nostril, you may actually alter your thoughts and emotional state over time.

Technique 2: The Spurt Technique

Many feel that emotions are typically less than 10 seconds in duration. The research of Dr. Paul Ekman demonstrates the relevance of this theory. His research on more than 200 different kinds of smiles shows that a person can actually alter his or her feeling state and immuno-efficiency by putting on a happy (or sad) face. When research subjects were trained to control their facial muscles and to form smiles voluntarily, their physiologies immediately changed and hormones circulating through their bodies altered drastically.

The "spurt technique" suggests that if our emotions are only seconds long, we can provide some emotional insurance for ourselves. Whether you feel like it or not, place your facial muscles in the smile position for 4 to 10 seconds as many times a day as possible. By doing this, you have actually altered your blood chemistry. The natural opiates in your system and the so-called neuropeptides also change. These opiates and neuropeptides are located not only in your brain but in your stomach and intestines as well, and the amount of these neuropeptides is increased by smiling. Perhaps this is why belly laughing feels so good.

To test the belly laugh theory, lay down on the floor with members of your family or a few very close friends. Have each person rest her or his head on another person's lower abdomen, and have one person begin to laugh. Use the phoniness-first principle if you have to. Laugh whether you feel like it or not. You will notice that the laughter immediately becomes contagious. You will feel better, and you will see that you do not need some poppy from Mesopotamia to "get high."

Technique 3: The Sip Technique

Dr. Aaron Ettenberg of the University of California has shown that being rewarded in today's society is dependent upon neurotransmitters, the brain chemicals described earlier. One specific chemical, called *dopamine*, is particularly related to the response to reward or positive signals from our environment. If drugs are used to switch off the dopamine system and lower the amount of dopamine in the brain, positive reinforcements do not work their "good stroke" effect. Recent research suggests that alcoholics and other persons who abuse drugs have reduced levels of dopamine and endorphins, the pleasure chemicals of the supersystem. For this reason, make sure you limit your intake of alcohol significantly, for drinking too much can lower your pleasure chemicals. Try sipping instead of gulping for a month, and you may find that things improve noticeably.

Technique 4: The Switch Technique

Researchers at the University of Texas are studying differences in gender and immunity function. They have discovered that women, due to their higher levels of estrogen, produce fewer T suppressor cells, the cells that help control the level of immune response as described earlier. While this helps women to be more resistant than men to many diseases, it also may make them more vulnerable to autoimmune disease as the immune system turns against itself, a finding that is now well documented.

Men, on the other hand, produce more testosterone, which causes an increase in T suppressor cells. This may leave the male more open to disease through a weakened immune system.

Since we know that thoughts can affect the brain and that the brain controls the hormones, perhaps a "switch" of thinking style periodically, attempting to think "like a man" or "like a woman," may balance the immune system. Manfred Porkert in his book *The Theoretical Foundations of Chinese Medicine* discusses the archetypical poles, the yin and yang that the Chinese believe underly the fundamental rhythm of the universe. Perhaps thinking like a man and thinking like a woman really relate to the constant flow of transformation and change, a movement back and forth between thoughts of nurturance, symbolism, freedom, and creativity and thoughts that are more abstract, concrete, and rational. Neither of these two states is better than the other; rather, they are both natural parts of a whole. Perhaps a new "androgyny" of thinking beyond our limited definitions of gender is a more healthy orientation to life.

2500-YEAR-OLD NEW IDEAS

To study Buddhism is to study the self.
To study the self is to forget the self.
To forget the self is to be one with others.
ZEN MASTER DOGEN

Historian Arnold Toynbee remarked that he considered the introduction of the principles of Buddhism to western cultures to be one of the most significant events of our time. Concepts such as altered states of consciousness, meditation, cognitive behavioral modification, state-dependent learning, mental training, ethicality, self-mastery, and commitment now fill the journals of modern psychology and psychiatry. These are all concepts that are hundreds of years old. I have restated some of these ancient principles to help you develop self-pledges regarding the possibility of enhancing your own immunity, for they all relate to beliefs, attitudes, and feelings.

Modern scientific thinking is evolving along lines very close to those established by ancient mystics and many of our most traditional cultures. These ancient ways of thinking saw mind and body as united and the practice of healing as a natural part of spiritual development. Chinese medicine has always stressed that all illness is related to the disruption of the natural flow of life energy and that teaching persons to restore that flow is central to holistic health. I have selected twelve concepts from eastern ways of thinking, Chinese medicine, and other historical conceptual frameworks and translated them to modern western psychological terminology in the hope that some of the ancient lessons have applicability to the enhancement of the immune system, and the strengthening of the B-A-FITER system.

1. Communication

The modern-day teacher Michael Jackson sang, "You've got to be startin' something." In terms of communication, the first rule is to begin.

You cannot wait for someone else. You must reach out, take a chance, and be vulnerable immediately.

Never respond to someone's statements about their feelings until you repeat that statement, reiterating it with sensitivity and feedback in regard to their emotions, not just their words.

Speak for yourself. Use "I" language: "I love," "I need," not "Do you want," "Would you like." Give the gift of self. Many angry moments are sadly related to failed attempts to please someone else. All ancient philosophers stress the importance of interpersonal exchange.

Set aside 15 minutes a day—just 15 minutes—using a timer if you have to, for some quiet discussion with someone. Sit comfortably and talk, not about work, kids, family, health, or problems, but about life, its meaning, the cosmos. Avoid *SSAADD* language: *s*arcasm, *s*urrender, *a*ssumption, *a*ccusation, *d*emands, and *d*emeaning statements. These communication errors always cause trouble in relationships.

You have learned that the brain is starving for input of information. Communication is a constructive way of feeding the brain. Without communication the brain will begin to talk to itself, causing problems in the body.

When I assign this 15-minute opportunity to my patients, they often report that they cannot find 15 minutes "just to talk." If they do find the time, the discussions become problematic, sometimes resulting in arguments. We are not used to talking *with* one another, but *to* and *about* each other. Through effective communication we merge with one another, we engage in meaningful intercourse.

Psychology principle 1: Research in modern-day psychiatry and psychology clearly indicates that the ability to speak for self, to listen effectively and with empathy, is one of the distinguishing traits of a person in good physical and mental health.

2. Vegetation

The market is flooded with books on exercise and diet. Most of them contain valid information. Keep moving and stretching; move intensely for short periods of time (about 20 minutes each period) at least every other day. Eat in moderation and avoid toxic substances. If you burn off more than you eat, you cannot gain weight. In spite of the variety of warnings presented in self-help books, these principles remain the one common thread that can be found in most books regarding our daily habits. They are also recommendations that are thousands of years old. We have been warned for years to avoid what I call the *CSSTAMM* products: *c*affeine, *s*ugar, *s*alt, *t*obacco, *a*lcohol, red *m*eat, and *m*ilk and dairy products. Increase fiber, reduce fats, and eat a rainbow, that is, foods in a variety of colors and textures. You are less likely to develop allergies or reactions to foods if you change the types of foods you eat in keeping with the above system. Fasting and other nutritional techniques have long been a part of ancient philosophies.

We know that food allergies or reactions to various foods do exist. Such reactions may account for a high percentage of hyperactivity and learning problems in children and adults and for the irritability and emotional states that can accompany this syndrome. Altering the food you eat is one way to avoid such problems.

The problem with all this material on vegetation is that most people do not follow this advice. We may read of a rat dying in a laboratory somewhere, and our diets are supposed to change in accordance with some proposed "rat-killing factor" determined by researchers. We have become suspicious, thinking "Oh well, who knows what they will find next. I might as well eat anything I want." One of my patients told me, "Next they are going to find that small amounts of saliva swallowed gradually over a lifetime can cause cancer. What the heck can you do about it anyway?"

What we have done about it is tended to turn to medications for our ills. As a test, go to your closet or medicine cabinet and count the different contents inside. These medications have been designed to accomplish what your body is supposed to do naturally. Whenever possible, it is wiser to make lifestyle changes than to take medications. Avoiding salt is better than taking a water pill. Exercising and relaxing are better for high blood pressure than eventually having to rely on medications with their serious side effects. Reducing weight can help significantly in some cases of diabetes.

Get rid of your bottles and drugs. More than 90 percent of the more than 1½ billion prescriptions written each year in this country are optional or unnecessary. There are now eight prescriptions for every man, woman, and child in the United States. For the elderly, the figure is likely to be much higher. In effect, we are putting sublethal dosages of lethal substances in our bodies to regulate what we should be able to regulate naturally if we could only take control of our brains.

Another recommendation under the vegetation concept is to go to sleep at the same time and awake at the same time, seven days a week.

There is a rhythm to the supersystem, and that rhythm, when disrupted, can cause problems for the efficiency of the supersystem.

We do not have to wait for more research to substantiate the above recommendations. We know it is important to eat slowly, without conflict or stress; to exercise regularly, but not to the point of ruining your enjoyment of that activity; to sleep consistently, in a pattern, at least 6 hours a day, but not more than 10. Sleeping more than 10 hours may signal depression or anxiety, emotionally unfinished business, or withdrawal from life. Our grandmothers were right. Eat well in moderation, sleep well, and exercise.

Psychology principle 2: Motivation always follows behavior; it does not precede it. You must change your behavior first; do not wait for the "mood to strike." The supersystem responds to teaching. Give it a chance to learn by altering your behaviors immediately.

3. Relaxation

Centuries of experience have taught us that if there is such a thing as stress response, there is certainly such a thing as relaxation response. Dr. Herbert Benson at Harvard Medical School has determined that a part of the hypothalamus, when stimulated, can produce activation of the whole-body system. Another part of that hypothalamus, however, when stimulated, can produce a relaxation of the entire body. This is the natural reflex of relaxation mentioned earlier, what Benson called the *relaxation response*.

Somewhere along the line we have lost our relaxation reflex. We are overburning or underburning, not "set" correctly. We run hot or cold. Our relaxation reflex can be relearned by readjusting our psychostats.

Dr. Benson suggests that we find a quiet place, breathe deeply, relax our muscles, and choose a mental focus such as a number or a prayer. During such times we can significantly lower our cholesterol levels and our blood pressure. We can also lower our blood lactate levels, which are a measure of the body's response to stress. Twice a day, for 20 minutes, practice this response and your supersystem will love you for it.

Another suggestion is to buy a small portable tape recorder with earphones. Play relaxing music to yourself during the 20 minutes if that helps you. Go out to your car and sit there during lunch if you are unable to get away from stress factors at work. This is one of the most important things you can do for yourself and for those who love you. Another idea would be to have a small container of a substance that emits an odor which you particularly appreciate. Smelling that substance during the time you are relaxing can condition your brain to relax automatically in response to the odor. Many researchers now carry small containers of peppermint to which they have taught their bodies to respond by pairing that odor with the relaxation response.

I know what you might be saying to yourself right now. "It's a good idea, but I don't have the time, there is no place, I'll never stick with it, and it's too hard to fit into my life." The third psychology principle will help you deal with this resistance.

Psychology principle 3: All attempts to change must be related to a system of measurement that assesses the success of that change. Feedback is necessary. Make posters, notes, and reminders to do the relaxation response. Record on a calendar the times that you have done it. Whether you fail or succeed, the effort itself will begin to teach your supersystem, and soon the response will become automatic. In my clinical experience, it takes several months to make such a technique a regular part of life. It is true, however, that you will become addicted to this relaxation response, and it will no longer take effort to find time for it once you teach yourself this positive addiction.

4. Simplicity

Thoreau's famous admonition to "simplify, simplify, simplify" has fallen on deaf ears in our modern society. More than 750,000 tourists and souvenir seekers visit Walden Pond each year. Bathhouses, piers, and concrete walls now surround this pond just west of Boston. Trees have been torn away, making room for parking lots, and tourist buses line the pond. But there is hope, even at Walden Pond. The Commonwealth of Massachusetts is attempting to return the pond to the state of simplicity and natural beauty described by Thoreau. We should be busy doing the same thing with our lives.

Think of the problems that confront you daily and of how they relate to the complexities of modern society. The number of decisions you must make in one day exceeds that of our ancestors by hundreds. Which car to take to which store, which lot to park in, which product to buy for which person, etc. Taking care of the lawn, the house, the water, the heater, the furnace, the phones, the carpet, the beds, the dishes—it is all so complex.

In his book *Voluntary Simplicity*, Donald Elgin describes what historian Arnold Toynbee called "the law of progressive simplification." Stated simply, this law suggests that the advancement and development of our society depends upon our ability to reflect on the simple, to focus our attention within ourselves on the more subtle realms of our experience. I explored this when we discussed the various strategies for stimulating a bored supersystem and the error that we make when we seek stimulation from outside rather than from within. Certainly, contemplating a dampened petal of a flower in the early morning dew is as stimulating as a professional football game. Even what we view as recreation is no longer relaxing, as in the case of football games characterized by war, aerial attacks, defensive lines, blitzing linebackers, and sudden death.

But how can we be simple when things are so complex in our day-to-day world?

Psychology principle 4: We are never victims unless we victimize ourselves. Life does not have to lead us. We can lead our own lives. We can make choices. Make an analysis of your home today, your work, and your daily schedule. See how much of that schedule is needlessly complex. Comedian George Carlin once said, "Home is where we leave our stuff while we go out to get more stuff." This "more and more stuff" approach only complicates our already muddled daily lives.

One of my patients told me that he and his family were "suffering in great comfort." He added that they were surrounded by complications, broken things, new purchases, time plans for buying more and more "stuff." I wondered then whether this comfort and its related complexities may not be the true cause of their suffering rather than a coincidental, coexisting factor. We have indeed failed to progress to simplicity and failed to stimulate our brains from within, with the result being dys-ease, a false sense of ease.

5. Sexuality

An assignment I use with patients has been very successful. Close your eyes and think of the best sexual encounter you have ever had. What were its characteristics? Were those characteristics haste, strangeness, alienation, fear, anxiety, and guilt, or were they freedom, enjoyment, mutuality, caring, sharing, and trust? Most likely your ideal experience was characterized by the second category of feelings.

A parallel between sexuality and our physical functioning is clear. As I stated earlier, the autonomic nervous system (the involuntary part of the nervous system) is subdivided into two categories: the sympathetic (SAM) and parasympathetic (PAC) nervous systems. The sympathetic system operates when we are under pressure or anxious, causing the stress hormones to be released. The parasympathetic system operates when we are relaxed, comfortable, self-assured. There is no sexual arousal without parasympathetic mediation and the hormones associated with parasympathetic functioning of the autonomic nervous system. If we are anxious, afraid, or guilty, we have sympathetic mediation where there should be parasympathetic, and sexual problems result.

Returning to our "just-right" phenomenon, it is also possible to have too much parasympathetic mediation. When this occurs, rather than having the comfort level necessary for sexual fulfillment, a form of anger and disgust occurs which is related to overstimulation of the parasympathetic nervous system. In this situation, a person may become sexually active but be unable to enjoy sex fully. Only through a trusting, open, warm interaction can this hormonal system stay in balance.

But what can you do about this? After all, it takes two persons, and where do you find a person who is truly sexually mature and willing to share responsibility with you? In societies without the inhibitions of our own, sexual frequency is much higher, sometimes two to three times per day. Sexuality is seen as communication and sharing, related to joy and personal fulfillment, not as a manipulative system or legal contract. All people in these societies consider themselves sexual. This is where you must begin. Take responsibility for your own sexuality. Express your needs directly and openly, and communicate freely about contraception, disease, responsibility, religious conviction, and expectations between yourself and your partner. We must all learn, and we must teach our children that sex is volitional, not exclusively emotional, that we can make responsible decisions and not just be victims of our impulses. We can take control and responsibility for our sexual lives.

One woman reported to me that men always asked her whether she was taking the pill after she experienced sex with them. She had decided from now on to say, "No, I can't take the pill because it only makes my sexually transmissible diseases much worse." Even though she had no such diseases, she felt that this would cause her partner to worry as much as he caused her to worry by expecting her to be responsible for the contraceptive issue. While this certainly does not reflect effective communication, it does reflect the failure to share responsibility for sexual satisfaction.

The idea is to make your sexuality congruent with your values and life system, to fit your sexuality into your spirituality.

Psychology principle 5: We should employ the *neutrality rule*, that is, "Never predict present or future based on the past." If you see each sexual encounter as a new opportunity for open communication with a partner, a new opportunity for closeness and sharing, sexuality will be more fulfilling. *Sexuality* means "intimate and human touching," and it is a touching that no one can do without. Just what type of touching, with whom, and how intimately or frequently are your own moral decision. Your health depends upon your ability to function within your own moral perspective, to make choices and to act in a personally enhancing fashion. A common teaching technique in this area is to require patients to spend time touching gently and slowly without talking. Using lotion, soft light, perhaps soft music, they are taught to communicate with their partners through their fingertips without demand, expectation, or some predetermined sexual sequence of events. Try this intense experience yourself, and end it without having sexual intercourse. Teach yourself and your body the importance of touch and closeness without goal directions, and sexual fulfillment may become a part of your life and enhance your wellness.

6. Equanimity

Psychologist Roger Walsh gives an example of equanimity in the following statement:

> Pleasure and pain
> Praise and blame
> Fame and shame
> Loss and gain
> Are all the same.

In this statement, he refers to the fact that we must learn to free ourselves from the automatic likes and dislikes that dominate our reactive pleasures and pains. We must become free of the automatic response to our environment. Psychologists know that one damaging factor to our health is *automaticity*, the tendency to react from prior biases to all situations.

I have pointed out earlier that the brain is bound by the rules of old physics. It seeks its fulfillment from stimulation at any cost. It tends to become "automatic," expressing its likes and dislikes through changes in the supersystem. It responds rapidly and prejudicially. However, if we assume control, if we learn to talk to our own brains, as I discussed earlier, by changing our self-talk, our brains will no longer be at the mercy of their environment but will actually be structuring and controlling that environment.

We give meaning to our lives through our perceptions. We become as we believe. One person is totally debilitated by an illness, while another person rallies in the face of the same illness. This is due in large part to the capacities that we have to form our own theories of life. There is no health without illness, no happiness without sadness. Learning to be free of our automatic prejudices and learning to relate intimately with all events is a goal that can enhance the supersystem.

Psychology principle 6: Reality is perception. Arguments about what reality is are a waste of time. The field of psychology called *phenomenology* has stressed that our views of phenomena, our perceptions, are the key to development. Taking control of your brain and practicing the 80 suggestions presented earlier can help you avoid reacting so that you may be more of an effective actor. You can develop a calm, disciplined brain under your own control, not under the control of some preconditioned reactivity. This is what is meant by *equanimity*.

Psychologist William James typified the view of equanimity and its relationship to our perceptions in his statement, "There is always more." What we see is dependent upon how we are, a concept sometimes referred to as *state-dependent learning*. We must be aware of how we are and of its effect on what we can be.

7. Integrity

Buddha instructed his son, "Never lie, even in jest." Being truthful to self and others is probably the most direct way to positively affect the supersystem. Lying, even in jokes, results in alterations of the supersystem. Such modifications are reflected in special instruments that can detect subtle body changes. These instruments are called *polygraphs* or lie detectors. Each of the small changes they detect are signals of disruption of the supersystem, of unhealthy responses to the world. Even lying about your name can cause the needle on a polygraph to jump, registering disruption somewhere inside.

But won't people hurt you if they always tell the truth? Won't they take advantage of you? "Business is built on the art of strategic and careful lying," said one successful businessman. He is wrong, of course. Business is built on integrity. Try for just 1 week to tell the complete truth, nothing but the truth, and see how it helps you. Our modern-day society's focus on lying is a sickness of our world. See how much better you feel when even the smallest lie is removed from your life.

One woman patient reported scolding her son about lying in school. "Never lie, it's just not right," she told him. She then announced that she was going to take a nap, but if anyone called her, her son was to state, "My mother isn't home; she will be home later." This double message is common in our society, and integrity toward self and others has eroded from lack of role models.

Politicians, in their attempts to avoid being caught in lies, have developed a strategy of clichés, of glaring generalities, that make one politician sound very much like another. This is not what is meant by the avoidance of lying. Telling the truth is taking the risk of giving the gift of self mentioned earlier, sharing openly your fears, concerns, and hopes; it is not avoidance but disclosure.

Psychology principle 7: The *cognitive-behaviorism* school of psychology studies the impact of our language and our thoughts on our daily behavior and general psychological wellness. Work from this field has indicated that words are powerful and that establishing a continual pattern of integrity results in positive body changes and reduction of anxiety, stress, and depression. Truth is simply the accurate sharing of your perceptions, without distortion to self or other.

8. Laughter

Norman Cousins, in his writings about wellness and combating disease, points out that laughter is a "jogging of the intestine." It is biochemically impossible to get sick or sicker when you are laughing. Dr. William Fry at Stanford University has developed the field of study called *gelontology* (from the Greek *gelus*, meaning "laughter"). He has demonstrated that an increase in dopamine accompanies laughter. This is the same important brain chemical related to wellness that responds to rewards.

When is the last time you laughed so hard your sides hurt? If they did hurt, it is probably because your laughter muscles are suffering from unemployment. Buy or rent some funny films. Borrow some funny books. Be around people with the type of laughter that causes everyone else to laugh.

Dr. Fry's work on tears, described earlier, demonstrated that crying, as well as laughing, is important to our health. Even animals enjoy tricks, jokes, and tickling. Dr. Fry has shown that tears of emotion wash away the body's remnants of toxic chemicals associated with stress. Tears of joy can do this job just as well as tears of sadness. We are indeed in a serious condition if we take ourselves too seriously.

When I present this fact in my lectures, I utilize a test joke to see whether the laughter quotient of my audience is intact. I present the joke as a test for you.

The fifth-grade teacher had finished her warning to her class. She had stated that only one person could talk in the classroom at a time, and everyone else should be a listener. She as teacher was ready now to talk, and all the class should listen. If there was any disruption, persons would be dismissed from class.

As the teacher turned to the board to write, the chalk slipped from her hand. As she bent to pick it up, a boy in the back of the room giggled quietly. The teacher stood up immediately and asked, "What's your problem?" The boy answered that he had seen the top of the teacher's stocking. The teacher pointed to the door angrily and stated: "Get out. You are out of here for one day." As the boy left, the teacher again attempted to retrieve her chalk. Another boy in the back of the classroom giggled softly. The teacher rose, even more quickly, and without commenting, stared directly at the boy. Without being asked, the boy responded, "Teacher, I saw your garter." The teacher said: "That does it. You are out of here. Three-day suspension. Get out of my classroom." By now the chalk had been kicked further under her desk, and as the teacher bent further over to retrieve it, a little boy in the back gathered his books and pencils, stood up, and began to leave the classroom. The teacher stopped him and asked, "Where do you think you are going?" The boy's response was, "Teacher, from what I have seen, my school days are over!"

If you were able to chuckle, even inside, then you are a little healthier for reading this. If you laughed out loud, you are really in good shape. I have found that suggesting a joke is a laughter test, an indication of wellness, causes my audiences to roar in approval, perhaps as a demonstration of wellness. Placing my jokes in the form of a test has never failed to guarantee a strong reaction to the jokes.

Psychology principle 8: The presence of humor is one of the strongest predictors of the absence of mental illness. The so-called psychiatric mental status exam assesses for appropriateness of humor. One of the most serious of psychiatric diseases, schizophrenia, contains as one of its most serious symptoms something called *anhedonia*, the absence of pleasure, laughter, and appropriate humor.

9. Spirituality

The idea that there are no atheists in foxholes, at times of life threat, was mentioned earlier. Most of us, in our modern-day world, are living in sociological foxholes. At a time when we have abandoned our belief systems, we need them the most. We all need a transcendent philosophy, a theory of meaning for the world and our place in that world. It matters less *what* we believe than *that* we believe. All religions are based on the dignity of men and women and their place in the cosmos. The contradictions of various religious groups are less important than the message about the eternal us. As Goethe said, "All religions are true in what they affirm, but wrong in what they deny."

If you used to go to church, go back immediately.

Recent research has indicated that those persons who attend church are less likely to be ill over time than those who do not attend church. I presented this finding at a recent meeting of members of the clergy. I noted that they have used this finding with some success in building their congregations and increasing the reliability of church attendance. Whether the stronger health of those persons who attend church is related to social support systems within the church or to the impact of their belief systems is not clear at the present time, but there is no use taking the chance. Go to church if it fits into your belief system.

Psychology principle 9: A strong faith, a strong belief, is a healing factor for any illness and an insulator against getting sick in the first place. As T. S. Eliot pointed out, "There is only the fight to recover what has been lost." Herbert Benson has written a book entitled *Beyond the Relaxation Response*, in which he refers to the "faith factor," or the importance of a belief system in enhancing the relaxation response.

10. Career

Occasionally I would start thinking how such dull people could make money. I should have known that money-making has more to do with emotional stability than with intellect.

J. P. MARQUAND

It is important to find meaningful work. It is dangerous to find meaning only through work. "Work" can be defined as doing what you do not want to do. A "career" is doing what you want to do for the common good of our world. Maintaining a home, putting doors on cars, sweeping streets, repairing teeth, and painting buildings are all potential careers. Second to sleeping, we spend more time working than doing anything else. We had best enjoy it and grow from it, or it can kill us.

The Hopi Indians view their society as a whole, a total system, with each part of it significant. If one member is sick, the entire society is seen as sick, and societal rites are used for healing. The Hopis embrace the same view regarding contributions of various tasks within their society. In our own society, we become trapped in specialty work, knowing more and more about less and less. Soon we will know almost everything there is to know about absolutely nothing. If you think about career, make plans for change. Many persons get stuck and feel trapped in their work, and this is one of the strongest contributors to illness.

Dr. Suzanne Kobasa has done comprehensive studies of what she calls the *stress-resistant personality*. She has found that people who see their work as a challenge, who see some sense of self-worth in their jobs, and who show a commitment to their work and have control and effectiveness in their workplaces are more immune to stress than people who do not have the "three C's" of challenge, commitment, and control.

As a minitest, ask yourself about the three C's in your own career. Do you experience all three? It has been said that a workaholic finds meaning through work while a person who is happy in his career finds meaningful work. Which state characterizes your career? If your work were a game, would you want to play?

Psychology principle 10: In a classic quote, Sigmund Freud states simply, "To work and to love." By this he meant that these two components of life must be intact if our wellness is to be intact. Stress in the workplace is a modern-day dilemma. Kenneth Pelletier in his book *Healthy People in Unhealthy Places* discusses the theory of the *performance zone*. This is the idea that too little challenge can result in illness, while too much challenge can lead to illness. Have you found the performance zone in your own career, in your day-to-day life?

11. Relationships

We have been talking about self, other, and us throughout this book. Taking care of the "us" in our lives is essential to our thriving. This is the second part of the "to work and to love" prescription offered by Sigmund Freud. Books on love are coming back into vogue, and I have been allowed to sneak this term into my lectures to even the most scientifically oriented audiences. I recently spoke on the topic "Love or Lust: Telling the Difference" to a large medical school audience. The answer was simple. Love is doing *with* someone else. Lust is doing *to* someone else. The ability to relate interactively with another person or persons is the keystone of our society's survival.

Mass lectures about love, followed by long lines of persons awaiting the opportunity to hug the lecturer, may be symptomatic of a need for relationships. Unfortunately, we have "McDonaldized" this need too. Waiting in lines for a "big hug attack" hardly replaces the personal need for intimacy.

I suggest that we prioritize relationships in our lives. Examine your relationship status today. Do you spend as much time enhancing and developing your relationship as you do in your work or with your children? Do you spend as much time on your work as you do on your relationships? If we spent as much time on our work as we do on our relationships, many of us would be bankrupt or unemployed. Many persons are interpersonally unemployed, and they have withdrawn from interpersonal interactions other than problem solving and day-to-day activities.

I have identified three basic forms of relationships: symmetrical, complementary, and adaptive. *Symmetrical relationships* are egalitarian, balanced, and nonsexist in role definitions. Competition and sameness can disrupt this type of interaction. *Complementary relationships* are based on strict role definitions, typically sexist, with "Mr. Outside" doing one set of tasks and "Ms. Inside" doing another. *Adaptive relationships* have a high *AC*, or alternating capacity, reacting to events in daily living rather than sticking with a static pattern of expectation. Ask yourself about your relationships and discuss which of the three patterns characterizes your interactions.

A special note of warning: Women are now entering the work force in increasing numbers. The illusion of the professional woman as a "wonder woman" stems from her adding to prior roles and not changing them. Serious and basic examination of our relationships as related to our health is a priority and a focus of my own research.

Psychology principle 11: Interdependence is as important as independence. For years psychology and psychiatry were dominated by *ego psychology*, the focus on self. We are finally learning that wellness is defined as much by our ability to interrelate as by our ability to function autonomously.

12. Celebration

We seem to have lost our ability to celebrate our humanness. We have fallen into the hands of receivers who execute our celebrations for us. We watch vicariously as others celebrate their successes. We sit alone in front of our televisions, watching a baseball team celebrate a season-ending championship. Our participation in the celebration is characterized by walking to the refrigerator for a snack or by cheering loudly at the TV screen.

Our parties have become exercises in social obligations and etiquette, rather than celebrations. The familiar scene of persons clustered around a game board in pursuit of the trivial bears witness to this fact.

Celebrate regularly. Laugh. Love. Dance. Cheer. Your wellness depends upon it. As Norman Cousins speculated, "If we could contemplate our own composite wonder, we would lose ourselves in celebration and have time for nothing else."

Psychology principle 12: We have institutionalized our celebrations and made them ceremonial. We have separated them from the spontaneity of our daily lives. Weddings, birthdays, and major events are the only causes that we accept for celebration. I suggest as an assignment that you have a built-in weekly celebration of being alive, of wellness, of being human. Developmental psychologists know the importance of appreciating the beauty and grace of humanness.

If we move toward the implementation of the first 11 principles of this "divine dozen," we deserve the twelfth. Try it now. At the end of this chapter, put this book down, gather your family together, and have one big family hug. Cheer together. Cheer for yourself, for others, for us, and for the universe. If you don't have a family available, stand up and cheer anyway. Stand up alone and run through the house singing. This is what we mean by thriving, by transcending health. It means freedom from the tyranny of fear of sickness and the ability to enjoy the moment-by-moment wellness of being human.

One of my medical students stated that he was looking forward to a TGIF party. As this was Monday, I was surprised and asked whether this was the traditional Thank God It's Friday party. He responded, "No Doc, I am just taking your advice. Our TGIF parties are Thank God I'm Fine parties." Maybe we will learn to have Thank God I'm Fantastic parties.

As Joseph Conrad wrote in *Victory*, "Woe to the man whose heart has not learned while young to hope, to love, to put its trust in life."

I have focused in this chapter on transcending the mere absence of symptoms toward a high-level wellness. But what about those times when we are hurt, experiencing dys-ease? Are there ways that we can enhance our wellness even at those times? Are there ways that the supersystem can learn at those times of crisis, can strengthen itself, and perhaps even save our lives? The next chapter of this book draws together the concepts I have outlined thus far in an attempt to help hurt people and their families.

Chapter Seventeen

GROWTH THROUGH CRISIS: HURTING AND LEARNING

God cures and the doctor sends the bill.
MARK TWAIN

Short, annoying beeps on the small paging device awakened the resident. He had completed a straight 36 hours of work and could barely raise his arm to switch off the tones. He struggled from the bed to the phone to discover that an elderly, chronically ill patient had died. A doctor was required to confirm this event and to initiate the legal requirements related to the dying process in our society.

The strict caste system in hospitals dictated that a doctor had to certify that a death had occurred. Any doctor would do, as long as the magical letters "M.D." or "D.O." followed the signature on the bureaucratic documents. The fatigued resident called one of his underlings, a young first-year resident who was obliged to follow any order from his superior.

"Go down to Unit 6 and pronounce Mr. Kane dead. I am too tired," said the senior resident. "He's been trying to die for days and you might know he'd pick tonight to get it done."

The first-year resident knew that his own survival depended upon his immediate compliance and on not asking any questions regarding this request. He hurried to the room where Mr. Kane lay dead. Three nurses were standing near the bed, and two other nurses were in the hall comforting relatives who had expected this loss for several months and were somehow both deeply saddened and deeply relieved at the old man's passing.

The young and inexperienced resident feigned a confident walk into the room and looked at the nurses standing near the bed. He realized that he was not at all sure what was expected of him. How do you pronounce someone dead? Medical school did not even acknowledge death other than as an enemy to be conquered or a sign of some failure in the attending physician. The nurses returned his questioning gaze, waiting for him to repeat tests that they had done themselves and to request the necessary forms for his signature. He checked for pulse, listened for heartbeat, and, remembering movies about physicians, even checked for breathing by placing his own cheek near the patient's mouth. The diagnosis was indeed accurate. The patient was dead. The confused student stood up and looked again at the nurses, who were now impatiently waiting for him to ask for the appropriate forms and to direct them to the next steps in preparing the body for removal to the morgue. They could not understand his hesitation as he again listened for heartbeat and attempted to look into the eyes of the dead man.

The young doctor felt panic. He had never before had the responsibility of declaring life or death but, rather, had served as an observer to these processes. Everything in hospitals is run by precedent, expectation, and cultural right. Orders are given along clearly established, traditional chains of command. Certainly, doctors always knew what to do and so did the nurses. Custom dictates clearly that doctors tell nurses to do what nurses almost always know to do anyway. To do it before they are told, however, is a breach of medical-cultural etiquette and is often met with disdain for or discipline of the nurse who has taken too much responsibility for the "doctor's patient," violating a medical "Simon says."

By now, everyone was feeling awkward. Relatives looked on curiously, nurses were becoming angry, and the young doctor repeated his tests for a third time, as if waiting for a return of life in this man who had been dead now for more than half an hour. He had to come up with something to reestablish his authority, to show his knowledge and expertise. He relied on his role models for guidance whenever he was confused, but he had not seen any of his idols do what he was now asked to do. All medical procedures are predicated on the idea "See one, do one," but he had never seen one to guide him at this most frightening moment. He relied on his instinct: "When in doubt, fake it." Although it is not listed on any curriculum guide sheet, all doctors are taught to act more confidently at those times when they have no confidence at all.

The student took a deep breath, stood up, and walked to the foot of the bed. He raised his right arm, looked at the patient, looked at the nurses and relatives, each in turn, and in his lowest, most clerical-sounding voice uttered softly, "I now pronounce thee dead." He bowed, turned, and walked from the room. The pronouncement was now complete. To this day, nurses raise their right arms when the more mature and still embarrassed physician passes the nursing station.

The helpless-observer status of health care professionals, in their attempts to intercede for our welfare (even though most of what they do is unnecessary or even dangerous), is illustrated by this true story. Almost all of us will get better or worse when we are ill no matter what the medical hierarchy does. Remember that 10 percent of us will be made worse by the institutional fumbling of the large and awkward medical establishment. Stories of abuse, neglect, and tragic error abound. That some of us will become better—why and how we become well, how we can survive being wounded, and how we can learn from the experience of illness and the faltering of the immune system—is the focus of this chapter. If we do not assume full responsibility for our own health and the maintenance of our own personal health systems, we may fall victim to institutional pronouncements of disease. The brain is the most complex and efficient health maintenance system, for it controls the supersystem constituting immunity and continued protection against internal invasion. It is the mind, not the doctor, that treats all illness.

DISEASES, ILLNESSES, AND PREDICAMENTS

There is a deep reciprocity at work, an unseverable linkage
between the hideousness of illness and the splendor of health.
LARRY DOSSEY

"Illness" is what we have on the way to the doctor's office. "Dys-ease" is what we end up with on the way home. Illness is our sense that something is wrong, those times when we just don't seem to feel well. Dys-ease is what our cosmopolitan medical system uses as a labeling system, the modern conceptualization of sickness. According to the dys-ease model, we are always ill because of some biological, metabolical disruption on the cellular level. The body is out of whack and needs to be put back in whack. Illness is seen as the opposite of health and is to be avoided at any cost. Wellness is what we have when we do not have an illness.

Dys-ease is always a theory, a way of explaining what has gone wrong with the body system and why some problem has occurred. The theory of sickness in our society is failing us. Mechanical aspects of our functioning are handled well by the old Cartesian-Newtonian mechanical model of disease. Bones are repaired, stones are removed, traumas are corrected, and most infectious diseases are controlled. The old theory of disease centers on the mechanical: the cell and the molecule. The mechanical theory fails, however, when it comes to cancer, cardiovascular disease, pain syndromes, stress management, obesity, drug addiction, and alcoholism—the so-called diseases of civilization. I have discussed a new approach (actually a reexamination of some very old approaches) to explaining dys-ease, a theory based on a systems view of the person within his or her world. This theory suggests that our thoughts, beliefs, and feelings, as well as our interaction with one another and with our entire universe, are important and that when some breakdown in the interaction within that system occurs, dys-ease results.

As one well-known umpire yelled back at a complaining batter who had protested that a called strike was actually a ball, "It ain't nothin' till I call it, and I called it a strike, so it's a strike." How umpires call things influences the whole game, and how we view sickness influences our whole lives and our whole world. I suggest that we must transcend the mechanical model in favor of a more inclusive explanation of dis-ease, or the lack of ease.

If illness is the feeling that something is wrong and dys-ease is a modern medical label for illness, then our "predicament" is the psychological and social impact of our illness and dys-ease. The supersystem becomes disrupted, and working, playing, and loving are impaired. Something has gone wrong from within, and even though we are typically looked at from without, our survival will depend upon resuming an inner balance.

Modern medicine treats individuals, not groups or communities. The principle of oneness with the universe suggests that when one of us is sick, all of us are sick. After an examination that reveals no cellular or mechanical disruption, one that shows completely normal, efficient body function, the typical statement from a physician is, "There are no remarkable findings." The statement should really be, "I found the usual, remarkable, extraordinary, complex, magnificent supersystem doing its job." The patient should learn much from his or her wellness state because it is truly a miracle.

Much has been written about our wellness, the idea of total balance of the mind, body, and spirit, congruent with the life choices of the individual. Unfortunately, this orientation to wellness has come to be seen by some as a state to be achieved or accomplished, something sought after by jogging, eating right, and purchasing an appropriate mantra. I have often wondered why it seems that so many persons who are seeking to achieve health with such vigor seem to experience so much illness while others who are more cavalier and casual in their lives and less goal-directed in their approaches to health seem to enjoy a form of spontaneous wellness. Perhaps the latter have learned to receive rather than pursue health?

I suggest that wellness is received, allowed to happen by self-talk, thinking, and feeling changes. Wellness is a state of the supersystem, a state of being in control of thought rather than simply being responsive to the changes of our world and the selfishness of our brains.

Some of the most "well" persons of our time have been sick according to the yardstick of modern medicine. This is because modern medicine continues to utilize objective measures rather than internal indicators for wellness. We get medical checkups to be declared healthy, failing to realize that we ourselves are the judge. It is possible to be very, very well, even though we experience "dys-ease." We can mobilize the supersystem to readjust and enhance the body itself. There is a healthy way to be ill and to experience and learn from disease. Talking to ourselves is everything, and talking gently, sensitively, and rationally helps us move toward wellness. Dys-ease is as much a part of us as is health, and if we take responsibility for both states and learn from both of these natural phenomena, perhaps we may be able to move toward a new, more humane view of thriving in our world.

When we visit a doctor, there is actually very little talking, very little assessment of our own self-talk patterns. Few of us have gone to our self-shamans before we seek advice from the medical experts. We are questioned about our bodies, we are picked, pulled, squeezed, and otherwise assessed mechanically. Seldom are we asked about our "self" and its relationship to "other," "us," and the "world." Seldom does the doctor help guide us to meet our world's greatest experts. The doctor may employ several different organizations to help him or her assess the products of our bodies and to help determine whether or not we are well. In fact, many of these long-distance assessments will be done without ever seeing us personally, by looking only at our waste products or other samples from our body systems. The blood lab, the urinalysis lab, and the x-ray lab will all send their partialistic mechanical reports to someone who will integrate and add up the scores and decide for us whether we have or do not have disease. Most of us who are ill do not have a serious dys-ease anyway, although we may be making our way towards one, maybe even "tested" into one. It is interesting to note how well some patients feel until they are told, upon integration of partialistic mechanical reports, that they are really sick.

One of my patients being treated for fertility arrived for her appointment with flowers. As she presented them to me, she stated, "You have made my life. You have helped my husband and I to accomplish something we have tried for years. You have helped us to understand that how we think and how we are as people is as much a part of fertility as those mechanical things we were going through before." I was pleased and proud with the patient's positive feedback, but I made one terrible mistake. I asked her, "Have you had any morning sickness yet?" She responded, "Absolutely not. I am feeling just fine. I can't believe how good the pregnancy is going."

The next morning I received a call from this same patient. She reported that she had spent most of the night experiencing terrible nausea and concluded, "I really have it now. Now I have the morning sickness." She had managed to live up to my expectations, my mechanical view of the process of pregnancy, and a self-fulfilling prophecy had taken place. She was a victim of what I call the "healer belief" effect.

I present below 20 questions that are seldom, if ever, asked by the medical establishment. It is important that you ask yourself these questions in the form of a home supersystem examination. It is important that you work with your physician in a team interaction, utilizing the test provided here and perhaps the help of your own world's greatest expert as you conduct this test of the supersystem. You must work toward a partnership with your physician, a partnership in which you hold most of the stock. The 20 questions that follow are key first steps in assessing your wellness and learning when your health stock is down.

Remember, in spite of immediate slack cycles and bear and bull markets, in the long view, the stock market continues to grow in value. So it is with your health.

THE HOME SUPERSYSTEM EXAMINATION

We fear our highest possibilities. We are generally afraid to become that which we can glimpse in our most perfect moments, under the most perfect conditions, under conditions of great courage.

ABRAHAM MASLOW

The examination you are about to take is an examination toward wellness, not to detect illness. It is an examination that will help you understand why you may be feeling ill. It is an examination designed to offer some suggestions to move beyond the absence of illness, beyond health and normality, to a higher state of exceptional well-being. I suggest that you do the campfire assignment with your self-shaman as you conduct the following examination.

QUESTION 1: How Are You Today?

First, categorize yourself regarding your health right now. Are you not feeling ill, but not feeling well either? Are you sort of in an in-between state? Are you hurt, or do you have an illness assigned to you currently, but seem to be feeling well in spite of this disease? Are you suffering from disease and, at the same time, not feeling well either, that is, chronically ill?

Most of us fail to take our wellness temperature. We are only aware of our wellness when we become sick, sensing its absence rather than presence. I suggest that four categories can serve as a wellness thermometer, a measure of "how we are" rather than how we could be or should be.

Category 1: Just Great

This is the category of exceptional wellness, of high-level functioning. You are cool, not cold, warm, not hot; you feel happy, growing, and alive.

This is a state not often studied in medicine. Most health care workers are taught very early in their careers to keep to themselves any discussion of the spirit, the soul, and its relationship to higher states of wellness that transcend the mere absence of illness. To function in the "just great" category, we must live in an interdependent coexistence with all others. *Holism* means "integration with others," not just within self.

The cancer cell cares only for itself. Since it can only live off the body of some "host," it eventually "kills" itself by its egocentric development and reckless destruction of the host upon which it depends. When we live egocentrically and narcissistically, we not only damage others but ultimately ourselves. Perhaps helping others teaches the supersystem a new way of "being," the altruistic egoism referred to by stress expert Hans Selye, thus reducing the chance of cancer and other selfish disease entities acting as invaders against the supersystem.

Category 2: So-So

This is the "fine, thank you" response to "How are you doing?" In this category you are not ill, but you are not completely well either. Although your own doctor may have declared you to be in "good health," you may simply be "making it."

More than 25 years ago, Dr. George Watmore at the University of Washington described a condition he called *dysponesis*. This is a bracing effect, a subtle tensing of the muscles in response to small hassles in a person's daily life. You may notice this bracing effect when someone pulls in front of you in traffic or when you feel pain if you cut your finger. Such bracing is counterproductive, for reduction of pain depends upon relaxation of muscles. Chronic bracing, or chronic dysponesis, eventually results in illness and disease. The person in the "fine, thank you" category may be unaware of the dysponesis, but persons around them may note the tense muscle triad referred to earlier (forehead, jaws, upper back).

Category 3: Down but not Out

This is the "not so good" response to "How are you?" In this category you are ill, but you may be well in terms of dealing with your illness effectively and constructively and learning from your illness.

As Alan Watts wrote in his book *The Wisdom of Insecurity*, "To understand this moment I must not try to be divided from it; I must be aware of it with my whole being.'' People who rally their strengths in the face of illness may ultimately thrive more than those who have never been fully aware of their illness, for awareness is the ultimate teacher. Some of my healthiest patients have had what the medical establishment calls ''the most serious of diseases.''

Category 4: Down and Out, Wounded

One patient jokingly referred to this state as the ''able to sit up and take nourishment'' state. In this category you are ill but not well. Unlike a person in category 3, who is rallying in the face of illness, you have panicked and withdrawn and your wellness quotient is low.

The imagery of people in category 4 is not healthy, but sick. Einstein once stated that time and space are not conditions under which we live, but ways in which we think. So it is with sickness and wellness. There is no reason to think sick just because we are not well, but people in category 4, the down and out, wounded people, fail to take responsibility for initiating positive thought processes that release the healing chemicals from the brain.

Remember that all of us go through all these categories at various times of our lives, or even within the same week or day. The supersystem is dynamic, changing as all elements of our universe change. If you are wounded, worried, hurt, or afraid because of a disease you are experiencing, you only worsen your disease. You must remember that you are never a patient in a hospital or a victim of a disease; you are a person in charge of your own life. You do not have a disease; you are ''dis-easing.'' You are in-process. This is the first step toward learning from your hurting. If you accept your disease as a pronouncement, you have surrendered some of the internal strength of your supersystem for coping with invasion.

It is well known that medications work best when people believe in their effects and that some medications do not work at all when people do not believe in their effects. The famous *placebo effect* is not some trick to fool us into wellness with a false pill, but an indication of the power of our own thinking and its impact on actual biochemical changes in our bodies. I have described some ways in which thinking affects the biochemical atmosphere within the body and the efficacy of the immune system. The placebo effect is simply a shorthand way of referring to this process. The historical meaning of the word "placebo" is "to please." Perhaps if we are pleased with the medications, our supersystems respond favorably, and if we are displeased (perhaps in reaction to some negative message given by the person providing the medicine), our supersystems may respond destructively, or at best skeptically. It is unfortunate that researchers often view the placebo effect as an indication of worthlessness, when in actuality the placebo effects of medications are at least equal to, if not in excess of, actual physiological impacts of medicines used today.

You may remember the cancer patient who had to decide between chemotherapy or no therapy at all and who felt that she had an unfortunate choice between two evils. She felt helpless, hopeless, and the victim of her situation. In cooperation with her physician, the woman responded by choosing chemotherapy. A significant difference in her chemotherapy, however, was that the patient also received relaxing music through earphones during the administration of the chemotherapy. Not only did this block out the mechanical and annoying sounds of the medical setting, but it also lowered her pulse rate, blood pressure, and respiratory rate. One day, when the tape player was broken and could not be used, severe nausea followed her chemotherapy. At the next session, with the return of music, only mild nausea accompanied her therapy. Her body was "more pleased" with the treatment during the playing of music, and it cooperated more effectively in the relaxed state that accompanied the music.

It is possible to teach our immune systems, just as Pavlov taught his dogs to salivate to a bell. I often provide a small tube of mint for my patients to inhale occasionally during the administration of their chemotherapy while soothing music is played. We have seen earlier that it is possible that the supersystem matches the odor to the relaxing music which, in turn, enhances the effects of the chemicals used for therapy. Eventually, doses of chemotherapy can be reduced, as if the music and the mint smell themselves are eliciting a response from the supersystem, helping it to attack the cancer cells and increasing the efficacy of the chemotherapy. While research in this area is just beginning, I have noticed my medical students and residents carrying small vials of various odors that they associate with relaxation and sniffing these before an examination. One of my students sniffed his relaxing mint several times while he was writing an essay answer criticizing the possibility of conditioning the immune system through the use of relaxing odors.

QUESTION 2: So Why Did You Get Sick?

If you are sick now, ask yourself about the cause of your sickness. If you are not aware of being sick at this moment, think back to when you were sick. Unfortunately, your doctor will seldom ask you why you think you are sick. Doctors tend to feel that you are paying them to determine the answer. Of course, they will not and cannot determine the answer for you. The answer lies within. Doctors have only their theories; they can determine only what is wrong mechanically and biologically. They detect perturbations in a system that have already been going on for months, perhaps years. They fail to talk to your self-shaman to detect disruption on the energy level. They are not physicists; they are biologists.

Whenever I ask my patients what they think caused their illness, they invariably answer in terms concerning emotions and human interactions. "I have had problems at work for years" is a typical answer. "My wife died three years ago and I don't think I ever have been right since" is another response. We do know the answer after all, and if we take the time, we will come up with an understanding of the processes affecting the immune system, not a description based on mechanical breakdown.

If you are in a hospital room as you read this book, ask for paper and pencil and draw a large circle. Start anywhere on this circle, and record a life event you think related to the reason for your illness. It doesn't matter how significant it is. Any little hassle that occurred in your life should be recorded. You are constructing what might be called a "hasslescope." Use pictures, words, short poems—anything that reminds you of life events and the hassles you have experienced. Place these hassles in some type of order around the circle. Remember, time is not linear, even though you are writing along a line that bends into a circle. This is not a picture of where you went wrong or of how you caused your own illness. It is a picture of some of the strains upon your supersystem that may have contributed to disruption, to the over-mobilization or demobilization of your immune system.

Your hasslescope should include hassles in the form of periods of boredom as well as stress and change. Cold and hot supersystems result from hot or cold stressors. You can suffer from "nothing-itis" as well as "everything-itis." If your hasslescope has large blanks on it, with no indications of anything having happened to you, this may have contributed to your illness as well, or you may be blind to events that are causing you difficulty.

It is complete "myth-information" to think that sadness creates cancer, that stress causes heart disease, that several years ago you failed to deal with something effectively and are now paying the price for it. Your hasslescope exercise provides an opportunity of putting your illness in the perspective of day-to-day living.

When your hasslescope is complete, you should have a feeling of "aha" as you look at it, thinking, "Now I have something to learn from that will help me mobilize my supersystem." You should not be thinking, "Oh no." That will only complicate future hasslescopes and the healing process. Life and wellness are processes, not events. The equanimity suggested earlier is important to remember here. Be careful that you do not attach value statements to your hasslescope. You are simply drawing a life sphere and attempting to trace contributions to your present functioning. This includes positives as well as negatives.

Now that your hasslescope is complete, talk into a tape recorder and record your reactions to it. How do the hassles and uplifts characterize your immune style? What events contributed to your present situation? How did they evolve? How are they still contributing? If you have tentatively placed yourself in the category of wellness and constructed a hasslescope, you are a long way along the process of self-healing, for you have taken responsibility and are asking questions of your total self, not simply analyzing a mechanical breakdown.

QUESTION 3: When Did This Happen to You Anyway?

During what life event do you feel your illness began? Study your hasslescope and look for some approximate "time frame." Time must be viewed not by "clock" hours, but in terms of processes such as having a child, going to school, losing a job. Translate these hassles to some frame of reference in your own life, such as problems raising a child, preparing to change jobs, studying for examinations during a particularly difficult semester. In terms of your life clock, not the wall clock, when do you think this illness may have started?

To answer this question fully, you must free yourself from thinking about when you first noticed your symptoms. By the time we are aware that something is wrong, it has been going on for a long time. Using this system of analysis will help you offer some guesses as to what processes may have been occurring when there was a change in your supersystem, some type of overheating or freezing of the immune system.

QUESTION 4: What Did You Say Was Wrong Again?

In the 20 questions of the supersystem exam, you will notice a built-in redundancy. Because it is impossible for you to answer the questions directly and openly the first time they are asked, questions will be repeated, but with slightly different wording. Each question has a different emphasis and reflects different techniques. We are looking for a pattern, not one concrete answer.

To determine accurately what exactly is wrong, you will have to use the most sophisticated instrument in the universe, the so-called self-scanner. *CAT scanners*, or computerized axial tomography scanners, are instruments that actually take computerized pictures of segments of your body from top to bottom. These are small pictures in search of breakdowns or abnormalities. Magnificent and helpful medical instruments, they pale in comparison to the personalized self-assessment scan, or the *PSA scan*.

Find a quiet place and time. Put on earphones from your tape player, but this time do not play the music. The earphones are intended to block out distractions and to remind you of the importance of doing so. Make sure the room is dark. Some persons do the PSA scan in a darkened bathroom, in a tub filled to the rim with warm bath water. Make sure you don't have any electrical devices nearby, lay back, and allow your arms to float up by their own buoyancy. Lie quietly and, starting at your hair, scan your entire system for wellness, not illness. This is not a stop-start technique or a checklist, but a slow flowing from hair down to toes, from toes back up to hair, and back down to toes again. Back and forth, scanning for wellness and good feelings in the body. You do not need a checklist; just search for positive areas. Even if you are seriously ill now, look for health.

One of my paralyzed patients who could not feel or move from the neck down, reported, "It's strange, but I seem to feel very well in the inside of my eyelids, the outside of my heart, the lining of my lungs, and the bottom of my stomach. Is that really possible?" Of course, the answer is that it is not only possible but a fact for this person. We have prematurely accepted the mechanical model of our bodies, ignoring the inner states that are so important for our wellness.

During your PSA scan you may have detected several wellness areas, and you may have noted that there are areas that are not doing so well at this time. We need our measurement techniques in medicine to allow us to talk with one another about the body. We need to be able to speak the language of cosmopolitan medicine, for many of its tools are most helpful to us, but the actual repair will have to come from the supersystem itself, which speaks its own symbolic language. Medicine can only help. You must learn to identify strong areas and weak areas, and you must understand their metaphor.

The table on the following pages illustrates one brief example of the way in which our bodies speak to us symbolically about our inner states. It is only a beginning, designed to start your own reading of the poems and symbolism of your supersystem. Remember, humor helps, so do not take this chart too seriously. Poems and metaphors are for learning and growing, not self-blame.

Now, try using the chart. Starting on the right side, find a dysease you have experienced. Look at the body system related to the dysease and see whether you can identify a metaphor and then a related emotion. Check back to see whether you have experienced a hot or cold emotion. You cannot be right or wrong in this opportunity; you are just looking for metaphors that may provide clues to whether you are over-mobilizing or demobilizing your immune system. Dr. Jeanne Achtenberg-Laulis and her colleagues studied 200 cancer patients in advanced stages of their disease and found that their prognosis related more to the patients' imagery and understanding of their immune systems than to any other measure. Dr. Achtenberg-Laulis states, "The immune system is a magnificent army which recreates health two billion times a minute." Mobilizing this army or putting the army on temporary rest and recreation depends upon learning the symbolic language of the supersystem. Remember, poems and paintings cannot be "wrong"; they just stimulate our imagination, and that is always right.

Many of my patients clearly indicate the metaphor of disease. One had enrolled in a computer class that he was finding excessively frustrating. He went to his car, turned the key in the lock, and sprained his wrist, rendering him unable to complete the computer class. Another of my patients, a woman gynecologist, had had problems in her practice, arguing with several of her colleagues, and had to "break the practice

Body System	Metaphor	Related Emotion	Sample "Dys-ease"
1. Hair	I feel like tearing my hair out. Get him or her out of my hair.	Frustration	Hair loss, folliculitis
2. Eyes	I can't believe my eyes. I got a real eyeful. Keep my eyes open.	Surprise	Sore eyes, cataracts, sties
3. Skin	It really gets under my skin. It makes my skin crawl. Jump right out of my skin. Skinned me.	Irritation	Rashes, sores, itching
4. Mouth	That's a mouthful. That's hard to swallow. Big mouthed.	Disappointment	Dental and gum disease, canker sores
5. Ears	That's a real earful. Stick it in his or her ear. Can't believe my ears.	Overwhelmed	Problems with balance, earaches, inner-ear problems
6. Neck	Real pain in the neck. Enough to feel like breaking his or her neck.	Fear and anger	Stiff neck, soreness in neck area
7. Nose	That really stinks. Stick my nose in. Nosey.	Distaste	Runny nose, repeated bloody noses, sinusitis
8. Back	Break my back. A real burden. Back-breaking effort. Get off my back.	Overburdened	Problems with lower back, back spasms

Body Part	Phrases	Emotion	Symptoms
9. Chest	Tear my heart out. Load off my chest. It hits me right here.	Remorse	Heart disease, heartburn, congestion of the chest
10. Arms	Twist my arm. Do some real arm twisting. Arms or hands full. Fall into someone's hands.	Insecure	Sprains, pains in the arm, strains, arthritis
11. Bones	Chilled to the bone. Bone-breaking effort. Feel it in my bones.	Contempt	Repeated breaks of the bone, aches as if located in bone area
12. Stomach	Sick to my stomach. Takes guts. A stomachful.	Repulsion	Nausea, ulcer, upset stomach, indigestion
13. Genitals	Pissed off. Various swearing phrases.	Unexpressed anger	Urethritis, kidney stones, kidney problems, gonorrhea
14. Rectum	Pain in the ass. Kick their asses. Up your ass.	Attacking or attacked	Bowel disease, diarrhea, irregularity, constipation
15. Legs	Knock the legs out from under me. Get my legs back.	Tricked, trapped, insecure, lack of direction	Leg cramps, numbness
16. Feet	Knocked off my feet. Stepped on someone's toes. Stepped on my toes. Get back on my feet.	Hurt, pursued, neglected	Sore feet, corns, callouses

apart,'' by her own report. The following day she fell from a footstool in her kitchen, shattering her pelvis. When she called me to report the injury, she stated, "Don't make a big thing out of this. I know how you think about this stuff, but my fractured practice has resulted in my fractured pelvis." A woman attorney had become frustrated with one of her clients who was not cooperating with any of her legal advice, causing considerable problems when in court. She had told me several times, "That client just gets under my skin." One week before the final court date, the attorney came down with chicken pox so severely that she had to miss almost 1 month of work. Certainly, it is not possible to predict dys-ease or explain dys-ease in these simplistic terms, but it is possible to understand the symbolism of dys-ease and to help understand our lives through such speculation. Such an approach places dys-ease and dis-ease in the perspective of life, not in the realm of random mechanical breakdown. It helps us see ourselves, not just our illness.

QUESTION 5: Why Did This Happen to You in the First Place?

All of us are exposed to "consternations," or the radiation from stress and change. Sometimes we get sick and sometimes we do not. If you are sick, why did you get sick? Is there anything unique about your life that seems to have made you particularly vulnerable?

You should have someone to help you in answering question 5. Your hasslescope and PSA scan can be done with your self-shaman, but it is also important to look at your relationships. It is not that any other person will have more accurate answers for you; it is just that another person will help you initiate some investigations in areas that you may be too close to yourself to fully see. Another person may help you ask different types of questions or at least listen more effectively to your own answers. Ask someone for an opinion on why you have become sick. The answer given may not be right, but it will offer some clues you may wish to pursue to form your "dys-ease theory." Why did your immune system over- or underreact?

Sometimes we give ourselves permission to get sick. Did you? We may get sick just when things are going very well and we never felt better. After all, being sick is a real challenge. All of us experience sickness, and what better time to experience it than when we are feeling well. We are most ready then. Of course, we can also get sick when our supersystems can least afford a challenge. The purpose of the question "Why did this happen to you in the first place" is to determine why you were fertile terrain for the invasion of germs and other causes of pathology. Question 5 asks about your theory and explanation of your vulnerability to dis-ease and dys-ease.

QUESTION 6: Why Did You Get This instead of That?

Why do you think you have this illness instead of some other illness? We have already learned that all disease is metaphor. The supersystem does not bother itself with the trivial, with mere chance. Although you may think you are both hot and cold, remember that we go back and forth between both systems in reaction to specific life situations. It is important for you to be aware of which way you are leaning at any given time.

Is it possible that some of your overgrowing cells are going unmonitored because of loss or boredom? Are your arteries clogged because of alienation from self? Is your back sore because of a burden that is too heavy? Continue to make up your own metaphors. Be a poet. Think symbolically in terms of the hot and cold scores you have achieved earlier. Have you learned the hot or cold adjustment strategy to the lifestyle that is causing you to suffer from the hot or cold diseases? Have you noticed that your scores change from one category to another, that you overlap both categories? I am talking about hot- and cold-running styles of immunity—your present temperature, not your character.

QUESTION 7: How Bad Is It?

How bad do you think your illness is? Have your doctors "pronounced" you sick or even told you how sick you are going to become in the future?

Comedians use a routine that illustrates this step. They tell a story about weather, stating that it is very hot outside. The audience is to respond, "How hot is it?" The answer is always a symbolic but humorous one, such as "It is so hot that people enjoy having muggers wave their guns in their faces to cool them off." As ridiculous as this may seem, it is important to find humor even though you are ill, to put humor into practice to help your supersystem. How sick are you? "I am so sick. . ." (and you finish the sentence). Make sure you are clever and as ridiculous as possible. Do not respond with laboratory results or from the left-hemisphere side of your brain. Be impulsive, be spontaneous, be funny. The response of one of my patient's was, "I'm so sick that I can't even study well for my blood test." Another responded, "I'm so sick that even my chemotherapy seems like a sexual experience by comparison." Another said, "I'm so sick that I had the delusion that my doctor actually spent some time with me." Each patient's worries were evidenced by his or her joke.

I am not suggesting that being sick is funny. I am suggesting that mobilizing positive emotions and the ability to laugh, to share illness through metaphor and humor, is as important as understanding illness from a mechanical point of view. We cannot deal with illness only within the modern medical framework. The supersystem is too complex to be limited by a one-track mechanical system that helps with some, but not all, dimensions of our illness and disease experience. Remember the emotion test that you took earlier, and try now to elicit as many of the positive emotions as possible through these 20 questions regarding the supersystem.

A word of warning: If you are in a hospital, staff and visitors may not be comfortable with your humor at first. They may call it "gallows humor" and view it as a sign of worsening illness. They expect somberness, subservience, and compliance as the pain or penance of getting well. Surprise them and help shock your supersystem into more action or settle it into more comfort. Do not let the environment deter you. Current research has shown that hospital rooms with a view toward trees and bushes typically are the rooms that contain the patients who respond most quickly from surgery and experience fewer complications. The environment outside and the environment you create inside are crucial factors in your response to disease.

What works well for one patient does not necessarily work well for another. Where one patient may benefit from a challenging view of nature outside his window, another may benefit from a calm, quiet environment without the distractions of a window looking out to beautiful scenery. It is important to understand your style of supersystem and your style of being ill and being well. Hot reactors may require cool environments; cool reactors may require hot environments. Sometimes the reverse may be true. You can know what is best for you only by taking this supersystem exam and understanding your style, a style that may be good for you at a given time, not in terms of a whole life.

Remember, you are paying a lot of money to stay in your hospital room. Make sure it is outfitted the way you like it. Bring in stereos, pictures, flowers, posters—things that make your room suitable to your own supersystem style. Require that people knock before entering your room. You are leasing this location for healing, and for now it belongs to you. While it is the temple within that will be the setting for your own magnificent healing system, the outside environment can help.

QUESTION 8: Why Is It So Bad?

I spoke earlier of the vegetation concept. Eating in moderation, sleeping with consistency of pattern, and generally caring for your body were stressed as a key part of keeping the supersystem in tune. If you are ill, why is it as bad or not as bad as you might expect? Have you neglected the vegetation part of your maintenance system, or does the problem lie with a lifestyle that violates some other supersystem principle?

Now is the time to recalculate your wellness quotient. This quotient changes continually, and it helps your supersystem if you recalculate it as often as possible, particularly when you are hurt.

It is never dys-ease that kills us, but the severity of the dys-ease in comparison to the rallying strength of the immunity system. If that supersystem is too hot or too cold, is functioning without our help, we may succumb prematurely. Why is aging more disabling for some people than others? Certain genetic, environmental, and other medical factors relate to this question. It is also true, however, that maintaining the supersystem can measurably impact on the aging process.

Check the 80 suggestions for cooling the hot system and warming the cool system, and you will see that there is much you can do to reduce the severity of dys-ease processes and retard the aging process. Remember that you were asked to generate some of your own ideas. The ideas that come from you will be much more important than any specific recommendations in this or any other book.

QUESTION 9: So How Long Is This Thing Going to Last?

"Every time I get a vacation, I get sick and then I get better when I go back to work." This statement came from one of the male patients in a discussion group of persons with heart disease. He seemed unaware that his supersystem was listening, perhaps just following his instructions and his self-expectations, his drawing of a map for his immune system.

In effect, we establish our own "illness sentence." Although we can learn from illness and learn to appreciate wellness even more from our experience of illness, we sometimes provide ourselves with prolonged illness penance through expectations, or acceptance of pronouncements from the medical profession. We do not have to wait to be healed; we must actively anticipate the process of healing and encourage it. We must allow ourselves to receive the natural gift of wellness.

Once again, remember that I am referring to time in terms of life events rather than clock hours, days, or months. Do you anticipate being "better" by the time your child starts school next week or by the time a work project is to be completed? You are not setting goals for improvement, but setting guidelines for effective points of reference that are bound not just by hours but by events. Provide your own time frame, allowing yourself to be ill. Learn from your illness. Don't rush yourself to wellness. Illness is as natural as being healthy. It too has a purpose. In fact, all illness may be an imposed pausing for reorganizing the supersystem, a time out from a hectic life, even a chance for the immune system to "do its thing," to stay in shape, a form of immune-system aerobics.

QUESTION 10: What Do You Get Out of This Illness?

What benefits do you derive from any illness you have had or have now? This may sound surprising at first, but I have already discussed the learning opportunity provided by illness. Other benefits accrue as well. We get time off from work, intensive caring from family members, attention from persons who used to ignore us. Gifts, flowers, and other tokens of caring arrive that are absent during times when we are well. As a matter of fact, we sometimes get much more attention and much more acknowledgment of our importance to others when we are sick than we do when we are well.

Where else but in a hospital can you lie on your back and have every single need attended to, including your breathing if necessary. There are persons who are regular hospital attendees, moving in and out of hospitals as if they were some form of "illness spa." The danger of this type of "vacationing," however, is that it can be very harmful

to your health. It may, in fact, kill you. Give hospitals enough opportunities and they are certain to find something seriously wrong with
you, and all treatments carry with them serious risks to your health.

Does a given illness provide a cooling-off period for the hot reactor
or a caring period for the cold reactor? Does illness provide a time for
introspection? Is it a time to reflect on the benefits of your life? Is it a
time to be aware of your humanness and vulnerability in relationship
to others? Psychiatry has typically called such benefits *secondary gains*,
but, in fact, they may be basic gains related to the transitional life
problems in our lives. Being aware of these gains from illness is important to the process of becoming well.

QUESTION 11: What Do You Think Should Be Done about Your Illness?

What kind of treatment do you think you should have or should have
had? The treatment for dis-ease and dys-ease is not something that is
done to you or for you; it is something you must do with yourself and
from within. It is not assigned to you; it is selected by you in consultation
with doctors, nurses, and your self-shaman. You form a partnership for
healing with the supersystem.

Do you choose strictly a medical treatment with chemicals, surgery,
and other mechanical intervention, or do you choose a treatment of the
spirit, the soul, of thought, feeling, and believing? Or do you choose
some compromise between these two? Remember, gardeners are just as
important as mechanics, and a continuum from outside ministrations to
internal imagery exists.

Modern medicine has become a system of dogma, not of option,
choice, and partnership. Indeed, the term "dogmatic" comes from the
name of a society formed by relatives of Hippocrates, the founder of
medicine, who were attempting to protect persons against untried theories and approaches to healing. You must remember that your doctor
and the hospital work for you. They are team members whom you have
hired to work with you, to help you understand your illness and move
toward wellness. Make sure your doctor presents to you all available
options. Present to your doctor your own treatment program. Read,
study, and listen to the rumor mill within the hospital. Do not be afraid
to raise the topic of even the most radical of healing systems. Remember,
our own medical system is seen as radical throughout most of the world.

Anyone who has worked in a hospital for very long learns that no treatment program works all the time. Different patients respond in different ways to different systems. This is because of the unique style of their supersystems. Health care professionals are trained to be compliant persons themselves, and they learn through a hazing system of deference and inhumane demands that are put upon them. They learn that rules are to be followed and that the system is to be adhered to. They learn that emulation equals matriculation. Our cosmopolitan medical system is not by its nature an open system. You must try to make it more so. You select your treatment program; you are not a victim of it.

QUESTION 12: How Were You Before You Got Sick?

How were you feeling before you became ill? Whenever I ask this question in my lectures, someone will respond, "Well, that's obvious. I was feeling healthy before I got sick." This is not always true. Ask yourself about your baseline condition. How were you feeling? Were you feeling very, very well, energized, happy, and in balance with all others? Put in its most simple form, the key question is, "Were you happy before you got sick?" If not, your treatment plan depends upon not only getting well but also figuring out ways to be more and more happy. The idea is not to treat the illness, but to treat the person, not to take care of the patient, but to care for the patient.

All medicine is too late. It is used when we are ill. Taking control of our supersystems offers the opportunity to care for ourselves while we are well. I was called in as a consultant to a tool and die plant where employees were suffering repeated injuries in the form of cuts and bruises on their jobs. The company hired a medical staff who repeatedly stitched up and salved the wounds of the employees, only to have them return again with the same types of bruises and cuts. New, more modern machines were installed and a new medical staff was hired, but the injuries continued.

After weeks of sitting and listening to the employees, I learned that there was no program to teach the employees how to use their machines. It was assumed by the personnel department that prior experience had trained the employees in on-the-job safety procedures. Management had also neglected the fact that once one employee is injured, others tend to be injured as well. The concept of oneness is at work in the workplace as well as in the home and community. Injury as well as safety is contagious.

My recommendation as consultant was that each employee, following an injury, should sit with uninjured employees and briefly discuss the impact of the injury and why he or she thought it occurred. In the months following this consultation, the injury rate was reduced 80 percent.

The medical system has functioned in much the same way as the business discussed above. Admit, diagnose, repair, and send back into the frey. No one is concerned with the *why* of the diagnosis. Perhaps we should be busier teaching people how to swim than teaching artificial resuscitation, teaching water safety rather than lifesaving.

QUESTION 13: How Does This Illness Differ from Your Other Illness Experiences?

Were your other illnesses more debilitating, more global, more frightening? Does any one illness seem to have affected your lifestyle more than any other? Does any one illness stand out in your mind? Do any of your illnesses relate to repeated patterns in your hasslescope? What changes did you make in response to your other illnesses, if you made any? Did you make dietary, eating, personal relationship changes? Is there a pattern to your development of illnesses? What did you learn that altered your illness pattern?

Every day in every way, are you getting sicker and sicker, or is there a steady upward trend of improvement and less-severe illnesses? What is your illness direction? Are there things which you should be doing to improve but which you have been reluctant to do? Are you suffering from the "Jonah" complex I mentioned earlier, avoiding or afraid of your ultimate potential?

QUESTION 14: So What Else Has Gone Wrong Lately?

What other problems in your life has being sick made you aware of? Illness can be a form of imposed introspection, and problems in your life can sometimes be seen more clearly while you are sick than when you are well. What new problems have occurred to you? Are there conflicts in the family that have long required attention but have been neglected because there is "just not enough time"? People who work in hospitals see family conflicts every day. As a matter of fact, such family conflicts are one of the major problems for hospital staff. Who comes to visit, how often do they come, who sends or does not send flowers or cards—all are issues raised daily. One woman patient told me, "Keep my youngest daughter and her husband out of here." When I asked why, she stated, "I have given them so much and all I got from them was a stupid, cheap card and a small bouquet of flowers."

One nurse reported to me that she had to break up a fistfight in the hall at the hospital. Visitors were fighting for the special privilege of being with their grandfather when he was dying. While they fought outside the room over who would go first and who would sit with the grandfather, the grandfather passed away, hopefully never knowing the conflicts surrounding him at this most significant of times.

Not only is illness related to change and strain but illness itself is one of the major forms of strain in our lives. While illness may represent a temporary disruption of the supersystem, or the fact that the super-system is doing intense battle at the moment, it is also a time that demands even more from the supersystem than coping with the given invader. In fact, we either get better and better or get worse and worse. The supersystem either grows from illness or diminishes from it. The supersystem is never static, and its direction depends upon how we think and feel about ourselves.

QUESTION 15: What Are You Afraid Of?

The woman was crying bitterly when I entered her room. She was scheduled for a radical mastectomy, the total removal of a breast. Her family had just left her after hours of sitting with her prior to the surgery scheduled for the early morning hours. I sat with her now and held her hand. She cried for several minutes and then stated, "I am so afraid." I asked her whether she had talked with her doctor and family about her prognosis, which was actually very positive. She responded, "Yes, I know that I have a good chance for a long life." I asked her what other fears she had. She answered, "I am afraid of how I will look to all those people in the surgery room. No makeup, no nothing." At this time when so much was on the line, this patient was most concerned about her appearance during surgery, her human dignity at a time when she felt very vulnerable. Reassurance and further education resulted in a surprisingly restful night for this woman. One nurse even provided a decorator version of a cap and gown for the big day.

Our fears are not always, perhaps seldom, rational, and they may not be the fears that the medical establishment thinks are priorities. No matter how simple, no matter how dumb, your fears may seem to you, ask about each and every one of them. Reassurance can do wonders. Remember, health care professionals are used to the torturous system of invasion taking place in your body. They may have forgotten your human dignity in the process. You cannot afford to do so. Ask!

QUESTION 16: Who Is Going to Help You with All This?

Aside from yourself, who can help you get well? All healing comes from within, but the "others" in your life are also important parts of the healing process; they are a part of that "within."

Even under the deepest anesthesia, the brain is capable of detecting not only the words of the surgery team but the mood in the surgical room. Each unit in the hospital has its own sense of morale and unity or lack of morale and togetherness. Patients are keenly sensitive to these factors.

Several years ago, I did patient rounds with several medical students. We passed one room where a patient had been in a coma for several weeks. I would always enter with the students and say to the patient, "This is Thursday, it's sunny, and it's early in the morning. I am Dr. Pearsall and I will see you at the same time tomorrow." The whole interchange took just seconds. The medical students would ask why I wasted my time on a patient who obviously could not hear. My response was, "I guess it doesn't hurt, just in case she can hear." I am sure these medical students snickered behind my back. Some months later I received a letter from the patient. She misspelled my name, but the note follows:

Dear Dr. Pershall:
You were the only one who talked to me. I will always remember you. I came out of my coma and have always thought of how much you did for me just by stopping by to touch my shoulder.
                                        (Signed) Down, but not out.

The supersystem responds to the minutest changes in the environment, to caring or lack of caring, to vocabulary, to tone of voice, to expressed feelings. To deny this is to deny the existence of the human spirit. It is important that you take responsibility for this yourself. Hospitals need fewer intensive care units and many more intensive caring people. It is important during your illness that you provide such caring as a role model and not wait for it. Send flowers to people who are not in the hospital while you are hospitalized yourself. Order flowers for your nurses. Remember the concept of altruistic egoism: Doing for others is one of the best ways of doing for self. Offer support and interest to the lives of those who are the healers, for it is likely that they are wounded as well. You cannot afford, for your own survival, to be a recipient of "health care." You must be a partner in the healing process. Patients get better much less frequently than do persons.

Being in a hospital can resemble a hostage situation. Researchers tell us that you must be a person to your captor in such a situation. Let the terrorists see your eyes. Let them know you as a person. Don't become a nameless face that can be easily dismissed, perhaps killed. The same rules hold for a hospital. Although the health care workers are certainly not terrorists, you are being held hostage by a system of ineffective bureaucracy and accelerated inefficiencies. For a ransom that can drive you into bankruptcy, you are held in a hospital seemingly against your will. Health care workers are victims themselves, becoming captors without being aware of their role. To break that cycle, you must give, as well as receive, care when you are in the role of patient. You must nurture as well as succor. A balance between give and take must be established.

Another word of caution: As cruel as it may seem, there tends to be a counterreaction to persons who are ill. While we initially may feel sorry for them and offer our caring, over time sick people become a burden to us. They frighten us by their own patterns of illness, suggesting their own mortality and vulnerability and, therefore, our own. We may show our fear by anger and disgust. This happens not only with relatives but with hospital staff as well.

While it is difficult to do so, it is important to understand that the abruptness, the distance, and the impatience shown by the hospital staff sometimes mask a deep concern, a caring just waiting to come out. As Marguerite Yourcenar wrote in *Memoirs of Hadrian*, "The mask, given time, comes to be the face itself." The best way to encourage sharing by members of the hospital staff, their transcendence of their assigned role of objectivism and professional distancing, is by showing a patience and tolerance yourself, showing a caring for the healer as well as the person hoping to be healed. Physician Larry Dossey writes of "wounded healers," persons who are victims of the fallout of our medical system, working as health care workers who are jeopardizing their own welfare. Even as a patient, you must realize your responsibilities for the hospital system, for you are a part of it, not just a project within it.

QUESTION 17: What Have You Learned about You?

What have you learned about yourself from your illness? This question has been asked in different forms throughout this 20-question examination. Have you come up with any better answers at this point? Ask to see your chart in the hospital, your hospital record. Read it with one of the nurses or your own doctor present to explain things to you. It will do no good to read it alone, for it is written in a secret code known only to the priesthood of the temple. Look not only for mechanical factors and treatment strategies but at the nursing notes in particular. What kind of patient have you been in the eyes of the staff? Remember, the so-called "sweetheart, compliant, nice patient" can be at risk. Does the record show you to be in charge of your treatment?

　　Ask your family how you behave as a patient. Are you hostile, demanding, accusatory, and uncooperative or are you a coordinator and facilitator of a treatment team? I am not suggesting that you seek approval of the hospital staff. You have already seen that patients who seek such approval actually heal slower than those who are more assertive and self-responsible. I am, however, suggesting that you look to your chart not only as a record of mechanical intervention but as a record of interpersonal interactions of your status as a member of the team. If all growth comes from crisis, you can learn as much about your growing in the hospital as you can anywhere else.

QUESTION 18: How Is Your Healing Power?

How do you think and feel about your own healing power? Are you proud of your supersystem? Are you proud of the way your immunity operates? Does it do good work? Is it doing good work for you right now? Has it responded to the challenges of illness? Can you rely on your supersystem for the future, or are you concerned that it will fail you? These are questions that will help you learn about your vulnerability to illness and your potential for wellness.

All the hospitals in the world cannot do what the smallest component of your supersystem does reliably and beautifully. A replica of the kidney, for example, would require a city block of space. While there are dialysis machines that can help the kidney, it would take countless numbers of them to give the consistency, reliability, and around-the-clock service that one of your kidneys can accomplish. Even then, the machines would not have the staying power, strength, and self-healing capacity of the human kidney. Have you congratulated that magnificent kidney system lately? Have you congratulated your entire immune system lately?

Do you realize now, even if you are lying sick and frightened in your hospital bed or sick at home, that your supersystem is willing and ready to help? Do you realize that all you have to do is take control and understand that the strategies suggested in this book can help you mobilize not only the strengths of yourself but of the entire universe as well. As I said in earlier chapters, you are not a separate being rotating around the perimeter of the universe, looking inside. You are part of a system. You are not separate from that system because you are ill; in some ways your illness may make you more keenly aware of your relationship to the world.

Tell your immune system that it is fantastic, and you will be all the better for it. It is important to talk to yourself, and contrary to mythology it is important to listen as well.

QUESTION 19: When Do You Think This Might Happen Again?

When and with what disease will you be ill again in the future? What do you think you will do about it then? Try to imagine what illness you expect next. When will it occur? Take action now to minimize the likelihood that your illness will occur or to guarantee that your supersystem will be ready to help you with that illness.

We live in a time when the multibillion-dollar contemporary medicine industry has frightened us. We have been warned that without more spending, more instruments, more cutting, and more drugs, we will get sicker and sicker. We have developed a hypochondriacal society, jogging madly down highways away from the monsters of heart disease, shopping carefully for the right food to insulate us against cancer. While lifestyle changes are significant in the prevention of illness, we must also learn to anticipate, not to fear, illness, and we must take active measures to enhance our supersystems from within far in advance of the certain challenges they will face.

We are living in a society of anticipation. Cholesterol levels of accountants go up in those time periods before their busy season, not just during their season of highest activity. While there are elevations in cholesterol levels at the busy season as well, they are equaled or excelled by elevations during anticipation of change and strain. This is because anticipation is a form of self-talk, and it is as disruptive as the actual event itself.

Although denial is a natural human emotion, it must not be a process that prevents us from realizing that illness and dys-ease are a part of living. Coping must not be something that takes place after the crisis occurs; it must be a continued life strategy. We will deal with our illness as we live, day to day.

An older patient was sitting in the hallway late one evening as I was leaving work. I stopped to talk to him. I said, "You look worried Mr. Smith." He responded, "Yes, I am an old man of many worries, most of which never happened." This is the price of our anticipation culture. We are always getting ready, somehow never "being." This is why the hot-reactor strategies of fighting and fleeing and the cold reactor strategy of flowing can lead to disease. It is important that we learn to *be*. As Seaborn Blair stated, "Everybody wants to change the world, but nobody wants to change his mind." We must change how we think now, and not focus on "later."

Preventive medicine has led us down the wrong road. If we are in a preventive strategy posture, we are in an anticipating posture, which is an orientation that is unhealthy for all of us.

QUESTION 20: So How Have You Been Running Lately?

Did you become hotter or colder as a reaction to your illness? Your supersystem is forever changing. Ask yourself what the illness experience has done to your system now. Where do your vulnerabilities lie? Are you more likely to fall victim to the hot diseases or cold diseases at this time in your life?

Extend this question beyond yourself to others. Do you see your friends, your lover, your family, your community, your state, even your country and our world as hot or cold? As hot reactors, are all of us in this world running faster and faster, head on into more illnesses? Have we gone beyond the race of legs to the arms race, and now to the most deadly race of all, the human race? Or are we in a cold world, a world understimulated, without a commonality of direction and mutual growth? Are we likely to seek more stimulation from outside, attempting to entertain ourselves to death through a mindless dash into the fire? Are we likely to create cosmic perturbations in a helpless attempt to stimulate a system that looks for answers from the outside rather than from within? Are we failing to see that we are all a part of one another, warm enough to be close and active and cool enough to be peaceful and steady?

Will we become a helpless, hopeless world of people looking back on what we lost? Or will we become an accelerated, impatient, hostile world of people looking so far ahead that we lose the meaning of life altogether? As Ralph Waldo Emerson said, "What lies behind us and what lies before us are tiny matters compared to what lies within us." The ultimate rescue, as well as the invasion, comes from inner space, a personal healing place.

Chapter Eighteen

A HEALING PLACE

Drugs are not always necessary. Belief in recovery always is.

NORMAN COUSINS

The nurse's small flashlight searched through the darkened hospital bed in an effort to find the little boy whose vital signs she was to assess. He was suffering from a usually fatal blood disease, and continued monitoring and sometimes nauseating medications were the physicians' orders. As a searchlight scans terrain, the small circle of light fell first on an empty pillow and then on deserted blankets. Distrusting her own eyes, the nurse felt with her hand around the bed, finding only a warm spot left by the body of the missing patient.

Finally, the nurse's light caught the image of the boy. He was sitting against the foot of the bed on the cold hospital floor. A surgical mask was drawn tight over his entire face.

"What in the world are you doing down there?" she asked. "It's freezing on that floor. Do you want to catch a cold?"

"So what?" responded the boy in muffled voice, the surgical mask puffing in and out with each word. "I'm dying anyway."

"Don't say that! You are not dying; you are just very sick."

"Well, I'm just trying to get better down here, then," answered the boy. "Ever since I got in that bed, I've been getting sicker. I'm not going to stay in it any more."

"Come on, be a good boy. Get back in bed, and take off that mask."

"No way!" shot back the boy. "The doctors wear these things to keep the sickness out of them and they never seem to get sick at all. From now on I wear this all the time. Just call me the masked patient. Who is that masked boy?"

"Being sick is not funny. Get back in that bed right now," was the nurse's ratchetlike response.

He refused to budge. The nurse called me at home to state, "Danny is becoming psychotic. He may need psychiatric consultation, even medications to calm him down."

I assured the night nurse that things could wait until the next morning and told her to let the boy sleep where he was. She answered, "Fine with me, but it's your responsibility."

On rounds the next day, I found Danny huddled inside an elaborate tent. His bed had been stripped bare to the mattress, and on a bedpan hung from the I.V. rack was a sign which read, "No germs or night nurses allowed." The spongy mat sometimes placed on hospital beds to prevent bedsores served as the floor of his tent. His supplies consisted of a pile of nurses' flashlights, hospital desserts stored over several days, and a box of surgical masks somehow pilfered from the supply room.

"Can I talk with you, Danny?" I asked.

"If you come into my secret healing place," he answered.

I crawled in, with three students peering down at my apparent regression "to his level." Danny had a surgical mask covering his face and surgical gloves on his hands.

"I know these gloves look dumb, but my hands get cold. Dr. Caster thinks my hands get cold because of my sickness, but these gloves work better than the medicine."

"Why are you living here now?" I asked.

"This is my healing place. I feel safe; I think I can get better here. My parents can come in, and you can come in, and Jeff the cleaning man can come in, but that's all."

"Can Dr. Caster come in?" I asked. I knew that special dispensation would be required to enter this newly erected temple.

"Only if he knows my new password," was Danny's response.

When I asked for the password, Danny slowly lowered his mask, leaned forward, placed his arm around my neck, and muttered into my ear the magical word to enter his new world.

Over the next 2 weeks, with continual grumbling by the hospital staff from dietary services to respiratory therapy, Danny conducted his hospital business from his healing place. He exited only for tests with those who knew the password. His laboratory results showed a rebound of his immunity faster than would have been expected. His blood disease had gone into remission.

Certainly, the medications, his care by the nurses and physicians, and the modern miracles of medicine had played a key role in saving Danny's life. But most of all he had taken control of his supersystem, rallied his own immunity, found his place to heal. He had become his own person, not a victim. He had accepted a diagnosis, but not a verdict. He had established his own world of intimacy, closeness, efficacy, and control.

It is the message of this book that we all need a healing place. I return to the B-A-FITER formula for a review and reminder that control of our supersystems is essential to the survival of all of us, for we are all a part of one another's healing place. A world of people, nations, governments, races, or religions that develops an intolerance to "other," that builds up defensively for anticipated attack from others and views all others as threats and self as victim, becomes open to invasion of the diseases of civilization, a world that is in parts and not whole. A world that becomes too defensive or hot, too lethargic or cold, becomes sicker and sicker. Again, "immune" does not mean isolated and safe. It means self-responsible and at one with the universe. B-A-FITER—not *against* disease—but *for* your own dignity and the dignity of humankind. Immunity is a balance, not a defensive position.

I (B) believe that we are living in the most exciting of times, a time when we can actually learn to control our own destiny, our own wellness, a time when we can learn from the metaphor of our immune systems the danger of over- or underpreparation for attack and the possibility of self-destruction by our own defense systems.

I have a positive (A) attitude toward courageous researchers who have broken from the restrictive theories that have limited the growth of our healing capacity, and I have confidence that their work will free us from much of our needless suffering.

I have an (F) feeling that we are entering a new time, a period of a different paradigm, or model, to explain the functioning of our supersystems and our world, a period of learning to run warm and cool, not hot and cold toward viruses, cells, and one another.

I see an (I) image of peace, joy, laughter, learning, and togetherness, an image of hospitals with plants, sun, healthy foods, and happy, caring people everywhere, with patients as directors of the system of health care, not as recipients of prescribed treatments, working with, not being worked on.

I (T) think it is all possible, for I look at the references supporting the material in this book and realize that each author of each article warns that the data is "only a beginning, an initial start," to what looks like one of the most exciting times in the history of our world, a time when we will not be victims of disease but will be much more responsible for our own destiny.

I have (E) experienced patients who have shown a limitless capacity for their own growth and development beyond the mere absence of symptoms to a new view of super health that does not separate illness from health but incorporates all experiences into meaningful life experiences.

But I also (R) remember that millions of people are still suffering far beyond even the most elementary of the mechanical aspects of our medical miracles. I remember that if any one of us is suffering, none of us can truly be well. I remember that there is, in effect, a global immune system that must develop a tolerance and acceptance, not a defensiveness and isolationism.

The real story of immunity is the development of a specificity for self-protection and at the same time the development of a tolerance that allows personal and world growth. Our world will become a sickness place or a healing place, the choice is ours.

If you have been wondering about Danny's secret password, you are not alone. For days the hospital staff tried to guess what the word was. Names of movie stars, heroes, weapons, clowns, and rock idols were immediately, and incorrectly, guessed. Those hospital members who knew the word guarded it carefully, relishing their special privilege.

What would your guess be? What would be the secret password for an isolated, frightened little boy who had had his identity taken from him by a mechanistic approach that crippled his supersystem, depersonalizing and dehumanizing to dangerous and vulnerable dimensions?

The secret password contained within it all the magic that can be mustered to bolster the supersystem. It was a word of pride, confidence, security, and faith. It was a word seldom used around this little boy, particularly when "his case" was being discussed. It was a word seldom used around this "patient."

The secret word was "Danny."

A GLOSSARY OF THE SUPERSYSTEM

Research is improving our understanding of the supersystem and the immune system every day. The following terms are some basic concepts related to the supersystem as we now understand it.

Acetylcholine (ACh). This is one of the most important neurotransmitters in the nervous system. It is related directly to arousal and tends to be present in largest amounts when we are sleeping. It may be that ACh serves to keep us alive while we are sleeping. The fatal poison curare works by blocking ACh transmission, resulting in paralysis and suffocation.

ACTH. Adrenocorticotropin. This hormone is secreted by the pituitary gland and acts on the adrenal cortex to produce the immune-suppressing corticosteroids.

Adrenal glands. These are the glands on top of the renals (the kidneys). They consist of two main parts. The inside of the adrenal gland is called the *medulla*; it secretes the hormones epinephrine and norepinephrine. Both these hormones tend to stimulate the cardiovascular system. The outside of the adrenal glands is called the *cortex*; it is involved in the release of the hormone cortisol, and it can have depressing effects on sex hormones. I hypothesize that hot-reacting people are characterized by dominance of the medulla of the adrenal glands, with the secretion of excess epinephrine and norepinephrine affecting nerve endings and thereby overstimulating the cardiovascular system. Cold reactors are characterized by dominance of the cortex of the adrenal glands, with the accompanying increase in cortisol and decrease in sex hormones, over time, depressing the immune system.

349

Alpha-melanocyte-stimulating hormone. This is a newly discovered healing chemical of the brain that is capable of fighting off fever 25,000 times more efficiently than aspirin. This internal fever fighter may be under the control of our own mental imagery.

Amygdala. This is a part of the limbic system, or the one-fifth of the brain that sits on top of the spine or "caps" the spine. It is related to anger, rage, and impatience. I hypothesize that this part of the brain tends to hyperfunction in the hot reactor, causing a part of the hypothalamus to interact with the pituitary gland for a hot hormonal pattern.

Angiogenisis. This process, unique to cancer cells, allows new blood vessels to "feed" the growing tumor. By the time cancer is detected, the tumor has increased to more than 10 billion cells due to this special "feeding process." The supersystem must be strong enough to battle on this numerical scale.

Antigens. These are substances that cause the immune system to produce antibodies. Antigens can come from outside the body or can be produced from within.

B and T cells. Both called *lymphocytes* because they are transported through a special clear medium called the *lymph fluid*. You have felt your lymph glands enlarge when you have had an infection. T and B cells are born inside the bones. The T cells move on to the thymus gland, where they are trained for their special jobs (see below). No one knows exactly where or how the B cells are trained, but we know their preparation is extensive, for their jobs are highly specific. Perhaps in hot reactors T and B cells are overtrained, overready, and overexcitable, while in cold reactors the training program is deficient and the student cells begin their careers unprepared and unmotivated.

> **T killer cells.** One of the three kinds of T cells, these cells hang around in the lymph glands and go to work killing viruses and foreign tissue with their potent poisons. The T killer cells are known to be involved in defense against cancer by scavenging normal cells that have gone awry. Perhaps a cold reactor has a depression of this scavenging function.

> **T helper cells.** A second type of T cell, these cells help the B cells, which have the complicated job of identifying and destroying unique and sometimes disguised invaders.

> **T suppressor cells.** These are cells designed to keep the immune system from getting out of control. The hormone testosterone, found in higher amounts in men, allows T suppressor cells to flourish and perhaps is related to the fact that the immune system of men is weaker than that of women. Perhaps the hot-reactor style causes the T suppressor cells to heat up, resulting in less efficient defense against some diseases. In women, the situation is reversed, and T suppressor cells are restricted by the presence

of estrogen. Women may have stronger immune systems because they have comparatively fewer T suppressor cells. Women are also known to be more prone to autoimmune disease, or the situation of uncontrolled immune function that results in the system's attack of itself.

B-cell differentiation factor (BCDF). Produced by T helper cells, this lymphokine signals some of the B cells to stop dividing and to start producing their antibodies.

B-cell growth factor (BCGF). Secreted by T helper cells, this protein causes B cells to multiply.

Catecholamines. These hormones from the adrenal medulla were among the first "stress chemicals" studied. The two catecholamines are epinephrine (called *adrenaline* in England) and norepinephrine. Over time, epinephrine particularly weakens the immune system.

Cell-mediated and humoral-mediated immunity. Usually involving the T cells, cell-mediated immunity is involved in the rejection of transplanted tissue; it is a type of immunity designed to fight off invasion from "other" elements entering the body. Humoral-mediated immunity is involved in protecting the body against bacteria and other toxic substances. It is humoral-mediated immunity that can sometimes go awry in autoimmune disease.

Cold cycle. This is a trend, not a personality. The pattern is characterized by right-hemisphere orientation in coordination with the hippocampus and relates to hypothalamus and pituitary stimulation, which directs the cortex of the adrenal glands to yield an increase in cortisol and to depress sex hormone levels, thus deenergizing the body and its defense system.

Corticosteroids (cortisol). These hormones from the adrenal cortex help regulate the immune system. Depression is a mood state associated with corticosteroids, and research suggests that depression impairs immune function.

Dopamine. The neurotransmitter dopamine connects the limbic system, or the lower part of the brain, to the cortex, or the higher part. It also serves a role in reward, and is particularly related to the control of motor activity. People with Parkinson's disease typically show severe shaking and tremors which are caused by a lack of the neurotransmitter dopamine.

Einstein's theory of relativity. In the chapter on time, we learned that time is a hypothesis and reflects our view of life more than do ticks on a clock. We discovered that time is relative. Research by psychologist Dr. Gary Schwartz suggests that by understanding Einstein's theory about the way in which time itself can change, we may actually be able to slow down the aging process. He suggests that clocks (and therefore time), relatively speaking, are slower at lower elevations than at higher ones due to the presence of gravity. This was theorized and proved by Einstein. Perhaps by focusing on our own centers, getting next to the earth, getting close to nature, and amplifying our own sense of gravity and oneness with the earth, we can slow the tick of our own life clocks and lead longer, healthier lives.

Endorphins, enkephalins, and lipotropins. Most scientists refer collectively to this family of natural opiates in the brain as the "endorphins." Enkephalins have been shown to enhance the activity of T killer cells in cancer patients. The lymphocytes probably have receptors on them to respond to and work with these miracle chemicals. Research has shown that some forms of music can lead to a "thrill" accompanied by secretions of endorphins. Any activity producing a reported "high" is accompanied by endorphin increase and, therefore, enhancement of immune function. Recent research has shown that endorphins not only invigorate the attack against cancer by T killer cells but also increase the number, percentage, and effectiveness of the immune cells. As with all opiates, it is possible to get hooked even on these natural opiates, and the Goldilocks "just-right" emphasis is just as important with these brain chemicals as it is with all other body systems.

Epinephrine. This is a catecholamine from the adrenal medulla that can impair the immune system.

Gamma interferon (IF). This protein does the same job as IL-2 and BCDF, and it also keeps the macrophages working at the site of the battle.

Hippocampus. A part of the old brain, the hippocampus is located near the temporal lobe of the human brain. It is related to novelty, challenge in life activities, and memory. Research indicates that memory may depend more on novelty and challenge than on simple reward or pleasure. I hypothesize that this area of the brain is deprived of stimulation or malfunctions in some way in the cold reactor, thus resulting in a disruption of the pattern of stimulation of the supersystem.

Hormones and stress. For the hot reactor, the principle neurotransmitters tend to be epinephrine and norepinephrine. In the cold reactor, adrenocorticotropic hormone enters the blood and stimulates the adrenal cortex (the outside of the adrenal glands) to release different hormones, the mineral corticoids, and the glucocorticoids. I hypothesize that the mineral corticoids are hormones related to the hot reaction, while the glucocorticoids are present in more abundant quantities in cold reactors who are attempting to flee rather than fight. The interaction between mineral corticoids and glucocorticoids is very complex, and much more needs to be learned regarding this interaction.

Hot cycle. Remember that we are all hot and cold and that we are talking about daily orientation and behaviors, not personalities. The hot cycle of response is essentially a left-hemisphere dominance pattern, resulting in an alarm state mediated through the amygdala and hypothalamus, which, in turn, causes the pituitary (master) gland to secrete excess stimulation to the medulla of the adrenal glands. This results in hormones which raise blood pressure and generally prepare and sometimes overprepare the body for defense.

Hypothalamus. You have learned that this part of the brain is the brain of the head brain. It literally directs the brain in daily activities. When some parts of the hypothalamus are stimulated in research programs, immune function decreases (stimulation of the medial hypothalamus in rat brains), while stimulation of other parts of the hypothalamus tends to have positive effects on the immune system.

Immune cells. About 1 trillion of the following white blood cells: macrophages, T helper cells, T suppressor cells, T killer cells, B cells, and memory cells (these cells circulate in the blood or lymph, storing remnants of prior immune reactions).

Immunoglobulins. These are long, complex, folded chains of protein that are on the surface of B cells. There are many types of immunoglobulins, for example, immunoglobulin A (IgA), which is related to defense against respiratory illness and tends to decrease in persons who are more "power-oriented" than "people-oriented."

Interleukin-1 (IL-1). Secreted by the macrophages, this protein activates T helper cells and causes the brain to raise the body's temperature which, in turn, increases the efficiency of the immune system.

Interleukin-2 (IL-2). Secreted by the T helper cells, this protein signals for production of T killer cells.

Left hemisphere and right hemisphere. Some research has shown that the left hemisphere controls the reaction of T killer cells and that right-hemisphere dominance may relate to problems with the immune system and depletion of T killer cells. I hypothesize that hemisphere dominance is partially under our control and, therefore, that our immunity can be enhanced by learning hemispheric control. It is no longer correct to assume that left- or right-hemisphere dominance is superior. Utilizing the entire body and brain working together seems to be the most healthy orientation.

Lymphocytes. Special white blood cells from the lymph system. A T cell is a lymphocyte.

Lymphokines. Proteins by which immune cells communicate with each other.

Macrophages. These are giant white blood cells that serve primarily as the mop-up crew of the immune system. (*Macro* means "large," and *phage* means "to eat.") These cells clean up after T killer cells have injected any abnormal cells with deadly toxins. Once the toxin is injected, the abnormal cells begin to look as if they were barbequed, and eventually they explode. The debris from the explosion is cleaned up by the macrophages. The surveillance theory of cancer suggests that in cold reactors' immune systems, T killer cells and macrophages are too sluggish to keep control of the millions of abnormal cells that are developed every day, particularly if the hypothesis is correct that the bored brain creates even more abnormal cells for the body to "play with."

Mast cells. Concentrated in the skin and respiratory system, these translucent cells play a key role in allergies, which are overreactions of the immune system.

Monoclonal Antibodies. Hybrid cells made from healthy B cells joined with cancerous B cells, these experimental cells called *Hybridomas* divide rapidly and can attack and destroy cancer cells while leaving healthy cells intact.

Neurotransmitters. It is likely that the brain has several hundred neurotransmitters, chemicals which are the lubricators of our dealings with our environment and one another. Rather than seeing the brain as an electronic organ, it is helpful to see it as a large chemical factory with millions of spurts from perfumelike bottles taking place every millisecond. Neurotransmitters help messages cross the *synapse*, or the connection between neurons, the basic cells of the brain. Neurotransmitters are stored in little pouches called *synaptic vesicles* and are emitted when communication between neurons is necessary.

Neutrophils. Over half the army of white blood cells designed to fight disease is made up of these special cells born in the bone marrow. About 100 billion of these warriors are produced every day. When called upon by chemicals released at the sight of invasion, they immediately change shape to fit better through the vessels of the body. Once on the scene, they stick a tiny foot (called a *pseudopod*) through any convenient crack that may exist, engulfing the invader with their own bodies. They then digest the invader quickly and efficiently. The neutrophils come in wave after wave of attack until the job is done. They do their work every day in healthy and sick people, sometimes overworking in hot reactors and perhaps underworking in cold reactors. I hypothesize that the stickiness developed in the vessels to help the neutrophils get a foothold (in this case, a pseudopodhold) may relate to the clogging of the arteries in the "heart allergy" of hot reactors. I also hypothesize that neutrophils become sluggish in cold reactors, perhaps not attending fully to the summons from problem areas.

Norepinephrine. This neurotransmitter is related to memory and the reward system in the brain, and it is secreted during states of pleasure. Norepinephrine is found in the autonomic nervous system outside the brain.

Null cells. Neither T nor B cells (therefore called "null"), these cells include the NK or "natural killer" cells that attack abnormal cells, tumors, and cells infected with viruses.

Phagocytes. Special white blood cells on constant patrol for any material that is dangerous to the body. These cells eat the invader (the word "phagocyte" literally means "cell eater").

Pituitary gland. This is the master gland of the body. It works in close interaction with the hypothalamus to regulate our hormonal environments and our dealing with day-to-day challenges. I hypothesize that interaction between the pituitary, hypothalamus, hippocampus, and amygdala is different in hot- and cold-reaction styles.

Plasma cells. Specially prepared and trained B cells divide into these plasma cells, which can produce and secrete the specific antibodies required for specific jobs of destruction. Sometimes these cells secrete a substance that coats invaders so that macrophages can ingest and destroy them. Lymphokines are the poisons from the T cells that destroy invaders, while the plasma cells secrete substances specially designed to do the same job on other and sometimes more devious and unique invaders. Cell-mediated immunity has to do with lymphokines, while humoral-mediated immunity has to do with plasma-cell secretions.

Serotonin. The neurotransmitter serotonin controls sleep and many of the activities that are related to sleeping. When we have insufficient serotonin, we tend to suffer from insomnia. This neurotransmitter actually slows communication between the neurons, and when it is not present in sufficient quantity, the activity level tends to increase greatly.

Smile muscles and frown muscles. It appears that a special muscle group, the *zygomatic region muscle*, is related to smiling and that another muscle group, the *corrugator region muscle*, is related to frowning. Research suggests that the left hemisphere of the brain controls the zygomatic region and that the right hemisphere controls the corrugator region. Perhaps changing thinking styles and even nostril breathing can lead to happy or sad faces.

Specificity. This concept refers to the unique response of the immune system to each invader. The system is designed to identify invaders, prepare for attack, and rid the body of invasion by matching immune-system forces with each unique invader, fitting them together as specifically as a key fits a lock. B cells have antibody molecules on their surface which are long, folded chains of protein that fit only with other molecules, and when this fit "works," or matches, immune response is more effective.

Sympathetic and parasympathetic nervous system. These parts of the nervous system belong to a subpart called the *autonomic nervous system*. I hypothesize that the hot reactor is characterized by sympathetic mediation, which, in turn, is related to an increase in blood pressure and an alerting of body systems, while the cold reactor is characterized by parasympathetic mediation, resulting in gastric changes and a general slowing down of the nervous system and the body defense system. SAM refers to the hot sympathoadrenomedullary system; and PAC refers to the cold parasympathoadrenocortical system.

Thymus gland. You have read about the uniqueness of this gland as a training site for T cells. Researchers have shown that the thymus gland is responsive to changes in thinking and imaging. Perhaps we can help train our training center by thinking and feeling more rationally and positively, a form of teaching the immunity teacher.

Tolerance. Molecules that are identified by the immune system as "not self" are called *antigens*. Tolerance refers to the immune system's ability to attack and rid the body of antigens, or non-self molecules, only and to accept "self."

Triune brain. Dr. Paul MacLean suggests that the brain is actually composed of three levels, with the outer, or *neomammalian* (new mammalian), layer composed of the most recent brain structures and having to do with thinking and rationale. The paleomammalian layer, or limbic system, where the amygdala and hippocampus are located, has to do with emotions. Finally, the reptilian brain, or R complex, has to do with prototypical patterns of behavior common to all our ancestors. I have hypothesized that according to the triune-brain concept, the hot reactor tends to be highly intellectualized, functioning on the neomammalian level, while the cold reactor tends to be frustrated on the emotional, or the paleomammalian, level.

White blood cells. Immune cells produced in the bone marrow, liver, and spleen. They are also called leukocytes.

There are many other terms, some very technical and some describing as yet unclear processes of immunity. In this glossary, and in this book, I have attempted to provide a simplified outline of the relationship between immunity and thinking. If you are curious enough to learn more and to keep an eye out for continuing developments in this exciting field, my goal has been met.

REFERENCES

INTRODUCTION

p. xii   The supplement to the August issue of the *Journal of Immunology* provides an introduction and current updating of the new field of neuroimmuno- modulation. See E. Goetzl (Ed.), "Proceedings of a Conference on Neu- romodulation of Immunity and Hypersensitivity."

p. xii   The clearest description of Chinese medicine is in Manfred Porkert, *The Theoretical Foundations of Chinese Medicine*. He suggests that all of us should be able to benefit not only from the latest advances in modern western medicine but from all the history of the healing arts, what he calls, "the pool of universal science." My book is intended to help in this effort.

p. xii   For a balanced review of alternative models of health and healing, see Richard Grossman, *The Other Medicines*.

p. xii   For a contrast between "dualist" or the mind-body split orientation and "monism" or the view that feelings and thoughts relate directly to our physiology, see H. Feigl, *Concepts, Theories, and the Mind-Body Problem*.

p. xii   For an interesting, although technical, debate of the issue of "pure im- munology," or the stance that the immune system is largely autonomous, and psychoneuroimmunology, which suggests that the immune system can be influenced by thoughts and feelings, see Theodore Melnechuk, "Why Has Psychoneuroimmunology Been Controversial? Proponents and Skeptics at a Scientific Conference."

p. xiii   The label *Type C* is related to emotional suppression, as contrasted to the more expressional, agitated Type A and comparatively easygoing Type B. See Meyer Friedman in *Treating Type A Behavior and Your Heart*. He had originally used the term *emotional stress* but adopted the term Type A in order to receive research grant support. Type C is used by Lydia Temoshok and her colleagues at the University of Chicago.

p. xiii   For a realistic and cautious summary of the issues related to the personality- immunity issue, see David F. Cella, "Psychological Adjustment and Cancer Outcome: Levy vs. Taylor."

357

p. xiii   For a discussion of the theories behind the psychosocial etiology of cancer, see B. Fox, "Current Theory of Psychogenic Effects on Cancer Incidence and Prognosis."

p. xiv   For an interesting discussion of the relationship between psychological and physical factors, see Edward Whitcomb, *Psyche and Substance*.

CHAPTER ONE

p. 5   For a discussion of mind-body dualism and the effect of that view on our society and culture, see Pitirim Sorokin, *Social and Cultural Dynamics*.

p. 5   Clarification of the impact of cosmopolitan medicine on health is provided by René Dubos, *Mirage of Health*.

p. 6   The quote from Francis Bacon and additional information on the evolution of psychosomatic medicine is found in J. J. Schwab, "Psychosomatic Medicine: Its Past and Present."

p. 6   Support for the notion of mind-body connection in prehistorical times is found in H. I. Kaplan, "History of Psychosomatic Medicine," in *Comprehensive Textbook of Psychiatry*, vol. 4.

p. 6   Further information on Ayurveda may be found in Dennis Cherin and F. Manteuffel, *Health: A Holistic Approach*.

p. 7   A study of early attitudes and later disease is found in C. B. Thomas et al., "Family Attitudes Reported in Youth as Potential Predictors of Cancer." See also the following: P. J. Dattore et al., "Premorbid Personality Differentiation of Cancer and Non-cancer Groups: A Test of the Hypothesis of Cancer Proneness." R. P. Greenberg et al., "The Relationship between Dependency and the Development of Cancer." R. J. Grossarth-Maticek et al., "Interpersonal Repression as a Predictor of Cancer." R. Shekelle et al., "Psychological Depression and 17-Year Risk of Death from Cancer." These studies are prospective research, or work that follows or examines the personal development of individuals in search for patterns that may relate to cell disease.

p. 7   Animal studies offer evidence of stress relating to tumor growth. See R. C. La Barba, "Experimental and Environmental Factors in Cancer. A Review of Research with Animals." See also B. H. Fox and B. H. Newberry (Eds.), *Impact of Psychoendocrine Systems in Cancer and Immunity*. See also V. Riley, "Mouse Mammary Tumors: Alteration of Incidence as an Apparent Function of Stress."

p. 8   An excellent review of the literature on the supersystem or the brain-immune system connection is found in Michael Fauman, "The Central Nervous System and the Immune System."

p. 9   A view of the mind as holographic, totally interactive within itself, with each part a representation of the whole, is described in Karl H. Pribram, "Holonomy and Structure in the Organization of Perception," in John M. Nicholas (Ed.), *Images, Perception, and Knowledge*. A protégé of Albert Einstein, David Bohm, suggested that the universe is a hologram, in effect more perception than thing. Pribram saw the relationship between his work and that of Bohm, stating, "Maybe the whole world is a hologram!" Such speculation relates to the importance of perception in health. See David Bohm, *Wholeness and the Implicate Order*.

p. 9   The concept of supermind was developed by Barbara B. Brown in *Supermind: The Ultimate Energy*.

p. 9   Documentation of the fact that thoughts can affect a single cell is in J. V. Basmajian, "Control of Individual Motor Units."

p. 9   The curing of the skin disease of the 16-year-old is reported in A. A. Mason, "Ichthyosis and Hypnosis." This work is verified and replicated in C. A. S. Wink, "Congenital Ichthyosiform Erythrodermia Treated by Hypnosis: Report of Two Cases." Further verification came 5 years later in C. B. Kidd, "Congenital Ichthyosiform Erythrodermia Treated by Hypnosis."

p. 10   Research supporting imagery changing breast size is found in G. J. Honiotes, "Hypnosis and Breast Enlargement: A Pilot Study." See also J. E. Williams, "Stimulation of Breast Growth by Hypnosis," and R. D. Willard, "Breast Enlargement through Visual Imagery and Hypnosis."

p. 10   Research supporting the use of imagery and belief in removing allergic reaction can be found in A. A. Mason and S. Black, "Allergic Skin Responses Abolished under Treatment of Asthma and Hay Fever by Hypnosis." See also Y. Ilkemi, "Psychological Desensitization in Allergic Disorders," in J. Lassner (Ed.), *Hypnosis and Psychosomatic Medicine*.

p. 10   The power of suggestion related to well-being is described in K. Platonov, *The Word as a Psychological and Therapeutic Factor*.

p. 10   Imagination influencing the Mantoux reaction is found in S. Black et al., "Inhibition of Mantoux Reaction by Direct Suggestion under Hypnosis."

p. 10   An excellent overview of the mind-body connection is found in A. A. Sheikh (Ed.), *Imagination and Healing*.

p. 11   Data on the treatment of warts by imagery is found in R. H. Rulison, "Warts: A Statistical Study of Nine Hundred and Twenty-One Cases." See also M. Ullman and S. Dudek, "On the Psyche and Warts: II, Hypnotic Suggestion and Warts." Note that research supporting the relationship between warts and imagery has existed for more than 50 years.

p. 11   "Dr. Wart's" magic machine is described and results documented in B. Block, "Über di Heilung der Warzen durch Suggestion."

p. 11   The idea that the mind can heal the body through our direct control of our own thinking is far from new. One historical discussion of this material is found in D. H. Tuke, *Illustrations of the Influence of the Mind upon the Body and Disease Designed to Elucidate the Action of Imagination*.

p. 11   As an illustration of the generalization of the mind-body integration to other fields of medicine, see A. P. French, "The Treatment of Warts by Hypnosis," published in a gynecology and obstetrics journal more than 12 years ago.

p. 11   Extensive documentation of such phenomena as reducing dermatitis produced by ivylike plants, causing and reversing skin inflammation, minimizing bleeding, and lessening the effects of burns is provided in Theodore

X. Barber, "Changing 'Unchangeable' Bodily Processes by (Hypnotic) Suggestions: A New Look at Hypnosis, Cognitions, Imagining, and the Mind-Body Problem."

p. 14   The field of psychobiology is defined and discussed in Richard M. Restak, *The Brain: The Last Frontier*. Understanding the mind-body connection is never fully possible, for as St. Francis of Assisi pointed out, "What we are looking for is what is looking." This "looking" is the field of psychobiology.

p. 14   Reference to the football stadium phenomenon and similar emergency room examples to the one mentioned in this chapter can be found in Norman Cousins, *The Healing Heart: Anecdotes to Panic and Helplessness*. Cousins outlined several key issues in the mind-body-spirit realm in his lecture "New Dimensions in Healing," at the Sixth Annual Esther B. Mellon Memorial Lecture, Sinai Hospital of Detroit, Nov. 12, 1984. Reprints of Cousins' address are available by contacting Sinai Hospital of Detroit, Community Relations Department, Detroit, Mich. 48235.

p. 14   The concept of superintelligence is presented in Lewis Thomas, *The Lives of a Cell*. See also his work "On the Science and Technology of Medicine," in John H. Knowles (Ed.), *Doing Better and Feeling Worse*.

p. 15   The example of the two students is based on research by David C. McClelland. He identified the *inhibited-power motivation* triad of a high personal need for power, a sense of frustration of that need, and a comparatively lower need for relationships than control. He found that the coexistence of these three factors related to a diminished immunity, specifically a lowering of immunoglobulin A, a component of the immune system which protects us from colds and that tickle in the back of the throat, reported by the two students. See his work "Stress Power Motivation, Sympathetic Activation, Immune Function, and Illness."

CHAPTER TWO

p. 18   The first description of the field of psychoneuroimmunology is credited to R. Ader (Ed.), *Psychoneuroimmunology*. Two books related to this book are scheduled for publication. See Steven Locke and D. Colligan, *The Healer Within*. See also S. E. Locke et al., *Foundations of Psychoneuroimmunology*.

p. 18   A pioneering work in drawing together findings on immunity and the brain is G. F. Solomon and R. H. Moos, "Emotions, Immunity, and Disease. A Speculative Theoretical Integration."

p. 18   Further information on the function and structure of the brain may be found in the following sources: R. Restak, including *The Brain*; Peter Russell, *The Brain Book*; C. Pribram, *Languages of the Brain*.

p. 18   The study on the immunity of cadets at West Point is described along with other studies documenting the link between emotions, the mind, and immunity in Stephen P. Maier and M. Laudenslager, "Stress and Health: Exploring the Links."

p. 19   Research on learned helplessness and the idea that perception of control over life events leads to more effective immune function than perception of no control is found in M. L. Laudenslager et al., "Coping and Immunosuppression: Inescapable Not Escapable Shock Suppresses Lymphocyte Proliferation."

p. 19   The work on decrease in natural killer-cell activity as related to perception of stressful events rather than stress itself is reported in Stephen E. Locke, "Stress Adaptation and Immunity: Studies in Humans."

p. 19   The relationship between cell disease and emotions is reviewed in Sandra M. Levy, "Emotions and the Progression of Cancer."

p. 19   Specific changes in suppressor cells related to cancer is found in S. Broder and T. Waldman, "The Suppressor-Cell Network in Cancer." See also J. Cohen et al. (Eds.), *Psychosocial Dimensions of Cancer*.

p. 19   The link between cancer and emotional state has not been finally established. For an opinion contrary to the view of Sandra Levy, see S. Taylor.

p. 19   Data supporting the neurochemical interaction between the central nervous system and the immune system is found in the following sources: M. Stein et al., "The Hypothalamus and the Immune Response," in M. Weiner et al. (Eds.), *Brain, Behavior and Bodily Disease*; Ruth Lloyd, "Possible Mechanisms of Psychoneuroimmunological Interactions"; H. Besodovsky and E. Sorkin, "Network of Immunoneuroendocrine Interactions."

p. 19   That the immune system can be taught to be effective or ineffective is documented in R. Ader and N. Cohen, "Behaviorally Conditioned Immunosuppression." See also M. Stein et al., "Influence of Brain and Behavior on the Immune System."

p. 20   Documentation of the relationship between emotions and heart rhythms is found in J. A. Herd, "Behavioral Factors in the Physiological Mechanisms of Cardiovascular Disease," in S. M. Weiss et al. (Eds.), *Perspectives on Behavioral Medicine*. This reference contains Dr. Herd's shorthand *SAM* designation used throughout this book, representing the sympathoadreno-medullary system. See also C. D. Jenkins, "Recent Evidence Supporting Physiologic and Social Risk Factors for Coronary Disease."

p. 20   The metaphor of disease has been discussed by researchers, poets, and musicians. Marilyn Ferguson wrote, "So the broken 'heart' may become coronary disease, the need to grow may become a tumor, ambivalence a 'splitting headache,' the rigid personality arthritis. Every metaphor is potentially a literal reality," *The Aquarian Conspiracy*, p. 253. My emphasis is that, while metaphor can help us understand disease, it may be misused as blame or self-recrimination. Looking toward how we can learn to heal, rather than how we might have caused ourselves to get sick, is the focus of this book. For further information on this issue of blame versus hope as we work toward an understanding of the mind-body-immunity connection, see Susan Sontag, *Illness as Metaphor*.

p. 20   The reference to the work at Cambridge University on counting brain cells in a simple worm can be found in Peter Russell.

p. 21   The concept of the brain functioning as a "gland" in a two-way interaction with the endocrine system may be found in R. Bergland and R. B. Page, "Pituitary-Brain-Vascular Relations: A New Paradigm."

p. 21   Information on the evolution of the human brain, including interesting teaching examples, may be found in R. Ornstein, *Psychology: The Study of Human Experience*.

p. 21   Material on the selfishness of the human brain is in A. T. W. Simeons, *Man's Presumptuous Brain: An Evolutionary Interpretation of Psychosomatic Disease*.

p. 21   The theory of the triune brain is described by Paul MacLean, "On the Evolution of Three Mentalities," in S. Arieti and G. Chrzanowki (Eds.), *New Dimensions in Psychiatry: A World View*, vol. 2.

p. 21   An interesting description of MacLean's theory is found in Carl Sagan, *The Dragons of Eden*.

p. 22   A description of the body-mind relationship as revealed by posture and other external physical signs is found in Ken Dychtwald, *Body-Mind*.

p. 22   The theory of our bodies as visual representations of our orientation to life is discussed in Gay Hendricks and B. Weinhold, *Transpersonal Approaches to Counseling and Psychotherapy*.

p. 22   The concept of *sanpaku* eyes is discussed in George Oshawa, *You Are All Sanpaku*.

p. 22   For a controversial discussion of techniques for "reading" the body for sources of allergies and illness, see John Diamond, *Your Body Doesn't Lie*.

p. 23   The reference to the brain's responsiveness while under anesthesia is in Henry L. Bennett and H. S. Davis, "Nonverbal Response to Interoperative Conversation."

p. 24   Research on the chemical composition of tears and their role in voiding the waste of the stress reaction is reported in W. H. Fry et al., "Effect of Stimulus on the Chemical Composition of Human Tears."

p. 25   For one of the clearest descriptions of the neuroendocrine cycle related to stress, and the effect of the adrenal cortex (increase in corticosteroids) and the adrenal medulla (increase in catecholamines), see Joan Borysenko, "Stress, Coping, and the Immune System," in J. D. Matarazzo et al. (Eds.), *Behavioral Health*.

p. 25   Dr. David Goodman reported his findings on the role of tears in altering hormonal levels at the 1984 Annual Meeting of the Society for Neuroscience. See Jeffrey L. Fox, "Crying Mellows Some, Masculinizes Others," for a review of this material.

p. 26   Research on the importance of newness and novelty to healthy human development is reported in Collin Wilson, *New Pathways in Psychology*.

p. 26   The brain's attempt to avoid automation and boredom by disrupting body functions and cell division processes is hypothesized in Augustin M. de la Pena, *The Psychobiology of Cancer*.

p. 27   For information on Dr. James Prescott's theory of the importance of movement to brain and personality development, see "Phylogenetic and Ontogenetic Aspects of Human Affectional Development," in Robert Gemme and Connie Wheeler (Eds.), *Selected Proceedings of the 1976 International Congress of Sexology.*

p. 27   The effort required to transcend our present limits of development is described in E. O. Wilson, *Sociobiology: The New Synthesis.* This work represents another controversial approach to understanding the relationship between mind, body, and human development.

p. 27   An excellent description of the mind-body-stress interaction is found in Kenneth Pelletier, *Mind as Healer: Mind as Slayer.* This reference describes the fight or flight response in detail.

p. 28   Information on the nature of the two sides of the human brain may be found in Mark Brown, *Left Hand, Right Hand.* See also Stuart Diamond, *The Double Brain.*

p. 28   Sexually dimorphic imprinting of the human brain, or the idea that there is a male and female hormonal influence on brain cells before birth that plays itself out in later male-female patterning, is found in Jerry Levy, "Possible Basis for the Evolution of Lateral Specialization of the Human Brain."

p. 28   I have adapted some of the concepts and analogies for explaining the development and function of the brain from the lectures and writings of Dr. Robert Ornstein. See his *Psychology of Consciousness,* 2d ed.

p. 29   Data on immunity and hemisphere orientation are reported by Dr. Pierre Flore-Henry of the University of Alberta, Canada. He suggests a natural oscillation of mind style. For more information, see G. Renoux et al., "The Production of T-Cell Inducing Factors Is Controlled by the Brain Neocortex." It is possible that an "oscillation" of mind style relates to the hot-cold cycle of life orientation.

p. 29   Work on neocortical lateralization and killer-cell activity is found in P. Bardos et al., "Neocortical Lateralization of N-K Activity in Mice."

p. 30   The relationship between higher brain structures and immunity received support from the work of K. Bulloch and R. Y. Moore, "Innervation of the Thymus Gland by Brainstem and Spinal Cord in Mouse and Rat."

p. 30   Differences between the genders in terms of relationship style, cognitive development uniqueness, and affective distinctions are described in Carol Gilligan, *In a Different Voice.*

p. 31   Some of the ideas in the cognitive style test were adapted from Barbara Meister, *Unicorns Are Real: A Right-Brained Approach to Learning.*

p. 32   The issue of handedness is not as simple as it would seem. For example, there is evidence that ambidexterity is different than an ambiguity of handedness and that this difference relates to emotional problems. Dr. Paul Satz has shown a relationship of ambiguity of handedness and left-handedness to certain types of autism. While ambidextrous people can perform skilled tasks with both hands and are consistent as to which hand is used for which task, ambiguous people perform skilled tasks poorly and show no preference for which hand is used for which task. See John Bales, "Hand Dominance as a Factor in Autism."

p. 33   An interesting discussion of the mind is found in Marilyn Ferguson, *The Brain Revolution*. Ferguson also edits the *Brain/Mind Bulletin*, an updating of new research related to the body-mind health issue.

CHAPTER THREE

p. 34   A detailed discussion of the issues of immunity described in this chapter may be found in S. M. Weiss et al. (Eds.), *Perspectives in Behavioral Medicine*.

p. 34   A description of the functioning of the immune system is in J. T. Matarazzo et al. (Eds.), *Behavioral Health*.

p. 35   The thymus gland has long been controversial in medicine. Beard, writing in 1902, stated, "Has it yet fallen to the lot of any writer upon the thymus to write the truth and be believed?"

p. 35   For a complete annotated bibliography on the immune system and the mind, see S. E. Locke and M. Hornig-Rohan, *Mind and Immunity: Behavioral Immunology*.

p. 35   The complex interaction between the brain and the immune system is demonstrated in H. O. Besedovsky et al., "Hypothalamic Changes during the Immune Response."

p. 35   The surveillance theory of cancer is described in F. M. Burnet, *Immunology, Aging, and Cancer*. See also his work in "A Modern Basis for Pathology."

p. 36   New evidence suggests that the *endorphins*, the term used by scientists to refer to a class of natural compounds discovered between 1969 and 1973 in the human body, not only help reduce pain and relate to joy and euphoria but actually promote effectiveness of the immune system. Macrophagelike cell response was induced by injecting endorphins directly into the brains of rats. See L. C. Saland et al., "Acute Injections of Opiate Peptides into the Rat Cerebral Ventricle: A Macrophage-like Cell Response."

The T cells taken from cancer patients were enhanced when they were exposed to endorphins. See N. P. Plotnikoff as reported in Achterberg. Specific receptors for the endorphins, actual message centers for communication between the immune system and our thinking and feeling, have been demonstrated by E. Hazum, "Specific Monoplate Receptors for Beta-Endorphins."

p. 36   Brain-immune system response and hormone changes are documented in H. O. Besedovsky et al., "Lymphokine-Containing Supernatants from Con A-Stimulated Cells Increase Corticosterone Blood Levels."

p. 36   Herbert Spector, at the National Institute of Health, did the work pairing odors with changes in the immune system. His work and the work by Dr. Norman Geshwind, who studied the effects of left-handedness on immunity, as well as the work of Drs. Ruff and Pert on brain chemicals and immunity, are reported in H. M. Schmeck, "By Training the Brain, Scientists Find Links to Immune Defenses."

p. 39   An enlightening and challenging discussion of the body-universe connection is found in Larry Dossey, *Space, Time, and Medicine*. He refers to a "biodance," the infinite and perpetual interaction between every element of our bodies and the planets and stars.

p. 40   The relationship between mental health and physical health is demonstrated in George Vaillant, "Natural History of Male Psychologic Health: Effects of Mental Health on Physical Health." See also his book *Adaptation to Life*, which outlines the intellectual and emotional defense systems described in the hot- and cold-reactive styles.

p. 40   The response to stress as related to hormone changes is discussed in J. W. Mason, "Emotions as Reflected in Patterns of Endocrine Integration," in L. Levy (Ed.), *Emotions: Their Parameters and Measurement*.

p. 40   A well-written textbook on the immune system is I. M. Roitt, *Essential Immunology*. This is a good source for a more in-depth description than the outline of immunity provided in this chapter.

p. 40   Researchers are focusing specifically on how changes in daily living affect the immune system. One research team recently studied the stress of the Three Mile Island nuclear reactor crisis on area residents. See M. A. Schaeffer et al., "Immune Status as a Function of Chronic Stress at Three Mile Island."

For a study of occupational stress and the immune system, see D. Corian et al., "Occupational Stress and Immunity."

p. 40   The *SAM* and *PAC* systems I use as shorthand designations for complex neurohormonal phenomena are derived from the early work of Walter Cannon in his *Wisdom of the Body*, and from Hans Selye in his *The Stress of Life*. The SAM system was described by J. A. Herd, and the PAC system is my own designation for complex parasympathetic neurohormonal mediation.

Both these systems work together but are separated in this book for emphasis of the hot- and cold-running times of our lives. The sympathetic system mediates when we are running cold, just as there is parasympathetic mediation during our hot times. However, SAM and PAC tend to dominate at hot and cold times, respectively. Some researchers would change the PAC designation from parasympathoadrenocortical to the "pituitary adrenal cortical" system, because of the dominance of the pituitary gland during the cooler physiological states.

For a complete description of the immune system, see Peter Jaret, "Our Immune System. The Wars Within." See also Jaret's co-authored work with Steven Mizel, *In Self Defense*.

p. 41   As we age, so do our immune systems. This is discussed by pioneer researcher R. Ader in his "Developmental Psychoneuroimmunology."

p. 41   A discussion of the negative effects on the immune system of ineffective coping techniques is in G. H. B. Baker, "Stress, Cortisol, and Lymphocyte Subpopulations."

p. 42   The Achterberg quote is in her book *Imagery and Healing*.

CHAPTER FOUR

p. 46   A review of the data documenting the role of a narrow, limited self-concept strongly defended by the person in the development of cardiovascular disease is provided by Larry Schkerwitz et al., "Self Involvement and the Risk Factors for Coronary Heart Disease."

p. 46   The effect of the orientation to life on the heart is shown in S. J. Zyzanski et al., "Psychological Correlates of Coronary Angiographic Findings."

p. 46   The concept of "I-thou" as opposed to an "I-it" orientation to life is described in M. Buber, *I and Thou*.

p. 46   The 12 items in the pretest for hot-running times are derived from an integration of research findings on thinking, feeling, and heart disease. See T. M. Dembroski et al., "Moving beyond Type A." See also Jenkins.

p. 51   The two-component theory of emotion and other views of emotional development are described in a clear and entertaining book by Sarah Cirese, *Quest: A Search for Self*.

p. 53   The cognitive styles described in this chapter and the chapter on cold style are adapted from the work of A. T. Beck, *Depression: Causes and Treatment*. See also Beck, *Cognitive Therapy and Emotional Disorders*.

The most readable and helpful book in the area of a more rational approach to life's challenges is David Burns. *Feeling Good: The New Mood Therapy*. My patients find this book to be very useful, and the cognitive styles Dr. Burns suggests are an outline for some of the thinking styles described in this book. He includes specific and practical techniques for changing cognitions, and I have modified many of his original ideas for the thinking style labels I use with my patients.

p. 56   The breakdown of the immune system into afferent (labeling), central (preparing), and efferent (executional) is described in G. G. Solomon, "Emotions, Stress, the Central Nervous System, and Immunity."

p. 56   The immune system's capacity to react as a sensory organ—to identify, learn, remember, and forget—is documented in J. E. Blalock, "The Immune System as a Sensory Organ."

p. 57   The relationship between the SAM system and the inhibited-power motivation triad is documented in D. C. McClelland, "Inhibited Power Motivation and Blood Pressure in Man."

p. 57   Stress impacts on the immune system are documented in A. A. Monjan et al., "Stress-Induced Modulation of the Immune Response."

p. 58   The defense systems of the hot and cold reactions are adapted from the work of G. E. Vaillant, *Adaptation to Life*.

p. 58   The contrast between neurosis (hot reaction?) and character disorder (cold reaction?) is drawn by Scott Peck, *The Road Less Traveled*. My patients have found Dr. Peck's best-selling book to be helpful in understanding their own struggles with life's daily setbacks. While some of the material in Peck's book is not clinically up to date, it is none the less a source for inspiration and support.

p. 62   The original Type A material is found in M. Friedman et al., "The Relationship of Behavior Pattern A to the State of the Coronary Vasculature."

p. 62   For a thorough and easily read explanation of the Type A and Type B theory, see M. Friedman and R. Rosenman, *Type A Behavior and Your Heart.*

p. 62   Techniques for the behavioral modification of Type A behavior are in M. Friedman, "The Modification of Type A Behavior in Post-infarction Patients."

p. 62   Further work on the relationship between self-involvement and heart disease is found in L. Scherwitz et al., "Type A Behavior, Self-Involvement, and Cardiovascular Response."

p. 62   The fight or flight response was originally described in Cannon. The general adaptation syndrome was originally described in H. Selye.

p. 62   The relationship between the mind, body, heart, and immune system is alluded to by Nobel Prize winner Nicholas Tinbergen, who stated, "The more that is being discovered about the psychosomatic diseases, and in general about the extremely complex two-way traffic between brain and the rest of the body, the more obvious it has become that too rigid a division between mind and body is of only limited use to medical science." This reference is found in N. Tinbergen, "Etiology and Stress Diseases," p. 85.

p. 62   I use the term *hot reaction* from the work of Robert S. Eliot, *Is It Worth Dying For?* This is an excellent reference for the layperson for understanding the physiology of the hot reaction and for learning some specific techniques for change. My patients have found this book helpful.

p. 64   The Apollonian cognitive style is described in Bernard Speigel and R. Speigel, *Trance and Treatment: Clinical Uses of Hypnosis.*

p. 64   Further discussion of the power motivation orientation as related to health is in Joan Borysenko, "Healing Motives: An Interview with David C. McClelland."

Dr. McClelland is quoted in this source as stating directly the theme of this book: "The most exciting thing scientifically right now is the exploration of the relationship of these deeper motives (power, relationships, caring, etc.) to the whole area of hormones and neurotransmitters, and how motives and physiology interact to produce learning and memory and health and disease" (p. 40).

p. 64   The ideas of ego-centrism and eco-centrism are developed in Fritjof Capra, *The Turning Point.* This book also contains an excellent section on wholeness and health. I suggest that it is the balance between the yang, or self, ego-centric orientation to life and the yin, or more altruistic, eco-centric orientation that results in superimmunity. The ego-centrism, or yang of the self-absorbed hot reaction, and eco-centrism, or yin of the self-depreciating cold reaction, may contribute to their own unique weakening of the supersystem, and what the Chinese call the yang or diseases of overfullness and the yin or diseases of emptiness are the hot and cold diseases, respectively.

CHAPTER FIVE

p. 68   Research suggests that stress-induced catecholamine (epinephrine, norep-inephrine) release, related to the hot style of reaction, is atherogenic, or a cause of atherosclerosis. This is because free fatty acids and other lipids are produced in high levels when we are running hot. These fatty acids are then taken up by arterial walls or converted to triglycerides, which, in turn, are deposited in arterial walls. See M. E. Carruthers, "Aggression and Atheroma."

p. 68   An excellent review of cardiovascular disease as related to psychological factors is in David S. Krantz and Stephen B. Manuck, "Acute Psycho-physiologic Reactivity and Risk of Cardiovascular Disease: A Review and Methodologic Critique."

I have divided hot and cold patterns of feeling and thinking as related to unique vulnerabilities to disease. Heart disease, indeed, all wellness and disease, is a multifactorial process related to adrenomedullary *and* pituitary adrenocortical activity. I hypothesize, however, that over time, a propensity to SAM mediation results in a different impact on the immune system than PAC mediation.

p. 68   The report by Dr. Eliot is in his book *Is It Worth Dying For?*

p. 68   The report by Norman Cousins in his book *The Healing Heart.*

p. 69   A complete discussion of Type A theory and research may be found in Theodore M. Dembroski et al., "Moving beyond Type A."

p. 69   Support for my hot-cold cycle hypothesis is found in work on *situational stereotype*, material on characteristic physiological patterns. See J. I. Lacey, "Somatic Response Patterning and Stress: Some Revisions on Activation Theory," in M. H. Appley and R. Trumble (Eds.), *Psychological Stress.*

This approach suggests that different physiological reactions to stress are elicited depending on whether or not the person is actively (hot) or passively (cold) coping with that stress. For further documentation, see K. C. Light, and P. A. Orbist, "Cardiovascular Response to Stress: Effects of Opportunity to Avoid Shock Experience, and Performance Feedback."

p. 69   The relationship between internal dialogue and cardiovascular reactivity is found in a case study of a man who experienced angina when asked to count during a stress test, but no such angina when free from such a perceived stressor. See Bernard Lown, "The Verbal Conditioning of Angina Pectoris during Exercise Testing."

p. 69   Data supporting the elevation of cholesterol during times of anticipation of stress is found in R. Eliot and in L. Dossey.

p. 69   The relationship between foods and emotions is summarized in David Gelman et al., "The Food-Mood Link: New Studies Explore How Diet Affects Our Feelings."

p. 74   The social readjustment rating scale, which measures the impact of major life events and changes, is in T. H. Holmes and R. H. Rahe, "The Social Readjustment Rating Scale."

p. 74   The theory of hassles and uplifts was first proposed and discussed in Richard Lazarus, *Psychological Stress and the Coping Process*.

p. 74   More information on the importance of placing life's day-to-day struggles in perspective can be found in D. Goleman, *Vital Lies, Simple Truths*.

p. 76   The study on the effect of touch on the development of arteriosclerosis in rabbits is described in L. Dossey. It originally appeared in *Science*, 1980.

p. 76   For information on heart disease and its sexual impact, see R. F. Klein et al., "The Physician and Postmyocardial Infarction Invalidism."

p. 79   A source which explains the evolution of the label Type A and also suggests further behavioral changes related to Type A behavior is M. Friedman and D. Ulmer, *Treating Type A Behavior and Your Heart*. I have found this book helpful to my patients, but only when paired with work on their own internal dialogue and interpersonal relationships, their hot selves.

p. 81   The existence of lucid dreams, the actual control of our dreams, is reported in S. P. Laberge et al., "Lucid Dreaming Verified by Volitional Communication during REM Sleep."

p. 83   References on the relaxation response include H. Benson, *The Relaxation Response*, and his work attending more to belief systems as related to the relaxation response, *Beyond the Relaxation Response*.

p. 84   The effectiveness of meditation as a therapeutic tool is described in I. J. Z. Kutz et al., "Meditation and Psychotherapy: A Rationale for the Integration of Dynamic Psychotherapy, the Relaxation Response, and Mindfulness Meditation."

p. 84   A debate exists in the research literature as to whether or not meditation is a special, beneficial, unique state different from "simple resting." *The American Psychologist* contains a series of exchanges over several issues regarding this point (1984–1985).

p. 84   For a simple and immediately useful technique for lessening the hot reaction, see Charles Stroebel, *The Quieting Reflex*.

p. 84   Some researchers warn that meditation, contemplation, and even willful attempts at relaxation can sometimes have a negative impact on the hot-running person, producing a relaxation-induced anxiety. This may be related to the occurrence of unfamiliar body states induced by relaxation or perhaps the encroachment of disruptive thoughts brought about by the "time to think." Dr. David Sobel, a pioneer in the mind-brain research area and the self-responsibility for wellness movement, describes this issue and many other interesting findings, including material on "inner sense of health or illness" and its predictability of sickness, in a series of audiotapes entitled *The Healing Brain*. These are available through the Institute for the Study of Human Knowledge, P.O. Box 176, Los Altos, CA 94022. Professionals and novices will find these tapes by respected leading researchers to be helpful and fascinating.

CHAPTER SIX

p. 87   The concept of Type A behavior is attacked by critic Peter Shaw in "A Type A Behavior Modification Sampler." He points out that life is an ever-changing cycle, with our orientation to life beyond the limits of a single label or description. So it is with the cold cycle.

p. 88   A review of the emotional states related to cancer can be found in E. R. Rosenbaum (Ed.), *Can You Prevent Cancer?*

p. 88   The Type C factors are discussed in B. H. Fox, "Premorbid Psychological Factors as Related to Cancer Incidence." Remember again that Type C behaviors are like a temperature reading. When we say it is cold outside, we know that, except for rare cases, it is never cold forever.

p. 88   I am suggesting two systems, oscillating rhythmically to life events. While the SAM (sympathoadrenomedullary) system dominates at hot-running times, the PAC (parasympathoadrenocortical) system dominates at cold times. These cycles are present in all of us and resemble the ebb and flow of the tides more than personality structures.

We tend to experience short periods of hot and cold orientation, transitional periods of more moderation in lifestyle (warm and cool) and *eras*, or prolonged phases of orientation to life that persist sometimes for years. For a discussion of such a developmental scheme for adult development, see Daniel J. Levinson, "A Conception of Adult Development." This concept is important for understanding hot and cold cycles, for researchers may be sampling life orientations at atypical times, times of transition, brief cycles, or "eras," and drawing conclusions about types and personalities that do not exist.

p. 89   The concepts of isolation, withdrawal, and familial factors as related to cancer are discussed in C. B. Thomas et al., "Family Attitudes Reported in Youth as Potential Predictors of Cancer."

p. 89   Description of the Dionysian orientation is in Speigel and Speigel.

p. 89   The Livingstone reflex is described and the quote from Dr. Livingstone appears in D. D. Kelly, "Somatic Sensory System IV: Representations of Pain and Analgesia," in J. E. Kandel and J. Schwartz (Eds.), *Principles of Neural Science*.

p. 95   Material on irrational thinking errors in the cold cycle is modified from David Burns and from A. Beck.

p. 98   The concept of character disorder is discussed in S. Peck.

p. 98   The defense systems employed at cold-running times are modified from G. Vaillant (1977).

p. 99   The radical hypothesis of the brain's boredom resulting in compensatory overstimulation by the brain is discussed in O. de la Pena (1983).

p. 99   The impact of the isolation experienced in the cold reaction is discussed in E. O. Wilson, *Sociobiology*. See also J. R. Averill, "Grief: Its Nature and Significance."

p. 100   The three phases of the immune system's organization are described in G. Solomon (1964).

p. 100   For a discussion of some of the emotional factors related to cell disease, see L. Sklar and H. Anisman, "Stress and Cancer."

p. 100   That the SAM (catecholamines adrenaline and noradrenaline) and PAC (cortisol) systems are capable of functioning independently and have an alternating inhibitory effect on each other is documented in N. J. Russo, II, et al., "Passive Avoidance and Amygdala Lesions: Relationship with Pituitary-Adrenal System."

See also G. R. Van Loon et al., "Evidence for Central Adrenergic Neural Inhibition of ACTH Secretion in the Rat."

p. 100   The relationship between the SAM and PAC systems as dependent on one another for regulation is documented in R. L. Conner et al., "Stress, Fighting, and Neuroendocrine Function."

p. 101   The contrast between the hot and cold physiological responses was described more than 50 years ago in W. B. Cannon, *Bodily Changes in Pain, Hunger, Fear, and Rage: An Account of Recent Researches into the Function of Emotional Excitement*. Cannon identifies the "vigilance" response (cold reaction?) as contrasted to the "alarm response" (hot reaction?). See also D. H. Funkenstein, "The Physiology of Fear and Anger."

CHAPTER SEVEN

p. 104   The association between bereavement and illness is discussed in James E. Birren and J. Livingston (Eds.), *Cognition, Stress, and Aging*.

p. 104   The concept of the importance of affectional bonding is described in J. Bowlby, *The Making and Breaking of Affectional Bonds*.

p. 104   Documentation of mortality among the bereaved is found in M. Young et al., "Mortality of Widowers." See also W.D. Rees and S. G. Lutkin, "Mortality and Bereavement."

p. 104   Statistics indicate that bereaved men have higher mortality rates than bereaved women. This may be due to the fact that men have fewer affectional bonds than women, and loss of a bond leaves them more vulnerable to illness. This viewpoint is discussed by Joan Stoddard and J. P. Henry, "Affectional Bonding and the Impact of Bereavement."

p. 104   Documentation of the relationship between depression and a change in lymphocytes, particularly the T-4 and T-8 ratio as discussed in this chapter, is found in R. B. Krueger et al., "Lymphocyte Subsets in Patients with Major Depression: Preliminary Findings."

p. 104   The speculation on the relationship between boredom, overstimulation, and shutdown, resulting in a compensatory overstimulation, is in O. de la Pena.

p. 104   For a general discussion of the importance of cognitive stimulation and its influence on our attentiveness, see J. Allison, "Cognitive Structure and Receptivity to Low Intensity Stimulation."

p. 106   The relationship between feelings of ineffectiveness and another cold disease process, arthritis, is examined in K. Lorig et al., "Arthritis Self-Management: A Study of the Effectiveness of Patient Education for the Elderly."

p. 108   For material on aging and immunity, see L. Hayflick, "What We Are Discovering about Your Body's Amazing Immune System." See also L. Hayflick, "Current Theories of Biological Aging." For a complete and thoroughly documented review of aging and health, see K. Pelletier, *Longevity: Fulfilling Our Biological Potential*.

p. 109   For a clear and precise overview of the complex immune system related to biological changes, see N. K. Jerne, "The Immune System"

p. 109   The decline in the competence of the immune system is related to changes in the T and B cells themselves as well as the general state of the body system. See T. Makinodan, "Mechanism, Prevention, and Restoration of Immunologic Aging."

If the T and B cells are directly implicated in the decline of immunoefficiency with aging, then another direct link between our thinking and feeling and immunity is established. I have pointed out that T cells are derived from cells from the bone marrow under influence from the thymus gland which is, in turn, influenced by the hypothalamus, or "brain of the brain," as I described in Chapter Two. Changes in our psychosocial situation along with aging influence the brain which influences the hypothalamus which influences the thymus which influences particularly the T cells, and so the holistic aspects of immune aging may be determined.

Many researchers would argue against the above reasoning, even questioning whether or not the thymus is a part of the endocrine system. Others suggest that the thymus gland is "master gland of the immune system." See J. L. Marx, "Thymic Hormones: Inducers of T Cell Maturation."

p. 109   The possibility of rejuvenation of the immune system, in effect reversing the aging process, has been raised. Life spans of mice have been lengthened and shortened by surgically altering the function of the thymus gland. See A. R. Favazza, "The Day of Our Years." Certainly, removing strain on the immune system would seem to increase the chances for a healthier, longer-living supersystem.

p. 110   Data on groups experiencing a lower frequency of cell disease is found in J. Achterberg et al., "A Possible Relationship between Cancer, Mental Retardation, and Mental Disorder."

p. 110   For further information on groups experiencing immunity to certain diseases, see D. Gregg, "The Paucity of Arthritis among Psychotic Patients." See also H. Newman, "Health Attitudes: Locus of Control and Religious Orientation."

p. 111   A helpful book on techniques for healing from within is Dennis T. Jaffe, *Healing from Within*. This easy-to-read and well-documented book has been found useful by many of my patients.

p. 112   Four hundred cases of spontaneous remission from cancer were reported by Eric Pepper and Kenneth Pelletier through their computer search and subsequent bibliography. An analysis of this material and its relevance for hope and belief in healing is in E. Green and A. Green, *Beyond Biofeedback*.

p. 114   The concept of self-actualization through balance of care of self and others is described in the classic work by A. H. Maslow, *Religions, Values, and Peak Experiences*.

p. 114   The percentage of active T cells is increased by the presence of the natural opiates. As mentioned earlier in this reference section, hope and joy may lead to higher levels of immunity through the influence of the endorphins. See J. Wybran et al., "Suggestive Evidence for Receptors for Morphine and Methinone-Enkephalin on Normal Human Block T Lymphocytes."

p. 117   A clear and balanced discussion of alternative cancer therapies is found in M. Lerner and R. Naomi, "A Variety of Integral Cancer Therapies."

p. 123   The concept of disautomatization, or the disruption of the autonomic nervous system (the SAM and PAC dominance cycles), is discussed in Hans Selye.

p. 124   For a comprehensive and easy-to-administer "self-test" for stress factors in all areas of life (eating, sleeping, work, etc.), see C. N. Shealy, "Total Life Stress and Symptomatology."

p. 124   For a review of data on survival after breast cancer, see H. C. Nauts, *Breast Cancer: Immunological Factors Affecting Incidence, Prognosis, and Survival.*

p. 124   For further information on depression and its impact on immunity, see Paul Willner, *Depression: A Psychobiological Synthesis.*

p. 124   The finding on women's reaction to breast cancer is in J. Polivy, "Psychological Effects of Mastectomy on a Woman's Feminine Self-Concept."

CHAPTER EIGHT

p. 132   Ingelfinger's quote and information on the limitations of our modern medical model may be found in F. J. Ingelfinger, "Health: A Matter of Statistics or Feeling."

p. 133   A discussion of the Wallenda factor, or the possibility of a negative, fearful, anticipatory orientation to life limiting the fulfillment of our personal potential, is found in Warren Bennis, *More Power to You.*

p. 133   A biopsychosocial model of medicine, integrating the advances of modern medicine with the spiritual dimensions of ancient forms of healing, is outlined in G. I. Engel, "The Need for a New Medical Model: A Challenge for Biomedicine."

p. 133   The phrase "In the absence of certainty, there is nothing wrong with hope" has been adopted from therapists Carl and Stephanie Matthews Simonton by Dr. Bernard Siegel in his care program Exceptional Cancer Patients, in New Haven, Connecticut.

p. 133   Pioneering work in the sensitive, holistic approach to cancer patients is in O. C. Simonton, S. Simonton, and J. Creighton, *Getting Well Again.*

p. 134   Further information on imagery such as the camp fire opportunity described in this chapter can be found in J. S. Singer, *Imagery and Daydream Methods in Psychotherapy and Behavior Modification.*

p. 137   Support should be in the form of educated support, or an effective balance between tolerance of the hot reactors' tendencies and limit setting and protection of the home environment from overheating from hot reaction. For a clear discussion of a program and suggestions for couples' communication, see Richard Stuart, *Helping Couples Change: A Social Learning Approach to Marital Therapy*.

p. 157   The book on juggling is by John Cassidy and B. C. Rimbeaux, *Juggling for the Complete Klutz*.

p. 157   A clear discussion of the control we have over our own health is in R. Dubos, "Bolstering the Body against Disease."

p. 158   For a discussion of the application of the principles of self-responsibility for the supersystem as applied to business and management, see John D. Adams (Ed.), *Transforming Work: A Collection of Organization Transformation Readings*. See also Charles F. Kiefer and Peter M. Senge, "Metanoic Organizations." The term *metanoic* refers to a fundamental shift of mind, the reawakening of intuition and vision. It is with such a reawakening that we reassume control of our supersystems.

CHAPTER NINE

p. 160   The orientation to reversing from the despair of the cold reaction to a new hope for personal and social change is described in Norman Cousins, *Human Options*.

p. 160   Two hopeful, helpful, optimistic sources for reversing the cold reaction are Edward Bauman et al. (Eds.), *The Holistic Health Handbook: A Tool for Attaining Wholeness of Body, Mind, and Spirit*, and Edward Bauman et al. (Eds.), *The Holistic Health Lifebook: A Guide to Personal and Planetary Well-Being*.

p. 160   A collection of stories by the Sufi masters that entertain and teach a new process of thinking, breaking out of the cold pattern, is by Idries Shah, *Tales of the Dervishes*.

My patients have found the following sources helpful in changing both hot- and cold-running styles:

Early work on assuming control of your own health is in H. Benson, *The Mind/Body Effect: How Behavioral Medicine Can Show You the Way to Better Health*.

For support for the importance of avoiding blame, see A. Smith, *Powers of the Mind*. See also D. Burns, *Feeling Good*.

For suggestions regarding social support at cold-running times, see Leslie Cameron-Bandler, *Solutions: Practical and Effective Antidotes for Sexual and Relationship Problems*.

For suggestions of problem-solving techniques at apparently hopeless times in the cold reaction, see A. Newell and H. A. Simon, *Human Problem Solving*.

For more suggestions for accomplishing change, see Edward T. Hall, *The Dance of Life*.

The importance of laughter and joy is documented in W. F. Fry Jr et al.,

"Mirth and Oxygen Saturation Levels of Peripheral Blood." See also W. F. Fry Jr., "The Respiratory Components of Mirthful Laughter."

A collection of poems that my patients find helpful for reversing their own cold times is *The Best of Robert Service*.

For a collection of readings of eastern thought and its potential for helping us at times of challenge, see John Welwood (Ed.), *Awakening the Heart: East/West Approaches to Psychotherapy and the Healing Relationship*.

Many of my patients find the work by Alice Steadman, *Who's the Matter with Me?* to be inspirational at times of cold reaction.

CHAPTER TEN

p. 186   See David Burns, *Feeling Good*.

p. 188   For an explanation and additional ideas on imagery, see A. Sheikh (Ed.), *Imagery: Current Theory, Research, and Application*.

p. 189   For a review of the "grandma rules of health," see L. A. Breslow, "A Quantitative Approach to the World Health Organization Definition of Health: Physical, Mental, and Social Well-Being." See also L. A. Breslow, "A Positive Strategy for the Nation's Health."

p. 189   A good medical self-help guide, including a unique flowchart approach to self-help on medical matters, is Donald M. Vickery and James F. Fries, *Take Care of Yourself: Consumer's Guide to Medical Care*.

p. 191   For a positive approach for moving beyond health to high-level wellness, see R. Walsh and D. Shapiro (Eds.), *Beyond Health and Normalcy: Exploration of Exceptional Psychological Well-Being*.

p. 192   An album of healing music is by Kay Gardner, *A Rainbow Path*. This album includes acoustic arrangements matched with suggested meditations as related to various *chakras*, or levels of the body and spirit.

Ancient Pythagorean and Hindu teachings suggest that various musical tones, colors, and charas (Sansrit for "wheels,") which relate to the endocrine system) can be combined for healing. Research suggests that largo movements (50 to 60 beats per minute) from baroque music, when played for cardiac patients, actually can help correct irregular heart rhythm.

Gifted composer Kay Gardner writes on her album cover, "These are difficult times. Because fear runs rampant in the world, it's important to remember that there's an even stronger force in the universe, a healing force we all may tap into. That healing power is love."

I have found it helpful to suggest that my patients' lie on the floor on a rug or pad, with speakers on the floor nearby, so that the vibrations of the music may have a more profound effect.

p. 192   For an interesting source for more information on the music-healing connection, see Bart Barlow, "As Wolves Howl and Whales Sing, Listen to the Music." See also Helen Bonny and Louis M. Savary, *Music and Your Mind*.

p. 192   For research supporting the music-healing connection, see *Brain/Mind Bul-*

letin, "Music Issue," Interface Press, Dec. 13, 1982. See also MacDonald Critchley, *Music and Brain*.

p. 194   For some funny reading, see M. Eastman, *The Enjoyment of Laughter*.

p. 194   For a book about the value of lightheartedness, see Laurence J. Peter and B. Dana, *The Laughter Prescription*.

p. 194   Documentation of the importance of laughter is in W. F. Fry Jr. See also H. A. Paskind, "Effect of Laughter on Muscle Tone."

p. 194   For more material on mirth, see E. B. White and K. S. White, *A Subtreasury of American Humor*.

p. 197   The importance of invisible means of support is discussed in J. Frank, "The Faith That Heals."

p. 200   Diet and nutrition are two different concepts. For information on healthy nutrition, see Jeffrey Bland (Ed.), *Medical Applications of Clinical Nutrition*. See also William G. Crook, *Tracking Down Hidden Food Allergy*. See also David Sheinkin, M. Schachter, and Richard Hutton, *Food, Mind, and Mood*.

p. 201   For information on relaxing breathing, see E. A. Fletcher, *The Law of the Rhythmic Breath*.

p. 201   For realistic information on aerobics, see K. H. Cooper, *The New Aerobics*. See also M. Spino, *Beyond Jogging*.

p. 201   For an entertaining and helpful guide to exercise and nutrition, see J. W. Farquhar, *The American Way of Life Need Not Be Hazardous to Your Health*.

CHAPTER ELEVEN

p. 203   An accurate description of the isolation of the AIDS virus in France and the United States, as well as reasonable precautions against the spread of this disease, is in N. Patrick Hennessey, "AIDS: What the Family Physician Needs to Know."

p. 205   For a review of some of the controversial issues related to the treatment of AIDS, see Gary Null, "The AIDS Cover-Up."

p. 205   For reprints of articles on AIDS, write to the *New York Native*: Charles Ortleb, publisher, editor, and chief, *New York Native*, 249 West Broadway, New York, NY 10013.

p. 205   For material on the effects of stress as related to AIDS, see John L. Martin and Carole S. Vance, "Behavioral and Psychosocial Factors in AIDS."

p. 206   A brief and clear discussion of the issues of tolerance and specificity of the immune system is provided in *Investigations: A Bulletin of the Institute of Noetic Sciences*. Sausalito, Calif., 1984.

p. 209   A reference for information on the sexually transmitted diseases is Maria Corsara and Carole Korzeniowsky, *STD: A Commonsense Guide*. See also Jennifer Wear and King Holmes, *How to Have Intercourse without Getting Screwed*.

p. 210   For information on the evolution of holistic medicine, see Richard Gross-man, *The Other Medicines*. The word "holism" first appeared in 1926 in Jan Christiaan Smuts book *Holism and Evolution*, where it was used to designate the dynamic interaction between all parts of our humanness, our bodies, minds, spirits, and environment.

p. 211   The psychosocial aspects of AIDS and the Mandel study referred to here are found in G. F. Solomon, "The Emerging Field of Psychoneuroim-munology with a Special Note on AIDS."

p. 211   A leading spokesperson for the concepts of "dis-ease" and "dys-ease" is Dr. Gary E. Schwartz. See his work in "Behavioral Medicine and Systems Theory: A New Synthesis." See also G. Schwartz, "Psychobiology of Health: A New Synthesis."

The following sources discuss various controversies and new research related to AIDS:

For the personal dimension of the AIDS issue, see a series of letters written by an AIDS patient in Suzanne Dolezal, "A Death's Chronicle: AIDS Fight Told in Letters to a Friend."

For a technical discussion of the failure of the immune system caused by AIDS, see A. Friedman-Kein and L. Laubensterin (Eds.), *AIDS: The Opportunistic Epidemic of Kaposi's Sarcoma and Opportunistic Infections*.

In December 1984, the Institute for the Advancement of Health sponsored a program entitled "The Psychosocial Aspect of AIDS." One AIDS patient at that meeting reported that he personally knew of AIDS patients living far beyond the forecasted time and even some who had gone into remission. He stressed that in each case, the individuals had been able to mobilize their emotions for healing. See Eileen Rockefeller Growald, "Health and Wholeness: The Mind/Body Mystery."

Preliminary research of relevance to the AIDS-stress issue may be found in D. M. Miller et al., "A Pseudo-AIDS Syndrome Following from a Fear of AIDS" (in press).

A discussion of the complex psychological factors related to AIDS and PGL (an immune-suppressed condition characterized by persistent gener-alized lymphadenopathy) is presented in J. Green and D. Miller "Psy-chology and AIDS in Britain."

A sensitive approach to the counseling of AIDS patients is in J. Green and D. M. Miller (1985), *Psychological Support and Counseling in Acquired Immune Deficiency Syndrome* (unpublished monograph).

For an example of work in the area of the relationship between disease and social support systems, see W. E. Broadhead et al., "The Epidemiologic Evidence for a Relationship between Social Support and Health." See also J. Mandel, "Biopsychosocial Aspects of the Acquired Immune Deficiency Syndrome."

CHAPTER TWELVE

p. 215   A collection of articles on stress and coping is in A. Monat and R. S. Lazarus (Eds.), *Stress and Coping: An Anthology*. The classic work in the field of stress research is by Hans Selye, *Stress without Distress*.

p. 216   A clear and accurate discussion of stress is in Kenneth R. Pelletier, *Mind as Healer: Mind as Slayer*. See also K. Pelletier, *Holistic Medicine: From Stress to Optimum Health*.

p. 217   Work on stress in the workplace is in K. R. Pelletier, *Healthy People in Unhealthy Places: Stress and Fitness at Work*.

p. 217   Information on the physiology of the neuroendocrine response to stress is in S. Levine et al., "Expectancy and the Pituitary-Adrenal System."

p. 217   For an account of stress addiction, see Barbara Gordon, *I'm Dancing as Fast as I Can*. See also K. Lamott, *Escape from Stress*. The most popular book on learning how to relax through systematic muscle control is E. Jacobson, *You Must Relax*.

p. 220   For early work on personality related to response to stress, see R. S. Lazarus, "Personality and Psychological Stress."

p. 221   For information on gaining control over excessive response to stress, see D. Meichenbaum, *Cognitive-Behavioral Modification: An Integrative Approach*.

p. 222   For cautions in seeking help for dealing with stress, see Bernie Zilbergeld, *The Shrinking of America: Myths of Psychological Change*. See also Martin L. Gross, *The Psychological Society*.

CHAPTER THIRTEEN

p. 225   The concepts of "dis-ease" and "dys-ease" were developed by Gary Schwartz.

p. 230   Information on healing and "miraculous cures" is found in St. John Dowling, "Lourdes Cures and Their Medical Assessment."

p. 230   A classic source of information on women and healing is M. J. Gage, *Women, Church, and State*. See also M. Murray, *The Witch Cult in Western Europe*. See also M. Eliade, "Some Observations on European Witchcraft," in *Occultism, Witchcraft, and Cultural Fashions*. See also J. Achterberg.

The yin, or feminine dimension, has been separated from modern medicine. Concepts of healing, supporting, comforting, and caring have until recent times been left to the nursing profession, which has been predominantly a feminine profession.

p. 232   A discussion of the role of illness as teacher and enhancer of life for some of our most creative and productive people is found in B. Zilbergeld, *The Shrinking of America*.

p. 234   An interesting review of the role of disease in creativity is found in Philip Sandblom, *Creativity and Disease: How Illness Affects Literature, Art, and Music*.

CHAPTER FOURTEEN

p. 237   For an interesting discussion of the evolution of our concepts of time, see Lawrence LeShan, "Time Orientation and Social Class."

Additional information on time and disease can be found in the following sources:

A discussion of the relationship between consciousness and time is found in R. E. Ornstein, *On the Experience of Time*.

The amounts of cortisol and growth hormone in the blood can vary by as much as 100 percent in a 24-hour period. We actually have several rhythms of life. Circadian rhythms are daily rhythms (actually about 25 hours in length). Ultradian rhythms are shorter periods of cyclicity, such as heartbeat and electrical brain rhythms. Longer cycles are called *infradian* rhythms, and include menstrual cycles and seasonal changes in mood. The field of study of human time cycles is called *chronobiology*, a term coined by Dr. Franz Halberg. A review of the work can be found in Susan Cunningham, "Circadian Rhythms: Is It One Clock, or Several, That Cycle Us through Life?"

The number of white cells, or lymphocytes, in our blood may vary as much as 50 percent in one day. Some researchers are suggesting that the time of use of chemotherapy and other medical interventions might be more closely matched with individual biological, or immune, rhythms. This work is being done primarily by Dr. Franz Halberg at the University of Minnesota. See the review by Susan Cunningham.

p. 237   The new physics is explained in Fritjof Capra, *The Tao of Physics*. Research on the immune system indicates that the "laws" of the universe operate on the level of the smallest components of the supersystem, and understanding these laws is a prerequisite to learning the ways in which our immunity functions.

p. 238   The work on owls and larks is reported in Restak (1984).

p. 239   Controversial speculations on the effects of light on emotions and health can be found in John N. Ott, *Health and Light*. Dr. Norman Rosenthal's work on SAD (seasonal affective disorder) was done at the National Institute of Mental Health, where he has studied more than 70 patients for the suppression of the substance melatonin. This substance is controlled by the hypothalamus and pineal gland interaction in response to exposure to light. The use of "grow lights" used for plants helped many of these patients overcome their seasonal psychological hibernation. See R. Restak, *The Brain* (p. 121).

p. 241   Material on different levels of "reality," each with their equally valid rules of function, is described and illustrated by Lawrence LeShan, *The Medium, the Mystic and the Physicist*.

p. 241   For a creative view of the wellness-illness relationship as related to the new physics, see Larry Dossey, *Beyond Illness: Discovering the Experience of Health*.

p. 241   Current material on the new physics and a new paradigm of our world is found in Ken Wilbur, *The Spectrum of Consciousness*. Wilbur's new book will be entitled *Quantum Reality: Beyond the New Physics*.

p. 242   The type of learning stressing the importance of perceptual development is discussed in Jean Piaget, *Origins of Intelligence in Children*. Piaget stressed the concept of learning to believe before we see, and the flying squirrel example and many similar stories are found throughout Piaget's writings.

This perceptual approach is also emphasized by L. Kohlberg, "Stage and Sequence: The Cognitive Developmental Approach to Socialization," in D. A. Goslin, *Handbook of Socialization Theory and Research*.

p. 244   A creative approach to integrating relativity theory and quantum mechanics with the practicality of day-to-day life is in Lawrence LeShan and Henry Margenau, *Einstein's Space and Van Gogh's Sky: Physical Reality and Beyond*.

p. 245   Interesting speculation on the impact of the biological orientation of cosmopolitan medicine as opposed to a "physics" emphasis stressing energy flow and disruption is in Julian Kenyon, "The Segmental Electrogram: A Non-invasive Early Diagnostic Scanning Technique." The focus of the work is on detecting perturbations in energy fields of the body before resultant "biological" changes in the form of tumor or other disease.

p. 245   The concept of *biodance*, our relationship with the universe, is in L. Dossey, *Space, Time, and Medicine*.

CHAPTER FIFTEEN

p. 262   The importance of health care workers attending to the sexual dimensions of health and illness is discussed in Robert Kolodny et al., *Textbook of Sexual Medicine*.

p. 262   For a discussion of educational programs for professionals in the area of human sexuality, see N. Rosenzweig and P. Pearsall (Eds.), *Sex Education for the Health Professional*.

p. 263   For a discussion of the work of McClelland, see J. A. Borysenko, "Healing Motives: An Interview with David C. McClelland."

p. 264   For a description of mineralocorticoids and glucocorticoids from the adrenal cortex, see R. Ornstein (1985).

p. 264   For information documenting the lung cancer and personality link, see D. M. Kissen, "The Significance of Personality in Lung Cancer in Men."

p. 265   For further documentation of the relationship between bonding and disease, see R. S. Weiss, *Loneliness: The Experience of Emotional and Social Isolation*. See also Joan B. Stoddard and J. P. Henry, "Affectional Bonding and the Impact of Bereavement."

p. 265   For a sensitive discussion of "healthy" versus "unhealthy" love, see S. Peck (1978).

p. 267   The concept of sociobiology is developed by E. O. Wilson (1980).

p. 267   The concept of altruistic egoism is suggested and described by Hans Selye (1978).

p. 267   The self-involvement factor as related to disease is in Scherwitz et al. (1985).

p. 268   The pioneering work of William Masters and Virginia Johnson is in *Human Sexual Response*.

p. 269   A unique analogy between immune-system functioning and pair bonding is drawn by John Money. He states, "There is an analogy here [regarding imprinting and bonding] with an immune system that fails; the residual pathology that ensues when an immune mechanism is faulty may induce a lifetime's impairment." I suggest that the development of the immune system is profoundly interrelated with the capacity for successful bonding. See Money's *Love and Love Sickness: The Science of Sex, Gender Difference, and Pair-Bonding.*

p. 287   Helpful books for understanding the definition of sexual wellness presented in this chapter include L. Barbach, *For Yourself: The Fulfillment of Female Sexuality*; L. Barbach, *Women Discover Orgasm: A Therapist's Guide to a New Treatment Approach*; B. Zilbergeld, *Male Sexuality*.

p. 288   A source for information on "love cultures" versus "hate cultures" and their respective impacts on the individual is Reuben Fine, *The Meaning of Love in Human Experience.*

p. 288   For people with disabilities, a reference concerning sexual health and impairment is Alex Comfort, *Sexual Consequences of Disability.*

p. 288   For an interesting and controversial discussion of female sexuality, breast cancer, and wellness, see Peggy Boyd, *The Silent Wound: A Startling Report on Breast Cancer and Sexuality.*

CHAPTER SIXTEEN

p. 289   The work of Abraham Maslow is summarized in A. H. Maslow, *The Farther Reaches of Human Nature*. See also A. H. Maslow, *Motivation and Personality*, and his *Religions, Values, and Peak Experiences*. Maslow's work in the area of business is discussed in his *Eupsychian Management.*

p. 290   The Jerome Frank work is described in Jerome Frank, *Persuasion and Healing.*

p. 291   The case reference is found in R. B. Case and Stanley Heller, "Behavior and Survival of Type A Personalities after Acute Myocardial Infarction."

p. 291   This new field of psychoneuroimmunology and related controversial issues are described in George F. Solomon (1985).

p. 291   For a review of information on the impact of positive emotions on health, see a report on the Stanford University 1984 Conference, "How Might Positive Emotions Affect Physical Health?" See Brendan O'Regan, "Positive Emotions: The Emerging Science of Feelings."

p. 291   Information on the relationship between imagery, cancer, and the immune system is in H. R. Hall, "Hypnosis and the Immune System: A Review with Implications for Cancer and the Psychology of Healing."

          See also H. R. Hall et al., "Hypnosis and the Immune System: The Effect of Hypnosis on T and B Cell Function."

p. 295   The Royce quote regarding neglect of important issues is found in J. Royce, "Psychology Is Multi-methodological, Variate, Epistemic, World View, Systemic, Paradigmatic, Theoretic, and Disciplinary."

p. 295   A discussion of issues of normalcy and extreme well-being may be found in G. Bateson, *Mind and Nature: A Necessary Unity.*

p. 295   Maslow identified two dangers in the conflict between science and the new view of transcending wellness. He suggested that one mistake is to reject the scientific approach altogether, confusing impulsiveness with spontaneity. The other mistake is a belief in a value-free, concrete technology emphasizing only scientific approaches. See A. Maslow, *The Psychology of Science: A Reconnaissance.*

p. 300   A controversial discussion of emotional reactions to foods is found in Ben F. Feingold, *Why Your Child Is Hyperactive.*

p. 300   See D. M. Vickery and J. F. Fries (p. 37) for a discussion of the appropriate and inappropriate use of medications in our society.

p. 303   The concept of voluntary simplicity is introduced in D. Elgin, *Voluntary Simplicity.*

p. 310   The three C's of challenge, commitment, and control are presented in S. C. Kobasas et al., "Health under Stress." This work examines psychological hardiness, or a research focus on health and learning from high-level, well, and successfully adapting people.

p. 311   The concept of a performance zone, a balance between challenging, constructive stress or change and overwhelming, destructive stress is known as the *Yerkes-Dodson law* and evolved at Harvard University in 1908. See K. Pelletier (1984).

CHAPTER SEVENTEEN

p. 317   Systems theory is discussed in Ludwig von Bertalanffy, *General Systems Theory.*

p. 317   Arthur Koestler used the word "holons" to describe subsystems within the whole which both integrate with the system and assert their individuality. In maximizing immunity, a balance between self (egoism) and system ("eco-ism") is important, the altruistic egoism of Hans Selye. See Arthur Koestler, *Janus.*

p. 317   The concepts of "dis-ease" and "dys-ease" were developed by Gary Schwartz.

p. 317   Holism is traced from ancient to contemporary medicine in David S. Sobel (Ed.), *Ways of Health: Holistic Approaches to Ancient and Contemporary Medicine.*

p. 320   For a discussion of questions to be asked to elicit the patients' "model of their disease" and the cultural perspective of illness, see A. Kleinman et al., "Culture, Illness, and Care: Clinical Lessons from Anthropologic and Cross-Cultural Research."

p. 327   A detailed description of *dysponesis*, or generalized muscle tension (activation of the gamma efferent system), is found in George B. Whitmore and D. R. Kohli, "Dysponesis: A Neurophysiologic Factor in Functional Disorders," in Eric Pepper et al. (Eds.), *Mind/Body Integration.*

p. 327   A creative and helpful view of the symbolism of illness is in Alice Steadman (1969).

p. 327   Albert Schweitzer is quoted as stating, "The witch doctor succeeds for the same reason all the rest of us succeed. Each patient has [his own doctor within]." See the translation by C. T. Campion of A. Schweitzer, *Out of My Life and Thought: Autobiography*.

p. 327   Information on the placebo effect may be found in J. Turner et al., *Placebo: An Annotated Bibliography*.

p 327   For the different meanings of disease, see J. Lipowski, "Psychosocial Aspects of Disease."

p. 332   The view from the hospital room and its effect on healing has been researched by Roger Ulrich at the University of Texas. See S. R. Tessler, "Recovering? Get a Room with a View."

BIBLIOGRAPHY

Achterberg, Jeanne. *Imagery and Healing*. Boston and London: Shambhala Press, 1985.

_____, Collerain, I., and Craig, P. "A Possible Relationship between Cancer, Mental Retardation, and Mental Disorder." *Journal of Social Science and Medicine*. *12* (May 1978) 135–139.

_____, and Lawlis, G. F. *Imagery of Cancer: A Diagnostic Tool for the Process of Disease*. Champaign, Ill.: Institute for Personality and Ability Testing, 1978.

_____, and _____. *Bridges of the Bodymind: Behavioral Approaches to Health Care*. Champaign, Ill.: Institute for Personality and Ability Testing, 1980.

Adams, John D. (Ed.). *Transforming Work: A Collection of Organizational Transformation Readings*. Alexandria, Va.: Miles River Press, 1984.

Ader, Robert. "Developmental Psychoneuroimmunology." *Developmental Psychobiology*. *16* (1983) 251–267.

_____(Ed.). *Psychoneuroimmunology*. New York: Academic, 1981.

_____, and Cohen, N. "Behaviorally Conditioned Immunosuppression." *Psychosomatic Medicine*. *37* (1975) 333–340.

_____, and Cohen, N. "Behaviorally Conditioned Immunosuppression and Murine Systemic Lupus Erythematosus." *Psychosomatic Medicine*. *44* (1982) 127–128.

Allison, J. "Cognitive Structure and Receptivity to Low Intensity Stimulation." *Journal of Abnormal and Social Psychology*. *67* (1963) 132–138.

Averill, J. R. "Grief: Its Nature and Significance." *Psychological Bulletin*. *70* (1968) 721–748.

Bales, John. "Hand Dominance a Factor in Autism." *American Psychological Association Monitor*. *16* (December 1985) 14.

Barbach, Lonnie G. *For Yourself: The Fulfillment of Female Sexuality*. New York: Anchor/Doubleday, 1976.

_____. *Women Discover Orgasm: A Therapist's Guide to a New Treatment Approach*. New York: Free Press, Macmillan, 1980.

Barber, Theodore X. "Changing 'Unchangeable' Bodily Processes by (Hypnotic) Suggestions: A New Look at Hypnosis, Cognitions, Imaging, and the Mind-Body Problem." *Advances*. *1* (Spring 1984) 7–40.

Bardos, P., Degenne, D., Lebranchu, Y., Biziere, K., and Renoux, G. "Neocortical Lateralization of NK Activity in Mice." *Scandinavian Journal of Immunology*. *13* (1981) 609–611.

Barlow, Bart. "As Wolves Howl and Whales Sing, Listen to the Music." *Smithsonian*. (September 1981) 110–116.

Basmajian, J. V. "Control of Individual Motor Units." *Science*. *141* (1977) 834–836.

_____. *Muscles Alive: Their Functions Revealed by Electromyography*. 3d ed. Baltimore: Williams and Wilkins, 1979.

Bateson, George. *Mind and Nature*. New York: Dutton, 1979.

_____. *Steps to an Ecology of Mind*. New York: Ballantine, 1972.

Bauman, Edward, Brint, Ian Armand, Piper, L., and Wright, A (Eds.). *The Holistic Health Handbook. A Tool for Attaining Wholeness of Body, Mind and Spirit*. Berkeley, Calif.: And/Or Press, 1981.

_____, Brint, I., Piper, A., and Brint, A. (Eds.). *The Holistic Health Lifebook. A Guide to Personal and Planetary Well-Being*. Berkeley, Calif.: And/Or Press, 1981.

Beck, Aaron T. *Cognitive Therapy and Emotional Disorders*. New York: New American Library, 1979.

_____. *Depression: Causes and Treatment*. Philadelphia: University of Pennsylvania Press, 1972.

Bennett, Henry L., and Davis, H. S. "Nonverbal Response to Interoperative Conversation." *Anesthesia and Analgesia*. *63* (1984) 63.

Bennis, Warren. *More Power to You*. New York: William Morrow, 1983.

Benson, Herbert. *Beyond the Relaxation Response*. New York: Times Books, 1984.

_____. "Systemic Hypertension and the Relaxation Response." *New England Journal of Medicine*. *296* (1977) 1152–1156.

_____. *The Mind/Body Effect: How Behavioral Medicine Can Show You the Way to Better Health*. New York: Simon and Schuster, 1979.

_____. *The Relaxation Response*. New York: Morrow, 1975.

_____. "Your Innate Asset for Combatting Stress." *Harvard Business Review*. *52* (1974) 49–60.

_____, Alexander, S., and Feldman, C. L. "Decreased Premature Ventricular Contractions through the Use of the Relaxation Response in Patients with Stable Ischemic Heart Disease." *Lancet*. ii (1975) 380–382.

Bergland, Richard, and Page, R. B. "Pituitary-Brain-Vascular Relations: A New Paradigm." *Science*. *204* (1979) 18–24.

Besedovsky, H. O., Del Rey, A., and Sorkin, E. "Lymphokine-Containing Super-natants from Con A-Stimulated Cells Increase Corticosterone Blood Levels." *Journal of Immunology. 126* (1983) 385–387.

_____, and Sorkin, E. "Network of Immunoneuroendocrine Interactions." *Clinical and Experimental Immunology. 27* (1977) 1–12.

_____, Sorkin, E., Felix, D., and Haas, H. "Hypothalamic Changes during the Immune Response." *European Journal of Immunology. 7* (1977) 325–328.

Birren, James E., and Livingston, J. (Eds.). *Cognition, Stress, and Aging.* Englewood Cliffs, N.J.: Prentice-Hall, 1985.

Black, S., Humphrey, J. H., and Niven, J. S. F. "Inhibition of Mantoux Reaction by Direct Suggestion under Hypnosis." *British Medical Journal. 1* (1963) 1649–1652.

Blalock, J. E. "The Immune System as a Sensory Organ." *Journal of Immunology. 132* (1984) 1067.

Bland, Jeffrey (Ed.). *Medical Applications of Clinical Nutrition.* New Canaan, Conn.: Keats Publishing, 1983.

Block, B. "Über di Heilung der Warzen durch Suggestion." *Klinische Wochenschrift. 6* (1927) 2271–2275, 2320–2325.

Bohm, David. *Wholeness and the Implicate Order.* London: Routledge and Kegan Publishers, 1980.

_____, and Hiley, B. "On the Intuitive Understanding of Nonlocality as Implied by Quantum Theory." *Foundations of Physics.* Vol. 5 (1975) 93–109.

Bonny, Helen, and Savary, Louis M. *Music and Your Mind.* New York: Harper & Row, 1973.

Borysenko, Joan A. "Healing Motives: An Interview with David C. McClelland." *Advances. 2* (Spring 1984) 29–41.

_____. "Stress, Coping, and the Immune System." In Matarazzo, J. D., Weiss, S. M., Herd, J. A., and Miller, N. E. (Eds.) *Behavioral Health.* New York: Wiley, 1984.

Bowlby, J. *The Making and Breaking of Affectional Bonds.* London: Tavistock Publications, 1979.

Boyd, Peggy. *The Silent Wound: A Startling Report on Breast Cancer and Sexuality.* New York: Addison-Wesley, 1985.

Breslow, L. A. "A Positive Strategy for the Nation's Health." *Journal of the American Medical Association. 242* (19) (1979) 2093–2095.

_____. "A Quantitative Approach to the World Health Organization Definition of Health: Physical, Mental, and Social Well-Being." *International Journal of Epidemiology. 1* (1972) 347–355.

Broadhead, W. E., et al. "The Epidemiologic Evidence for a Relationship between Social Support and Health." *Journal of Epistemology. 109* (1979) 521–537.

Broder, S., and Waldman, T. "The Suppressor-Cell Network in Cancer." *New England Journal of Medicine. 299* (1978) 1281–1284.

Brown, Barbara. *Supermind: The Ultimate Energy.* New York: Harper & Row, 1980.

Brown, Mark. *Left Hand, Right Hand.* Newton-Abott, England: David and Charles Publishers, 1978.

Buber, M. *I and Thou.* New York: Charles Scribner and Sons, 1958.

Bulloch, D., and Moore, R. Y. "Innervation of the Thymus Gland by the Brainstem and Spinal Cord in Mouse and Rat." *American Journal of Anatomy. 161* (1981) 157–166.

Burnet, F. M. "A Modern Basis for Pathology." *Lancet. 1* (1968) 1383–1387.

Burns, David. *Feeling Good: The New Mood Therapy.* New York: Signet Books, 1980.

Cameron-Bandler, Leslie. *Solutions: Practical and Effective Antidotes for Sexual and Relationship Problems.* San Rafael, Calif.: Future Pace, 1985.

Cannon, W. B. *Bodily Changes in Pain, Hunger, Fear, and Rage: An Account of Recent Researches into the Function of Emotional Excitement.* 2d Ed. New York: Appleton, 1929.

_____. *The Wisdom of the Body.* New York: Norton, 1942.

_____. "Voodoo Death." *Psychosomatic Medicine. 19* (1957) 182–190.

Capra, Fritjof. *The Tao of Physics.* 2d ed. Boulder, Colo.: Shambhala Press, 1983.

_____. *The Turning Point.* Toronto and New York: Bantam Books, 1983.

Carruthers, M. E. "Aggression and Atheroma." *Lancet. 2* (1969) 1170–1171.

Case, Robert B., and Heller, Stanley. "Behavior and Survival of Type A Personalities after Acute Myocardial Infarction." *New England Journal of Medicine. 312* (March 1985) no. 12, 737–741.

Cassidy, John, and Rimbeaux, B. C. *Juggling for the Complete Klutz.* 2d ed. Stanford, Calif.: Klutz Press, 1977.

Cella, David F. "Psychological Adjustment and Cancer Outcome: Levy vs. Taylor." *American Psychologist. 40* (November 1985) 1275–1276.

Cherin, Dennis, and Manteuffel, G. *Health: A Holistic Approach.* Wheaton, Ill.: The Theophysical Publishing House, 1984.

Cirese, Sarah. *Quest: A Search for Self.* 2d ed. New York: Holt, Rinehart, and Winston, 1985.

Comfort, Alex. *Sexual Consequences of Disability.* Philadelphia: George F. Stickey Company, 1978.

Conner, R. L., Vernikos-Daniellis, J., and Levine, S. "Stress, Fighting, and Neuroendocrine Function." *Nature. 234* (1971) 564–566.

Cooper, Kenneth H. *The Aerobics Way.* New York: Bantam Books, 1977.

Corian, D., et al. "Occupational Stress and Immunity." *Psychosomatic Medicine. 47* (1985) 77.

Cousins, Norman. *Anatomy of an Illness*. Toronto and New York: Bantam Books, 1981.

_____. *The Healing Heart*. London: W. W. Norton and Co., 1983.

_____. *Human Options*. New York: Berkley Books, 1983.

Crook, William G. *Tracking Down Hidden Food Allergy*. Jackson, Tenn.: Professional Books, 1980.

Cunningham, Susan. "Circadian Rhythms: Is It One Clock, or Several, That Cycle Us Through Life?" *American Psychological Association Monitor*. *16* (September 1985) 24–26.

Dattore, P. J., Shontz, F. C., and Coyne, L. "Premorbid Personality Differentiation of Cancer and Noncancer Groups: A Test of the Hypothesis of Cancer Proneness." *Journal of Consulting and Clinical Psychology*. *48* (1980) 388–394.

de la Pena, Augustin M. *The Psychobiology of Cancer*. South Hadley, Mass.: J. F. Bergin, Publishers, 1983.

Dembroski, T. M., et al. "Moving beyond Type A." *Advances*. *1* (1984) 16–26.

Diamond, Stuart. *The Double Brain*. London: Churchill Livingstone Publishers, 1972.

Dolezal, Suzanne. "A Death's Chronicle: AIDS Fight Told in Letters to a Friend." *The Detroit Free Press*. (Oct. 20, 1985) 1L–4L.

Dossey, Larry. *Beyond Illness. Discovering the Experience of Health*. Boulder and London: Shambhala, 1984.

_____. *Space, Time, and Medicine*. Boulder and London: Shambhala, 1982.

Dowling, St. John. "Lourdes Cures and Their Medical Assessment." *Journal of the Royal Society of Medicine*. *77* (1984) 634–638.

Dubos, René. "Bolstering the Body against Disease." *Human Nature*. (August 1978) 68–73.

_____. *Mirage of Health*. New York: Harper, 1959.

Dychtwald, Ken. *Body-Mind*. New York: Jove Publishers, 1984.

Eastman, Max. *The Enjoyment of Laughter*. New York: Johnson Reprint Co., 1971.

Elgin, D. *Voluntary Simplicity*. New York: Morrow, 1981.

Eliade, M. "Some Observations on European Witchcraft." *Occultism, Witchcraft, and Cultural Fashions*. Chicago: Chicago University Press, 1976.

Eliot, Robert S., and Breo, Dennis L. *Is It Worth Dying For?* Toronto: Bantam Books, 1984.

Engel, George I. "The Need for a New Medical Model: A Challenge for Biomedicine." *Science*. *196* (1977) 129–136.

Farquhar, John W. *The American Way of Life Need Not Be Hazardous to Your Health*. New York: W. W. Norton, 1978.

Fauman, Michael. "The Central Nervous System and the Immune System." *Biological Psychiatry*. *17* (1982) 1459.

Favazza, A. R. "The Day of Our Years." *M.D.* (October 1977) 19–101.

Feigle, H. *Concepts, Theories, and the Mind-Body Problem.* Minneapolis: University of Minnesota Press, 1958.

Feingold, Ben F. *Why Your Child Is Hyperactive.* New York: Random House, 1975.

Ferguson, Marilyn. *The Aquarian Conspiracy.* Los Angeles: J. P. Tarcher, 1980.

————. (Ed.). *Brain/Mind Bulletin.* Box 42211, Los Angeles, Calif.

————. (Ed.). *The Leading Edge: A Bulletin of Social Transformation.* Box 42247, Los Angeles, Calif.

Fine, Reuben. *The Meaning of Love in Human Experience.* New York: Wiley, 1985.

Fletcher, Ella Adelia. *The Law of the Rhythmic Breath.* San Bernadino, Calif.: Bargo Press, 1980.

Fox, B. H. "Current Theory of Psychogenic Effects on Cancer Incidence and Prognosis." *Journal of Psychosocial Oncology. 1* (1983) 17–32.

————. "Premorbid Psychological Factors as Related to Incidence of Cancer." *Journal of Behavioral Medicine. 1* (1978) 45–133.

————, and Newberry, B. H. (Eds.). *Impact of Psychoendocrine Systems in Cancer and Immunity.* New York: C. F. Hogrefe, 1984.

Fox, Jeffrey. "Crying Mellows Some, Masculinizes Others." *Psychology Today. 19* (1981) 559–567.

Frank, Jerome. *Persuasion and Healing.* Baltimore and London: Johns Hopkins University Press, 1974.

————. "The Faith That Heals." *Johns Hopkins Medical Journal. 137* (1975) 127–131.

French, A. P. "The Treatment of Warts by Hypnosis." *American Journal of Obstetrics and Gynecology. 116* (1973) 887–888.

Friedman, M. "The Modification of Type A Behavior in Post-infarction Patients." *American Heart Journal. 97* (1979) 551–560.

————, Rosenman, R. H., Straus, et al. "The Relationship of Behavior Pattern A to the State of the Coronary Vasculature." *American Journal of Medicine. 44* (1968) 525–537.

————, and Ulmer, D. *Treating Type A Behavior and Your Heart.* New York: Alfred A. Knopf, 1984.

————, and Rosenman, R. *Type A Behavior and Your Heart.* New York: Knopf, 1974.

Friedman-Kein, A., and Laubensterin, L. (Eds.). *AIDS: The Opportunistic Epidemic of Kaposi's Sarcoma and Opportunistic Infections.* New York: Masson Publishers, 1984.

Fry, William H., Desoto-Johnson, D., Hoffman, C., and McCall, J. T. "Effect of Stimulus on the Chemical Composition of Human Tears." *American Journal of Opthomology. 92* (1981) 559–567.

_____, and Langeth, M. *Crying: The Mystery of Tears*. New York: Winston Press, 1985.

_____. "The Respiratory Components of Mirthful Laughter." *Journal of Biological Psychology*. *19* (1977) 39–50.

_____. "Mirth and Oxygen Saturation Levels of Peripheral Blood." *Psychotherapy and Psychosomatics*. *19* (1971) 76–84.

Gage, M. J. *Women, Church, and State*. Chicago, Ill. 1893.

Gardner, Kay. *A Rainbow Path. An Album of Healing Music*. Ladyslipper Records, Ladyslipper Inc., Durham, NC 27705.

Gelman, David, et al. "The Food-Mood Link: New Studies Explore How Diet Affects Our Feelings." *Newsweek*. *16* (1985) 93–94.

Gilligan, Carol. *In a Different Voice*. Cambridge, Mass.: Harvard University Press, 1982.

Goetz, E. (Ed.). "Proceedings of a Conference on Neuromodulation of Immunity and Hypersensitivity." *Journal of Immunology*. *135* (1985) 739s–863s.

Goleman, Daniel. *Vital Lies, Simple Truths*. New York: Simon and Schuster, 1985.

Goodman, David. Work reviewed in Fox, Jeffrey L., "Crying Mellows Some, Masculinizes Others," *Psychology Today*, op. cit.

Gordon, Barbara. *I'm Dancing as Fast as I Can*. New York: Harper & Row, 1979.

Green, E., and Green, A. *Beyond Biofeedback*. New York: Delta, 1977.

Green, John, and Miller, David. "Psychology and AIDS in Britain." *American Psychologist*. *40* (November 1985) 1273–1275.

_____, and Miller, D. *Treating Patients with a Fear of AIDS*. Unpublished manuscript. St. Mary's Hospital, London, England, 1985.

Greenberg, R. P., and Dattore, P. J. "The Relationship between Dependency and the Development of Cancer." *Psychosomatic Medicine*. *43* (1981) 35–43.

Gregg, D. "The Paucity of Arthritis among Psychotic Patients." *American Journal of Psychiatry*. (1939) 853–854.

Gross, Martin L. *The Psychological Society*. New York: Random House, 1978.

Grossarth-Maticek, R., Siegrist, J., and Vetter, H. "Interpersonal Repression as a Predictor of Cancer" *Social Science Medical Journal*. *16* (1983) 493–498.

Grossman, Richard. "Ecumenical Medicine. Notes on the History of a Possibility." *Advances*. *2* (1985) 39–50.

_____. *The Other Medicines*. New York: Doubleday, 1985.

Growald, Eileen Rockefeller. "Health and Wholeness: The Mind-Body Mystery." *Advances*. *2* (Fall 1985) 4–10.

Hall, Edward T. *The Dance of Life*. Garden City, N.Y.: Anchor Press/Doubleday, 1983.

Hall, H. R. "Hypnosis and the Immune System: A Review with Implications for Cancer and the Psychology of Healing." *Journal of Clinical Hypnosis*. *25* (2 and 3, 1982 and 1983) 92–103.

_____, Longo, S., and Dixon, R. "Hypnosis and the Immune System: The Effect of Hypnosis on T and B Cell Function." Paper presented to the *Society for Clinical and Experimental Hypnosis.* 33d Annual Workshop and Scientific Meeting, Portland, Oregon. October 1981.

Hayflick, L. "Current Theories of Biological Aging." *Federal Proceedings. 34* (1975) 9–13.

_____. "What We Are Discovering about Your Body's Amazing Immune System." *Executive Health. 15* (November 1978) 2.

Hendricks, Gay, and Weinhold, Barry. *Transpersonal Approaches to Counseling and Psychotherapy.* Denver and London: Love Publishing Co., 1982.

Hennessey, N. Patrick. "AIDS: What the Family Physician Needs to Know." *Medical Aspects of Human Sexuality. 19* (1985) 22–39.

Herd, J. A. "Behavioral Factors in the Physiological Mechanisms of Cardiovascular Disease." In Weiss, S. M., Herd, J. A., and Fox, B. H. (Eds.) *Perspectives on Behavioral Medicine.* New York: Academic, 1979, p. 62.

Holmes, T. H., and Rahe, R. H. "The Social Readjustment Rating Scale." *Journal of Psychosomatic Research. 11* (1967) 213–218.

Honiotes, G. J. "Hypnosis and Breast Enlargement—A Pilot Study." *Journal of the International Society for Professional Hypnosis. 6* (1977) 8–12.

Ilkemi, Y. "Psychological Desensitization in Allergic Disorders." In Lassner, J. (Ed.) *Hypnosis and Psychosomatic Medicine.* New York: Springer/Verlag Publishers, 1967.

Ingelfinger, F. J. "Health: A Matter of Statistics or Feeling." *New England Journal of Medicine. 296* (1977) 448–449.

Investigations. A Bulletin of the Institute of Noetic Sciences. "Psychoneuroimmunology: The Birth of a New Field." vol. 1, num. 2, 1983.

Jacobson, E. *You Must Relax.* New York: McGraw-Hill, 1978.

Jaffe, Dennis T. *Healing from Within.* Toronto and New York: Bantam Books, 1982.

Jaret, Peter, and Mizel, Steven B. *In Self Defense.* New York: Harcourt, Brace, Jovanovich, 1985.

Jaret, Peter. "Our Immune System. The Wars Within." *National Geographic. 169* (June 1986) 702–734.

Jenkins, C. D. "Behavioral Risk Factors in Coronary Artery Disease." *Annual Review of Medicine. 29* (1978) 543.

Jerne, N. K. "The Immune System." *Scientific American. 229* (1973) 52–60.

Kaplan, H. I. "History of Psychosomatic Medicine." In Kaplan, H. I., and Saddock, D. (Eds.) *Comprehensive Textbook of Psychiatry*, Vol. 4. Baltimore: Williams and Wilkins, 1985.

Kaplan, Helen Singer. *The New Sex Therapy.* New York: Brunner/Mazel, 1979.

Kelly, D. D. "Somatic Sensory Systems IV: Central Representations of Pain and Analgesia." In Kandel, J. E., and Schwartz, J. (Eds.) *Principles of Neural Science.* New York: Elsevier North Holland, 1981.

Kenyon, Julian. "The Segmental Electrogram: A Non-invasive Early Diagnostic Scanning Technique." *British Journal of Holistic Medicine. 1* (1984).

Kidd, C. B. "Congenital Ichthyosiform Erythrodermia Treated by Hypnosis." *Journal of the International Society for Professional Hypnosis. 6* (1977) 8–12.

Kissen, D. M. "The Significance of Personality in Lung Cancer in Men." *Annals of the New York Academy of Science. 125* (1966) 820–826.

Klein, R. F., et al. "The Physician and Postmyocardial Infarction Invalidism." *Journal of the American Medical Association. 194* (1965) 123–128.

Kleinman, A., Eisenberg, L., and Byron, G. "Culture, Illness, and Care. Clinical Lessons from Anthropologic and Cross-Cultural Research." *Annals of Internal Medicine. 88* (1978) 251–258.

Kobasas, S. C., Hilker, R. R., and Maddi, S. R. "Health under Stress." *Journal of Occupational Medicine. 21* (1979) 595–598.

Koestler, Arthur. *Janus.* London: Hutchinson, 1978.

Kohlberg, L. "Stage and Sequence: The Cognitive Developmental Approach to Socialization." In Goslin, D. A. (Ed.) *Handbook of Socialization Theory and Research.* Chicago: Rand-McNally, 1969.

Kolodny, R., Masters, W. H., and Johnson, V. *Textbook of Sexual Medicine.* Boston: Little, Brown and Company, 1979.

Korzeniowsky, Carole, and Corsara, M. *STD: A Commonsense Guide.* New York: St. Martin's Press, 1981.

Krantz, David S., and Manuck, S. B. "Acute Psychophysiologic Reactivity and Risk of Cardiovascular Disease: A Review and Methodologic Critique." *Psychological Bulletin. 96* (1984) 435–464.

Krueger, R. B., et al. "Lymphocyte Subsets in Patients with Major Depression: Preliminary Findings." *Advances. 1* (1984) 5–9.

Kutz, I., Borysenko, J. Z., and Benson, H. "Meditation and Psychotherapy: A Rationale for the Integration of Dynamic Psychotherapy, the Relaxation Response, and Mindfulness Meditation." *The American Journal of Psychiatry. 142* (1985) 1–8.

La Barba, R. C. "Experimental and Environmental Factors in Cancer. A Review of Research with Animals." *Psychosomatic Medicine. 32* (1970) 259–274.

Laberge, S. P., et al. "Lucid Dreaming Verified by Volitional Communication during REM Sleep." *Perceptual and Motor Skills. 52* (1981) 727–732.

Lacey, J. I. "Somatic Response Patterning and Stress: Some Revisions on Activation Theory." In Appley, M. H., and Trumble, R. (Eds.) *Psychological Stress.* New York: Appleton Century Crofts, 1967.

Lamott, K. *Escape from Stress.* New York: G. P. Putnam's Sons, 1975.

Laudenslager, M. L., et al. "Coping and Immunosuppression: Inescapable Not Escapable Shock Suppresses Lymphocyte Proliferation." *Science. 221* (1983) 568–570.

Lazarus, Richard. *Psychological Stress and the Coping Process*. New York: McGraw-Hill, 1966.

Lerner, Michael, and Naomi, R. "A Variety of Integral Cancer Therapies." *Advances*. 2 (1985) 14–33.

LeShan, Lawrence. *The Medium, the Mystic, and the Physicist*. New York: Rinehart, Winston, 1976.

————. "Time Orientation and Social Class." *Journal of Abnormal and Social Psychology*. 47 (1942) 582–589.

————, and Margenau, Henry. *Einstein's Space and Van Gogh's Sky: Physical Reality and Beyond*. New York: Macmillan, 1983.

Levine, S., Goldman, L., and Coover, G. D. "Expectancy and the Pituitary-Adrenal System." *Physiology, Emotion, and Psychosomatic Illness*. Elsevier, N.Y.: Ciba Foundation Symposium 8, Excerpta Medica, 1972.

Levinson, Daniel J. "A Conception of Adult Development." *American Psychologist*. 41 (January 1986) 3–13.

Levy, Jerry. "Possible Basis for the Evolution of Lateral Specialization of the Human Brain." *Nature*. 224 (1969) 614–615.

Levy, Sandra. "Emotions and the Progression of Cancer." *Advances*. 1 (1984) 10–15.

Light, K. C., and Orbist, P. A. "Cardiovascular Response to Stress: Effects of Opportunity to Avoid Shock Experience, and Performance Feedback." *Psychophysiology*. 17 (1980) 243–252.

Liipowski, Z. J. "Psychosocial Aspects of Disease." *Annals of Internal Medicine*. 71 (1969) 1197–1206.

————. "Psychosomatic Medicine in the Seventies: An Overview." *American Journal of Psychiatry*. 134 (1977) 233–244. (102 references.)

Lloyd, Ruth. "Possible Mechanisms of Psychoneuroimmunological Interactions." *Advances*. 1 (1984) 43–51.

Locke, Steven E. "Adaption and Immunity: Studies in Humans." *General Hospital Psychiatry*. 4 (1982) 49–58.

————, and Colligan, D. *The Healer Within*. New York: Dutton, 1986.

————, and Hornig-Rohan, Mady. *Mind and Immunity: Behavioral Immunology*. New York: Institute for the Advancement of Health, 1982.

Lorig, K., Laurin, K., and Holman, H. "Arthritis Self-Management: A Study of the Effectiveness of Patient Education for the Elderly." *The Gerontologist*. 24 (1984) 455–457.

Lown, Bernard. "The Verbal Conditioning of Angina Pectoris during Exercise Testing." *American Journal of Cardiology*. 40 (1977) 630–634.

MacLean, Paul. "On the Evolution of Three Mentalities." In Arieti, S., and G. Chrzanowki. (Eds.) *New Dimensions in Psychiatry: A World View*. Vol. II. New York: Wiley, 1977.

Maier, Stephen P., and Laudenslager, M. "Stress and Health: Exploring the Links." *Psychology Today. 19* (August 1985) 44–49.

Makinodan, T. "Mechanism, Prevention, and Restoration of Immunologic Aging." *Birth Defects. 14* (1978) 197–212.

Mandel, J. Biopsychosocial Aspects of the Acquired Immune Deficiency Syndrome. Paper presented at the 41st Annual Convention of the American Psychological Association, Anaheim, California, 1983.

Martin, John L., and Vance, Carole S. "Behavioral and Psychosocial Factors in AIDS: Methodological and Substantive Issues." *American Psychologist. 39* (November 1984) 1303–1308.

Marx, J. L. "Suppressor T Cells: Role in Immune Regulation." *Science. 188* (April 1975) 245–247.

————. "Thymic Hormones: Inducers of T Cell Maturation." *Science. 187* (March 1975) 1883–1885.

Maslow, Abraham. *Eupsychian Management.* Homewood, Ill.: Richard D. Irwin, Inc., and the Dorsey Press, 1965.

————. *Motivation and Personality.* 2d ed. New York: Harper & Row, 1970.

————. *Religions, Values and Peak Experiences.* New York: Penguin Books, 1976.

————. *The Farther Reaches of Human Nature.* New York: Viking Press, 1971.

Mason, A. A. "Ichthyosis and Hypnosis." *British Medical Journal. 2* (1955) 57.

————, and Black, S. "Allergic Skin Responses Abolished under Treatment of Asthma and Hay Fever by Hypnosis." *Lancet. 1* (April 1958) 887–880.

Mason, J. W. "Emotions as Reflected in Patterns of Endocrine Integration." In Levy, L. (Ed.) *Emotions: Their Parameters and Measurement.* New York: McGraw-Hill, 1975.

Masters, W., and Johnson, V. *Human Sexual Response.* Boston: Little Brown, 1966.

Matarazzo, J. T., et al. (Eds.). *Behavioral Health.* New York: Wiley, 1984.

McClelland, David C. "Stress Power Motivation, Sympathetic Activation, Immune Function, and Illness." *Journal of Human Stress. 6* (1980) 11–19.

————. "Inhibited Power Motivation and Blood Pressure in Men." *Journal of Abnormal Psychology. 88* (1979) 182–190.

Meichenbaum, D. *Cognitive-Behavioral Modification: An Integrative Approach.* New York: Plenum Publishers, 1977.

Meister, Barbara. *Unicorns Are Real: A Right-Brained Approach to Learning.* Rolling Hills Estates, Calif.: Jalmar Press, 1982.

Melnechuk, Theodore. "Why Has Psychoneuroimmunology Been Controversial? Proponents and Skeptics at a Scientific Conference." *Advances. 2* (1985) 22–38.

Miller, D. M., Green, J. U., Farmer, R., and Carroll G. "A Pseudo-AIDS Syndrome Following from a Fear of AIDS." *British Journal of Psychiatry.* (in press)

————. "Psychological Support and Counseling in AIDS Syndrome." *Genitourinary Medicine.* (in press)

Monat, A., and Lazarus, R. S. (Eds.). *Stress and Coping. An Anthology.* New York: Columbia University Press, 1977.

Money, John. *Love and Love Sickness: The Science of Sex, Gender Difference, and Pair-Bonding.* Baltimore and London: Johns Hopkins University Press, 1980.

Monjan, A. A., and Collector, M. I. "Stress-Induced Modulation on the Immune Response." *Science. 197* (1977) 307–308.

Murray, M. *The Witch Cult in Western Europe.* Oxford: Oxford University Press, 1921.

"Music Edition." *Brain/Mind Bulletin.* Los Angeles: Interface Press, Dec. 13, 1982.

Nauts, H. C. *Breast Cancer: Immunological Factors Affecting Incidence, Prognosis, and Survival.* New York: Cancer Research Institute, 1983.

Newell, A., and Simon, H. A. *Human Problem Solving.* Englewood Cliffs, N.J.: Prentice-Hall, 1972.

Newman, H. "Health Attitudes: Locus of Control and Religious Orientation." A master's thesis, University of Texas Health Science Center, School of Allied Health Sciences, Dallas, Tex., 1983.

Null, Gary. "The AIDS Cover-Up." *Penthouse.* (December 1985) 84.

O'Regan, Brendan. "Positive Emotions: The Emerging Science of Feelings." *Institute of Noetic Science Newsletter. 12* (1984) 5–18.

Ornstein, R. E. *On the Experience of Time.* London: Penguin Books, 1969.

————. *Psychology of Consciousness.* 2d ed. New York: Harcourt Brace Jovanovich, 1977.

————. *Psychology: The Study of Human Experience.* San Diego and New York: Harcourt Brace Jovanovich, 1985.

Ortleb, Charles. *New York Native.* 249 West Broadway, New York, NY 10013. For information on AIDS.

Oshawa, George. (Translated by Dufty, W.) *You Are All Sanpaku.* Secaucus, N.J.: University Books, 1965.

Ott, John N. *Health and Light.* New York: Pocket Books, 1976.

Paskind, H. A. "Effect of Laughter on Muscle Tone." *Archives of Neurology and Psychiatry. 28* (1932) 623–628. For an interesting comparison between this historical research and modern approaches to the study of laughter, see Black, D. W., "Laughter," *Journal of the American Medical Association, 252* (1984) 2995–2998.

Peck, Scott. *The Road Less Traveled.* New York: Simon and Schuster, 1978.

Pelletier, Kenneth. *Healthy People in Unhealthy Places.* New York: Delacorte Press/Seymour Lawrence, 1984.

————. *Holistic Medicine. From Stress to Optimum Health.* New York: Delacorte Press/Seymour Lawrence, 1979.

————. *Longevity. Fulfilling Our Biological Potential.* New York: Delacorte Press/Seymour Lawrence, 1981.

_____. *Mind as Healer: Mind as Slayer.* New York: Delacorte Press/Seymour Lawrence, 1977.

Pepper, Eric, and Pelletier, K. *"A Compilation of 400 Cases of Spontaneous Remission from Cancer."* Circulated Monograph. Sponsored by the Reynolds Foundation, 1976. This material is reviewed in Green, E., and Green, A., *Beyond Biofeedback*, op. cit.

Peter, Laurence J., and Dana, Bill. *The Laughter Prescription.* New York: Ballantine Books, 1982.

Piaget, Jean, *The Origins of Intelligence in Children.* New York: International Universities Press, 1952.

Platonov, K. *The Word as a Psychological and Therapeutic Factor.* Moscow: Foreign Language Publishing House, 1959.

Plotnikoff, M. P. "Responses of T Cells of Cancer Patients Enhanced by Exposure to Enkephalin." Reported at Second International Conference on Immunopharmacology. Washington, D.C., 1982. Quoted in Achterberg, J., *Imagery in Healing.*, op. cit. See also Plotnikoff, M., and Murgo, A. *Science News, 22* (July 24, 1982).

Polivy, J. "Psychological Effects of Mastectomy on a Woman's Feminine Self-Concept." *Journal of Nervous and Mental Disease. 164* (1977) 77–87.

Porkert, Manfred. *The Theoretical Foundations of Chinese Medicine.* Cambridge, Mass.: MIT Press, 1974.

Prescott, James. "Phylogenetic and Ontogenetic Aspects of Human Affectional Development." In Gemmer, R., and Wheeler, W. (Eds.) *Selected Proceedings of the 1976 International Congress of Sexology.* New York: Plenum Publishers, 1977.

Pribram, Karl H. "Holonomy and Structure in the Organization of Perception." In Nicholas, John M. (Ed.) *Images, Perception, and Knowledge.* Dordrecht-Holland: Reidel, 1977.

_____. *Languages of the Brain.* Monterey, Calif.: Brooks/Cole Publishing Co., 1971.

Rees, W. D., and Lutkin, S. G. "Mortality of Bereavement." *British Journal of Medicine. 4* (1967) 13–16.

Renoux, G., Biziere, K., Renoux, M., and Guillian, I. N. J. "The Production of T-Cell Inducing Factors Is Controlled by the Brain Neocortex." *Scandinavian Journal of Immunology. 17* (1983) 45–50.

Restak, Richard. *The Brain.* Toronto and New York: Bantam Books, 1984.

_____. *The Brain: The Last Frontier.* New York: Warner Books, 1979.

Riley, V. "Mouse Mammary Tumors: Alteration of Incidence as Apparent Function of Stress." *Science. 189* (1975) 465–467.

Roitt, I. M. *Essential Immunology.* St. Louis: C. V. Mosby, 1980.

Rosenbaum, E. R. (Ed.). *Can You Prevent Cancer?* St. Louis: C. V. Mosby, 1983.

Rosenzweig, Norman, and Pearsall, F. Paul. (Eds.). *Sex Education for the Health Professional.* New York: Grune and Stratton, 1978.

Royce, J. "Psychology Is Multi-methodological, Variate, Epistemic, World View, Systemic, Paradigmatic, Theoretic, and Disciplinary." In *Nebraska Symposium on Motivation, 1975. Conceptual Foundations of Psychology.* Lincoln, Neb.: University of Nebraska Press, 1976, 1–64.

Rulison, R. H. "Warts: A Statistical Study of Nine Hundred and Twenty-One Cases." *Archives of Dermatology and Syphilology. 46* (1942) 66–81.

Russell, Peter. *The Brain Book.* New York: E. P. Dutton, 1979.

Russo, N. J., II., Kapp, B. S., Homquist, B. K., and Musty, R. E. "Passive Avoidance and Amygdala Lesions: Relationship with Pituitary-Adrenal System." *Physiology and Behavior. 16* (1976) 191–199.

Sagan, Carl. *The Dragons of Eden.* New York: Ballantine Books, 1977.

Saland, L. C., van Epps, D. E., Ortiz, E., and Samora, A. "Acute Injections of Opiate-Peptides into the Rat Cerebral Ventricle: A Macrophage-like Cellular Response." *Brain Research Bulletin. 10* (1983) 523–528.

Sandblom, Philip. *Creativity and Disease: How Illness Affects Literature, Art, and Music.* Philadelphia: George F. Stickley Co., 1985.

Schaeffer, M. A., McKinnon, W., Baum, A., et al. "Immune Status as a Function of Chronic Stress at Three Mile Island." *Psychosomatic Medicine. 47* (1985) 85.

Scherwitz, Larry, Berton, K., and Leventhal, H. "Type A Behavior, Self-Involvement, and Cardiovascular Response." *Psychosomatic Medicine. 40* (1978) 593–609.

————, Graham, L. E., and Ornish, D. "Self-Involvement and the Risk Factors for Coronary Heart Disease" *Advances. 2* (1985) 6–18.

Schmeck, H. M. "By Training the Brain, Scientists Find Links to Immune Defenses." *New York Times.* (Jan. 1, 1985).

Schwab, J. J. "Psychosomatic Medicine: Its Past and Present." *Psychosomatics. 26* (1985) 583.

Schwartz, Gary E. "Behavioral Medicine and Systems Theory: A New Synthesis." *National Forum.* (Winter 1980) 25–30.

————. "Psychobiology of Health: A New Synthesis." *Master Lecture Series. Psychology and Health.* American Psychology Association, Washington, D.C.: (1983) 149–193.

Schweitzer, Albert. *Out of My Life and Thought: Autobiography.* Translated by Campion, C. T. New York: Holt, Rinehart, Winston, 1979.

Selye, Hans. *The Physiology and Pathology of Exposure to Stress.* Montreal: Acta, 1950.

————. *The Stress of Life.* New York: McGraw-Hill, 1956.

————. *Stress without Distress.* Philadelphia and New York: Lippincott, 1974.

Service, Robert. *The Best of Robert Service.* New York: Dodd, Mead and Company, 1953.

Shah, Idries. *Tales of the Dervishes.* New York: E. P. Dutton, 1970.

Shaw, Peter. "A Type A Behavior Modification Sampler." *The Wall Street Journal*. (July 24, 1985) 16.

Shealy, C. Norman. "Total Life Stress and Symptomatology." *Journal of Holistic Medicine*. *6* (1984) 112–129.

Sheikh, A. A. (Ed.). *Imagination and Healing*. New York: Baywood Publishing Co., 1984.

Sheinkin, David, Schachter, M., and Hutton, Richard. *Food, Mind, and Mood*. New York: Warner Books, 1979.

Shekelle, R., et al. "Psychological Depression and 17-Year Risk of Death from Cancer." *Psychosomatic Medicine*. *43* (1981) 117–125.

Silverman, S. *Psychological Aspects of Physical Symptoms*. New York: Meredith Corporation, 1968.

Simeons, A. T. W. *Man's Presumptuous Brain: An Evolutionary Interpretation of Psychosomatic Disease*. New York: Dutton, 1961.

Simonton, O. C., Simonton, S., and Creighton, J. *Getting Well Again*. Los Angeles: Tarcher, 1978.

Sklar, L., and Anisman, H. "Stress and Cancer." *Psychological Bulletin*. *89* (1981) 369–406.

Smith, A. *Powers of the Mind*. New York: Random House, 1975.

Sobel, David (Ed.). *Ways of Health. Holistic Approaches to Ancient and Contemporary Medicine*. New York: Harcourt Brace Jovanovich, 1979.

_____. "The Healing Brain: Audio Update I. A Review of Current Research on the Brain as a Health Maintenance System." *The Healing Brain*. Four volumes. The Institute for the Study of Human Knowledge, Los Altos, CA 94022.

Solomon, George F. "The Emerging Field of Psychoneuroimmunology." *Advances*. *2* (Winter 1985) 6–19.

_____. "Emotions, Stress, The Central Nervous System, and Immunity." *Annals of the New York Academy of Science*. *164* (1969) 335–343.

_____, and Moos, R. H. "Emotions, Immunity, and Disease. A Speculative Theoretical Integration." *Archives of General Psychiatry*. *11* (1964) 657–764.

Sontag, S. *Illness as Metaphor*. New York: Farrar, Straus, and Giroux, 1978.

Sorokin, Pitirim A. *Social and Cultural Dynamics*. Four volumes. New York: American Book Company, 1937–1941.

Speigel, Bernard, and Speigel, R. *Trance and Treatment: Clinical Uses of Hypnosis*. New York: Basic Books, 1978.

Steadman, Alice. *Who's the Matter with Me?* Marina del Ray, Calif.: DeVorss and Company, 1969.

Stein, M., Keller, S. E., and Schleiger, S. J. "The Hypothalamus and the Immune Response." In Weiner, H., Hofer, M., and Stunkard, S. (Eds.) *Brain, Behavior, and Bodily Disease*. New York: Raven Press, 1981.

_____, Schiavi, R. C., and Camerino, M. "Influence of Brain and Behavior on the Immune System." *Science*. *191* (1976) 435–440.

Stoddard, Joan B., and Henry, J. P. "Affectional Bonding and the Impact of Bereavement." *Advances*. 2 (1985) 19–28.

Stroebel, Charles. *The Quieting Reflex*. New York: Berkley Books, 1983.

Stuart, Richard B. *Helping Couples Change*. New York: The Guilford Press, 1980.

Taylor, S. "Adjustment to Threatening Events: A Theory of Cognitive Adaptation." *American Psychologist*. 38 (1983) 1161–1174.

Tessler, S. R. "Recovering? Get a Room with a View." *The Detroit News*. (Oct. 5, 1985).

Thomas, C. B., Duszynski, K. R., and Shaffer, J. W. "Family Attitudes Reported in Youth as Potential Predictors of Cancer." *Psychosomatic Medicine*. 41 (1979) 287–302.

Thomas, Lewis. "On the Science and Technology of Medicine." In Knowles, John (Ed.) *Doing Better and Feeling Worse*. New York: Norton, 1977.

_____. *The Lives of a Cell*. New York: Bantam Books, 1975.

Tinbergen, N. "Etiology and Stress Diseases." *Science*. 26 (1974) 85.

Tuke, D. H. *Illustrations of the Influence of the Mind upon the Body in Health and Disease Designed to Elucidate the Action of Imagination*. London: J. A. Churchill, 1872.

Turner, J., Gallimore, R., and Fox, C. *Placebo: An Annotated Bibliography*. Los Angeles: The Neuropsychiatric Institute, University of California, 1964.

Ullman, M., and Dudek, S. "On the Psyche and Warts: II. Hypnotic Suggestion and Warts," *Psychosomatic Medicine*. 22 (1960) 68–76.

Vaillant, George E. *Adaptation to Life*. Boston: Little, Brown and Company, 1977.

_____. "Natural History of Male Psychologic Health: Effects of Mental Health on Physical Health." *New England Journal of Medicine*. 301 (1979) 1249–1254.

Van Loon, G. R., Scapagnini, U., Moberg, G. P., and Ganong, W. F. "Evidence for Central Adrenergic Neural Inhibition of ACTH Secretion in the Rat." *Endocrinology*. 184 (1971) 1464–1469.

Vickery, Donald M., and Fries, J. F. *Take Care of Yourself*. Menlo Park, Calif.: Addison-Wesley, 1981.

von Bertalanffy, Ludwig. *General Systems Theory*. New York: Braziller, 1968.

Walsh, R., and Shapiro, D. (Eds.). *Beyond Health and Normalcy. Explorations of Exceptional Well-Being*. New York: Van Nostrand Rhinehold, 1983.

Wear, Jennifer, and Holmes, King. *How to Have Intercourse without Getting Screwed*. Seattle: Madrona Publishers, 1976.

Weiss, R. S. *Loneliness: The Experience of Emotional and Social Isolation*. Cambridge, Mass.: MIT Press, 1973.

Weiss, S. M., Herd, J. A., and Fox, B. H. (Eds.). *Perspectives in Behavioral Medicine*. New York: Academic, 1981.

Welwood, John. *Awakening the Heart*. Boulder and London: New Science Library, 1983.

Whitcomb, Edward. *Psyche and Substance*. Richmond, Calif.: North Atlantic Books, 1980.

White, E. B., and White, K. S. *A Subtreasury of American Humor*. New York: Capricorn Books, 1962.

Whitmore, George B., and Kohli, D. R. "Dysponesis: A Neurophysiologic Factor in Functional Disorders." In Pepper, Eric, et al. (Eds.) *Mind/Body Integration*. New York: Plenum Press, 1979.

Wilber, Ken. *The Spectrum of Consciousness*. Wheaton, Ill.: Theophysical Publishing House, 1977.

————. *Quantum Reality: Beyond the New Physics*. Boulder and London: New Science Library. (in press).

Willard, R. D. "Breast Enlargement through Visual Imagery and Hypnosis." *American Journal of Clinical Hypnosis*. *19* (1977) 195–200.

Williams, J. E. "Stimulation of Breast Growth by Hypnosis." *Journal of Sex Research*. *10* (1974) 316–326.

Willner, Paul. *Depression: A Psychobiological Synthesis*. New York: Wiley, 1985.

Wilson, Collin. *New Pathways in Psychology*. New York: Taplanger Publishing Co., 1972.

Wilson, E. O. *Sociobiology. The New Synthesis*. The abridged edition. Cambridge, Mass.: Belknap Press, 1980.

Wink, C. A. S. "Congenital Ichthyosiform Erythrodermia Treated by Hypnosis. Report of Two Cases." *British Medical Journal*. *2* (1961) 741–743.

Wybran, J., et al. "Suggestive Evidence for Receptors for Morphine and Methinone-Enkephalin on Normal Human Block T Lymphocytes." *Journal of Immunology*. *123* (1979) 1068–1070.

Young, M., Benjamin, B., and Wallis, C. "Mortality of Widowers." *Lancet*. *2* (1963) 454–456.

Zilbergeld, Bernie. *Male Sexuality*. New York: Bantam Books, 1968.

————. *The Shrinking of America: Myths of Psychological Change*. Boston and Toronto: Little, Brown and Company, 1983.

Zyzanski, S. J., Jenkins, D. D., Ryan, T. J., et al. "Psychological Correlates of Coronary Angiographic Findings." *Archives of Internal Medicine*. *136* (1976) 1234–1237.